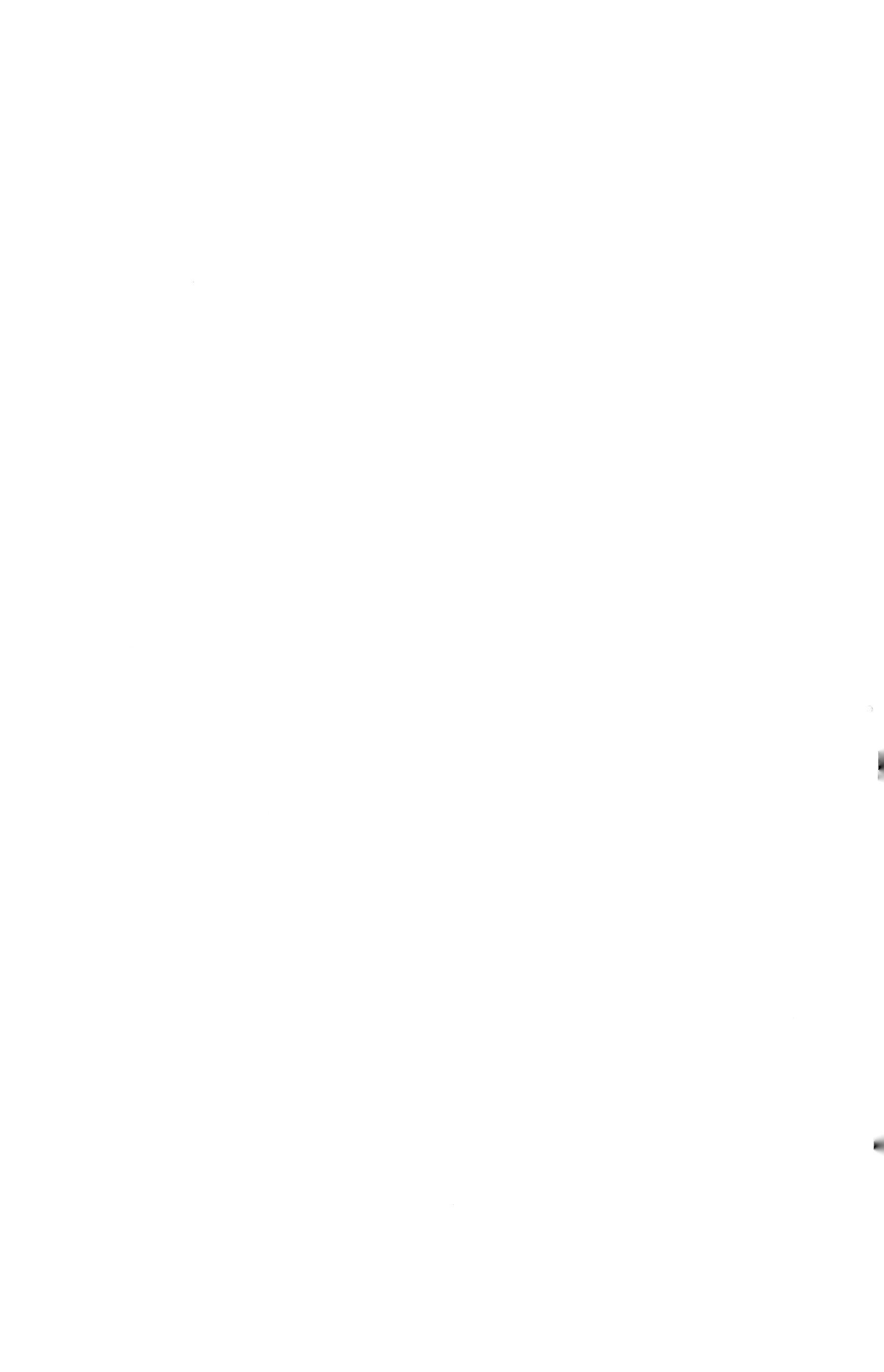

Endocrine and Neuroendocrine Cancers

Endocrine and Neuroendocrine Cancers

Editors

Alfredo Berruti
Vito Amoroso
Nicola Fazio

MDPI • Basel • Beijing • Wuhan • Barcelona • Belgrade • Manchester • Tokyo • Cluj • Tianjin

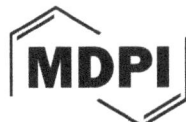

Editors
Alfredo Berruti
University of Brescia at ASST
Spedali Civili di Brescia
Italy

Vito Amoroso
ASST-Spedali Civili
Italy

Nicola Fazio
European Institute of
Oncology
Italy

Editorial Office
MDPI
St. Alban-Anlage 66
4052 Basel, Switzerland

This is a reprint of articles from the Special Issue published online in the open access journal *Cancers* (ISSN 2072-6694) (available at: https://www.mdpi.com/journal/cancers/special_issues/Endocrine_Neuroendocrine).

For citation purposes, cite each article independently as indicated on the article page online and as indicated below:

LastName, A.A.; LastName, B.B.; LastName, C.C. Article Title. *Journal Name* **Year**, *Volume Number*, Page Range.

ISBN 978-3-0365-5763-2 (Hbk)
ISBN 978-3-0365-5764-9 (PDF)

© 2023 by the authors. Articles in this book are Open Access and distributed under the Creative Commons Attribution (CC BY) license, which allows users to download, copy and build upon published articles, as long as the author and publisher are properly credited, which ensures maximum dissemination and a wider impact of our publications.

The book as a whole is distributed by MDPI under the terms and conditions of the Creative Commons license CC BY-NC-ND.

Contents

Preface to "Endocrine and Neuroendocrine Cancers" vii

Alfredo Berruti, Vito Amoroso and Nicola Fazio
Endocrine and Neuroendocrine Tumors: A Special Issue
Reprinted from: *Cancers* **2022**, *14*, 4994, doi:10.3390/cancers14204994 1

Chiara Alessandra Cella, Francesca Spada, Alfredo Berruti, Francesco Bertolini, Patrizia Mancuso, Massimo Barberis, Eleonora Pisa, et al.
Addressing the Role of Angiogenesis in Patients with Advanced Pancreatic Neuroendocrine Tumors Treated with Everolimus: A Biological Prospective Analysis of Soluble Biomarkers and Clinical Outcomes
Reprinted from: *Cancers* **2022**, *14*, 4471, doi:10.3390/cancers14184471 5

Mirco Bartolomei, Alfredo Berruti, Massimo Falconi, Nicola Fazio, Diego Ferone, Secondo Lastoria, Giovanni Pappagallo, et al.
Clinical Management of Neuroendocrine Neoplasms in Clinical Practice: A Formal Consensus Exercise
Reprinted from: *Cancers* **2022**, *14*, 2501, doi:10.3390/cancers14102501 19

Catherine G. Tran, Luis C. Borbon, Jacqueline L. Mudd, Ellen Abusada, Solmaz AghaAmiri, Sukhen C. Ghosh, Servando Hernandez Vargas, et al.
Establishment of Novel Neuroendocrine Carcinoma Patient-Derived Xenograft Models for Receptor Peptide-Targeted Therapy
Reprinted from: *Cancers* **2022**, *14*, 1910, doi:10.3390/cancers14081910 39

Angela Lamarca, Melissa Frizziero, Jorge Barriuso, Zainul Kapacee, Wasat Mansoor, Mairéad G. McNamara, Richard A. Hubner, et al.
Molecular Profiling of Well-Differentiated Neuroendocrine Tumours: The Role of ctDNA in Real-World Practice
Reprinted from: *Cancers* **2022**, *14*, 1017, doi:10.3390/cancers14041017 53

Rexhep Durmo, Angelina Filice, Federica Fioroni, Veronica Cervati, Domenico Finocchiaro, Chiara Coruzzi, Giulia Besutti, et al.
Predictive and Prognostic Role of Pre-Therapy and Interim 68Ga-DOTATOC PET/CT Parameters in Metastatic Advanced Neuroendocrine Tumor Patients Treated with PRRT
Reprinted from: *Cancers* **2022**, *14*, 592, doi:10.3390/cancers14030592 63

Alessandro Prete, Antonio Matrone, Carla Gambale, Valeria Bottici, Virginia Cappagli, Cristina Romei, Liborio Torregrossa, et al.
Active Surveillance in *RET* Gene Carriers Belonging to Families with Multiple Endocrine Neoplasia
Reprinted from: *Cancers* **2021**, *13*, 5554, doi:10.3390/cancers13215554 75

Iuliu Sbiera, Stefan Kircher, Barbara Altieri, Martin Fassnacht, Matthias Kroiss and Silviu Sbiera
Epithelial and Mesenchymal Markers in Adrenocortical Tissues: How Mesenchymal Are Adrenocortical Tissues?
Reprinted from: *Cancers* **2021**, *13*, 1736, doi:10.3390/cancers13071736 89

Arnaud Jannin, Alexandre Escande, Abir Al Ghuzlan, Pierre Blanchard, Dana Hartl, Benjamin Chevalier, Frédéric Deschamps, et al.
Anaplastic Thyroid Carcinoma: An Update
Reprinted from: *Cancers* **2022**, *14*, 1061, doi:10.3390/cancers14041061 103

Camilla Bardasi, Stefania Benatti, Gabriele Luppi, Ingrid Garajovà, Federico Piacentini, Massimo Dominici and Fabio Gelsomino
Carcinoid Crisis: A Misunderstood and Unrecognized Oncological Emergency
Reprinted from: *Cancers* **2022**, *14*, 662, doi:10.3390/cancers14030662 . . . . **129**

Camilo Jimenez, Gustavo Armaiz-Pena, Patricia L. M. Dahia, Yang Lu, Rodrigo A. Toledo, Jeena Varghese and Mouhammed Amir Habra
Endocrine and Neuroendocrine Tumors Special Issue—Checkpoint Inhibitors for
Adrenocortical Carcinoma and Metastatic Pheochromocytoma and Paraganglioma: Do They Work?
Reprinted from: *Cancers* **2022**, *14*, 467, doi:10.3390/cancers14030467 . . . . **143**

Charalampos Aktypis, Maria-Eleni Spei, Maria Yavropoulou, Göran Wallin, Anna Koumarianou, Gregory Kaltsas, Eva Kassi, et al.
Cardiovascular Toxicities Secondary to Biotherapy and Molecular Targeted Therapies in Neuroendocrine Neoplasms: A Systematic Review and Meta-Analysis of Randomized Placebo-Controlled Trials
Reprinted from: *Cancers* **2021**, *13*, 2159, doi:10.3390/cancers13092159 . . . . **159**

Tiziana Feola, Roberta Centello, Franz Sesti, Giulia Puliani, Monica Verrico, Valentina Di Vito, Cira Di Gioia, et al.
Neuroendocrine Carcinomas with Atypical Proliferation Index and Clinical Behavior: A Systematic Review
Reprinted from: *Cancers* **2021**, *13*, 1247, doi:10.3390/cancers13061247 . . . . **177**

Preface to "Endocrine and Neuroendocrine Cancers"

Endocrine and neuroendocrine tumors represent heterogeneous diseases. Many of these neoplasms are rare and may be included in genetic syndromes. Their treatment is often challenging and requires a multidisciplinary approach.

This Special Issue encompasses original papers and review papers regarding current state of the art and future prospects in (a) diagnosis, (b) genetics, (c) biology and genomics, (d) multidisciplinary approaches and the effectiveness of currently available therapies, and e) new molecular targeted therapies and immunotherapies.

Alfredo Berruti, Vito Amoroso, and Nicola Fazio
Editors

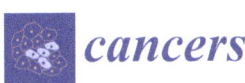

Editorial

Endocrine and Neuroendocrine Tumors: A Special Issue

Alfredo Berruti [1,*], Vito Amoroso [1] and Nicola Fazio [2]

1. Medical Oncology Unit, Department of Medical and Surgical Specialties, Radiological Sciences and Public Health, University of Brescia, ASST Spedali Civili of Brescia, 25123 Brescia, Italy
2. Division of Gastrointestinal Medical Oncology and Neuroendocrine Tumors, European Institute of Oncology, IEO, IRCCS, 20132 Milan, Italy
* Correspondence: alfredo.berruti@gmail.com

Endocrine and neuroendocrine tumors (NETs) represent a group of heterogeneous malignancies that have endocrine cell onset as a common denominator. They are relatively rare and may be classified within inherited syndromes. The prognoses are various and mainly related to tumor stage at diagnosis and tumor grade. The treatment of patients with these malignancies is often challenging and therefore requires a multidisciplinary approach. In recent years, we have witnessed an improvement in the biological and pathogenetic knowledge of these diseases, and new effective drugs have been identified [1,2].

This Special Issue, which comprises 12 papers (seven original articles and five reviews), addresses various aspects concerning the state of the art and future perspectives in the field of clinical and translational research of endocrine and neuroendocrine tumors.

As regards the original contributions, adrenocortical carcinoma (ACC) is an extremely rare and challenging malignancy [3]. The paper by Sbiera et al. [4] addressed an important topic: the epithelial to mesenchymal transition (EMT) as a potential mechanism associated with metastasis in adrenocortical carcinoma (ACC). The authors studied EMT in tissues from 138 ACC, 29 adrenocortical adenomas and three normal adrenal glands. The results showed that both normal and neoplastic adrenocortical tissues showed no expression of epithelial markers, but strongly expressed mesenchymal markers. The authors concluded that there is no indication of EMT in ACC as all adrenocortical tissues showed no expression of epithelial markers and exhibited closer similarity to mesenchymal tissues. However, they observed that the EMT marker SLUG seems to be associated with a more aggressive phenotype.

Multiple Endocrine Neoplasia-2 (MEN-2) has a very high penetrance in medullary thyroid carcinoma (MTC) patients, although with intra- and inter-familial variability. The paper by Prete et al. [5] reported results of a large prospective study that involved 189 gene carrier patients, of whom 67 were admitted to immediate thyroid surgery and 122 were followed-up and were sent to surgery only if they met pre-defined clinical and biochemical characteristics. In the follow-up group, only 22 patients underwent surgery, while 100 could spare their thyroid at least at the last examination visit. This important study demonstrated that a patient-centered surveillance approach permits postponing thyroid surgery in children until adolescence/adulthood.

Although peptide receptor radionuclide therapy (PRRT) is an effective therapeutic option in patients with metastatic NET, this treatment modality is inefficacious in about 15–30% of cases. The paper by Durmo et al. [6] was designed to retrospectively identify biomarkers able to predict responses to PRRT in metastatic NET patients with different primary malignancies. The results found that a high baseline tumor volume was the only parameter negatively associated with the disease response to PRRT and patient survival.

The study by Lamarca et al. [7] explored the feasibility of assessing circulating tumor DNA (ctDNA) in a cohort of 15 patients with advanced well-differentiated NETs. A cohort of 30 patients with non-WD NETs was utilized for comparative purposes only. In this study,

Citation: Berruti, A.; Amoroso, V.; Fazio, N. Endocrine and Neuroendocrine Tumors: A Special Issue. *Cancers* **2022**, *14*, 4994. https://doi.org/10.3390/cancers14204994

Received: 26 September 2022
Accepted: 8 October 2022
Published: 12 October 2022

Publisher's Note: MDPI stays neutral with regard to jurisdictional claims in published maps and institutional affiliations.

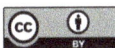

Copyright: © 2022 by the authors. Licensee MDPI, Basel, Switzerland. This article is an open access article distributed under the terms and conditions of the Creative Commons Attribution (CC BY) license (https://creativecommons.org/licenses/by/4.0/).

mutation-based ctDNA analysis, although feasible (with a non-evaluable sample rate of 27.8%), was of limited clinical utility.

Few cellular and patient-derived xenograft (PDX) models are available for testing new therapies and studying the heterogeneous nature of neuroendocrine neoplasms (NENs). Tran et al. [8] described the establishment and characterization of two novel neuroendocrine carcinoma (NEC) cellular and PDX models (NEC913 and NEC1452). NEC913 PDX tumors expressed somatostatin receptor 2 (SSTR2), whereas NEC1452 PDX tumors were SSTR2-negative. As a proof-of-concept study, the authors demonstrated how these PDX models can be used for peptide imaging experiments targeting SSTR2 using fluorescently labeled octreotides.

Several societies have issued guidelines for the diagnosis and treatment of NETs; however, there are still areas of controversy for which there is limited guidance. A group of experts met to formulate 14 statements regarding controversial issues relative to the diagnosis, treatment, and follow-up of NENs, which are presented in the paper by Bartolomei et al. [9]. The nominal group and estimate–talk–estimate techniques were used.

Despite the approval of new targeted therapies for pancreatic neuroendocrine tumors (PanNETs) over recent decades, the early identification of resistant tumors remains a major challenge. Cella et al. [10] evaluated a specific soluble angiogenesis panel as a possible predictor of efficacy/resistance to everolimus in patients with PanNETs. This study showed that none of the investigated categories of biomarkers had predictive value for everolimus resistance or efficacy. However, the data suggested that circulating endothelial progenitors might be surrogate biomarkers for angiogenesis activity in PanNETs during everolimus treatment, and their baseline levels might correlate with patients' survival outcomes.

Among the review papers, Feola et al. [11] performed a systematic literature review to explore the clinicopathological features and the treatment response according to the Ki-67 labeling index cut-off in NECs. A total of 268 NEC patients from eight studies were analyzed. The results showed that NECs with a low Ki-67 labeling index had a better prognosis than the subgroup with higher Ki-67 but worse than G3 NET patients. These results support the notion that NECs are heterogeneous, and their clinical behavior is different from NETs irrespective of the proliferative activity.

Aktypis et al. [12] presented the results of a systematic review and quantitative meta-analysis on the cardiovascular toxicity of biotherapy and molecular targeted therapies currently in use in the management of patients with advanced and/or metastatic NENs. They found that somatostatin analogs and tryptophan hydroxylase inhibitors appeared to be safer than mTOR and tyrosine-kinase inhibitors (TKIs) with regard to cardiovascular toxicity. The authors concluded that special consideration should be given to a patient-tailored approach with anticipated toxicities of targeted treatments for NENs together with the assessment of cardiovascular comorbidities, and early recognition/management of cardiovascular toxicities in order to preserve cardiovascular health and overall quality of life.

Whether immunotherapy is efficacious or not in the management of adrenal cancers is a controversial issue [13]. Jimenez et al. [14] reviewed the current literature to summarize the role of immunotherapy in these rare cancers. The results of clinical trials with immune checkpoint inhibitors (ICIs) for adrenocortical carcinoma or metastatic pheochromocytoma or paraganglioma demonstrated limited benefits; nevertheless, published trials also suggest interesting mechanisms that might enhance clinical responses, including the normalization of tumor vasculature, the modification of the hormonal environment, and vaccination with specific tumor antigens.

Carcinoid crisis is a severe adverse event that may rarely occur in patients with advanced NET. In their review paper, Bardasi et al. [15] discussed its potential etiopathogenetic mechanisms, clinical implications, potential treatments and prophylaxis.

Anaplastic thyroid carcinoma (ATC) is a very aggressive neoplasm and the patient prognosis is dismal [16]. However, a significant survival improvement might be possible in tertiary centers owing to the systematic use of molecular tests for targeted therapies and the integration of fast-track dedicated care pathways. Jannin et al. [17] reviewed the current knowledge on ATC and provided perspectives to improve the management of this deadly disease.

We hope this Special Issue may have responded to the clinical need for up-to-date and in-depth information for the optimal management of patients with NENs.

Author Contributions: Conceptualization, A.B., V.A. and N.F.; writing—original draft preparation, A.B.; writing—review and editing, A.B., V.A. and N.F.; visualization, A.B., V.A. and N.F.; supervision, N.F. All authors have read and agreed to the published version of the manuscript.

Funding: This research received no external funding.

Conflicts of Interest: The authors declare no conflict of interest..

References

1. Baudin, E.; Caplin, M.; Garcia-Carbonero, R.; Fazio, N.; Ferolla, P.; Filosso, P.L.; Frilling, A.; de Herder, W.W.; Hörsch, D.; Knigge, U.; et al. Lung and thymic carcinoids: ESMO Clinical Practice Guidelines for diagnosis, treatment and follow-up. *Ann Oncol.* **2021**, *32*, 439–451. [CrossRef] [PubMed]
2. Pavel, M.; Öberg, K.; Falconi, M.; Krenning, E.P.; Sundin, A.; Perren, A.; Berruti, A. Gastroenteropancreatic neuroendocrine neoplasms: ESMO Clinical Practice Guidelines for diagnosis, treatment and follow-up. ESMO Guidelines Committee. *Ann Oncol.* **2020**, *31*, 844–860. [CrossRef] [PubMed]
3. Cremaschi, V.; Abate, A.; Cosentini, D.; Grisanti, S.; Rossini, E.; Laganà, M.; Tamburello, M.; Turla, A.; Sigala, S.; Berruti, A. Advances in adrenocortical carcinoma pharmacotherapy: What is the current state of the art? *Expert Opin. Pharmacother.* **2022**, *23*, 1413–1424. [CrossRef] [PubMed]
4. Sbiera, I.; Kircher, S.; Altieri, B.; Fassnacht, M.; Kroiss, M.; Sbiera, S. Epithelial and Mesenchymal Markers in Adrenocortical Tissues: How Mesenchymal Are Adrenocortical Tissues? *Cancers* **2021**, *13*, 1736. [CrossRef] [PubMed]
5. Prete, A.; Matrone, A.; Gambale, C.; Bottici, V.; Cappagli, V.; Romei, C.; Torregrossa, L.; Valerio, L.; Minaldi, E.; Campopiano, M.C.; et al. Active Surveillance in RET Gene Carriers Belonging to Families with Multiple Endocrine Neoplasia. *Cancers* **2021**, *13*, 5554. [CrossRef] [PubMed]
6. Durmo, R.; Filice, A.; Fioroni, F.; Cervati, V.; Finocchiaro, D.; Coruzzi, C.; Besutti, G.; Fanello, S.; Frasoldati, A.; Versari, A. Predictive and Prognostic Role of Pre-Therapy and Interim 68Ga-DOTATOC PET/CT Parameters in Metastatic Advanced Neuroendocrine Tumor Patients Treated with PRRT. *Cancers* **2022**, *14*, 592. [CrossRef] [PubMed]
7. Lamarca, A.; Frizziero, M.; Barriuso, J.; Kapacee, Z.; Mansoor, W.; McNamara, M.G.; Hubner, R.A.; Valle, J.W. Molecular Profiling of Well-Differentiated Neuroendocrine Tumours: The Role of ctDNA in Real-World Practice. *Cancers* **2022**, *14*, 1017. [CrossRef]
8. Tran, C.G.; Borbon, L.C.; Mudd, J.L.; Abusada, E.; AghaAmiri, S.; Ghosh, S.C.; Vargas, S.H.; Li, G.; Beyer, G.V.; McDonough, M.; et al. Establishment of Novel Neuroendocrine Carcinoma Patient-Derived Xenograft Models for Receptor Peptide-Targeted Therapy. *Cancers* **2022**, *14*, 1910. [CrossRef]
9. Bartolomei, M.; Berruti, A.; Falconi, M.; Fazio, N.; Ferone, D.; Lastoria, S.; Pappagallo, G.; Seregni, E.; Versari, A. Clinical Management of Neuroendocrine Neoplasms in Clinical Practice: A Formal Consensus Exercise. *Cancers* **2022**, *14*, 2501. [CrossRef]
10. Cella, C.A.; Spada, F.; Berruti, A.; Bertolini, F.; Mancuso, P.; Barberis, M.; Pisa, E.; Rubino, M.; Gervaso, L.; Laffi, A.; et al. Addressing the Role of Angiogenesis in Patients with Advanced Pancreatic Neuroendocrine Tumors Treated with Everolimus: A Biological Prospective Analysis of Soluble Biomarkers and Clinical Outcomes. *Cancers* **2022**, *14*, 4471. [CrossRef]
11. Feola, T.; Centello, R.; Sesti, F.; Puliani, G.; Verrico, M.; Di Vito, V.; Di Gioia, C.; Bagni, O.; Lenzi, A.; Isidori, A.M.; et al. Neuroendocrine Carcinomas with Atypical Proliferation Index and Clinical Behavior: A Systematic Review. *Cancers* **2021**, *13*, 1247. [CrossRef]
12. Aktypis, C.; Spei, M.E.; Yavropoulou, M.; Wallin, G.; Koumarianou, A.; Kaltsas, G.; Kassi, E.; Daskalakis, K. Cardiovascular Toxicities Secondary to Biotherapy and Molecular Targeted Therapies in Neuroendocrine Neoplasms: A Systematic Review and Meta-Analysis of Randomized Placebo-Controlled Trials. *Cancers* **2021**, *13*, 2159. [CrossRef]
13. Grisanti, S.; Cosentini, D.; Laganà, M.; Volta, A.D.; Palumbo, C.; Massimo Tiberio, G.A.; Sigala, S.; Berruti, A. The long and winding road to effective immunotherapy in patients with adrenocortical carcinoma. *Future Oncol.* **2020**, *16*, 3017–3020. [CrossRef]
14. Jimenez, C.; Armaiz-Pena, G.; Dahia, P.L.M.; Lu, Y.; Toledo, R.A.; Varghese, J.; Habra, M.A. Endocrine and Neuroendocrine Tumors Special Issue-Checkpoint Inhibitors for Adrenocortical Carcinoma and Metastatic Pheochromocytoma and Paraganglioma: Do They Work? *Cancers* **2022**, *14*, 467. [CrossRef] [PubMed]
15. Bardasi, C.; Benatti, S.; Luppi, G.; Garajovà, I.; Piacentini, F.; Dominici, M.; Gelsomino, F. Carcinoid Crisis: A Misunderstood and Unrecognized Oncological Emergency. *Cancers* **2022**, *14*, 662. [CrossRef]
16. Filetti, S.; Durante, C.; Hartl, D.; Leboulleux, S.; Locati, L.D.; Newbold, K.; Papotti, M.G.; Berruti, A. ESMO Guidelines Committee. Thyroid cancer: ESMO Clinical Practice Guidelines for diagnosis, treatment and follow-up. *Ann. Oncol.* **2019**, *30*, 1856–1883. [CrossRef]
17. Jannin, A.; Escande, A.; Al Ghuzlan, A.; Blanchard, P.; Hartl, D.; Chevalier, B.; Deschamps, F.; Lamartina, L.; Lacroix, L.; Dupuy, C.; et al. Anaplastic Thyroid Carcinoma: An Update. *Cancers* **2022**, *14*, 1061. [CrossRef] [PubMed]

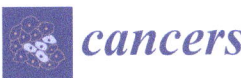

Article

Addressing the Role of Angiogenesis in Patients with Advanced Pancreatic Neuroendocrine Tumors Treated with Everolimus: A Biological Prospective Analysis of Soluble Biomarkers and Clinical Outcomes

Chiara Alessandra Cella [1,*], Francesca Spada [1,*], Alfredo Berruti [2], Francesco Bertolini [3,4], Patrizia Mancuso [3,4], Massimo Barberis [5], Eleonora Pisa [5], Manila Rubino [1], Lorenzo Gervaso [1,6], Alice Laffi [7], Stefania Pellicori [8], Davide Radice [9], Laura Zorzino [10], Angelica Calleri [11], Luigi Funicelli [12,13], Giuseppe Petralia [14,15] and Nicola Fazio [1]

1. Division of Gastrointestinal Medical Oncology and Neuroendocrine Tumors, European Institute of Oncology, IRCCS, 20141 Milan, Italy
2. Medical Oncology Unit, Department of Medical and Surgical Specialties, Radiological Sciences and Public Health, University of Brescia at the Azienda Socio Sanitaria Territoriale (ASST)-Spedali Civili, 25121 Brescia, Italy
3. Laboratory of Hematology-Oncology, European Institute of Oncology, IRCCS, 20141 Milan, Italy
4. Onco-Tech Lab, European Institute of Oncology IRCCS and Politecnico di Milano, 20019 Milan, Italy
5. Division of Pathology and Laboratory Medicine, European Institute of Oncology, IRCCS, 20141 Milan, Italy
6. Molecular Medicine Department, University of Pavia, 27100 Pavia, Italy
7. Medical Oncology and Hematology Unit, Humanitas Cancer Center, IRCCS Humanitas Research Hospital, 20089 Rozzano, Italy
8. Oncology Department, Azienda Ospedaliera di Lodi, 26900 Lodi, Italy
9. Division of Epidemiology and Biostatistics European Institute of Oncology, IRCCS, 20141 Milan, Italy
10. Division of Laboratory Medicine, European Institute of Oncology, IRCCS, 20141 Milan, Italy
11. Division of Diagnostic Haematopathology, European Institute of Oncology, IRCCS, 20141 Milan, Italy
12. Division of Medical Imaging and Radiation Sciences, European Institute of Oncology, IRCCS, 20141 Milan, Italy
13. SIRM, Italian College of Computed Tomography, Italian Society of Medical and Interventional Radiology, 20122 Milan, Italy
14. Department of Oncology and Hemato-Oncology, University of Milan, 20122 Milan, Italy
15. Precision Imaging and Research Unit, Department of Medical Imaging and Radiation Sciences, European Institute of Oncology, IRCCS, Via Ripamonti 435, 20141 Milan, Italy
* Correspondence: chiaraalessandra.cella@ieo.it (C.A.C.); francesca.spada@ieo.it (F.S.); Tel.: +39-02574298 (C.A.C.); +39-02574298 (F.S.)

Citation: Cella, C.A.; Spada, F.; Berruti, A.; Bertolini, F.; Mancuso, P.; Barberis, M.; Pisa, E.; Rubino, M.; Gervaso, L.; Laffi, A.; et al. Addressing the Role of Angiogenesis in Patients with Advanced Pancreatic Neuroendocrine Tumors Treated with Everolimus: A Biological Prospective Analysis of Soluble Biomarkers and Clinical Outcomes. *Cancers* **2022**, *14*, 4471. https://doi.org/10.3390/cancers14184471

Academic Editor: Girolamo Ranieri

Received: 28 July 2022
Accepted: 5 September 2022
Published: 15 September 2022

Publisher's Note: MDPI stays neutral with regard to jurisdictional claims in published maps and institutional affiliations.

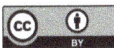

Copyright: © 2022 by the authors. Licensee MDPI, Basel, Switzerland. This article is an open access article distributed under the terms and conditions of the Creative Commons Attribution (CC BY) license (https://creativecommons.org/licenses/by/4.0/).

Simple Summary: Despite the approval of new targeted therapies for pancreatic neuroendocrine tumors (PanNETs) over the past decades, the early identification of resistant tumors remains the major challenge, mainly because clear signs of tumor shrinkage are rarely achieved by imaging assessment. Starting from the hypothesis that angiogenesis can be implicated in the resistance to mTOR inhibitors, we evaluated a specific angiogenesis panel (through the measurement of soluble biomarkers for angiogenesis turnover, circulating endothelial cells, and circulating progenitors) as possible predictors of resistance to everolimus or everolimus efficacy in PanNETs. Our study showed that none of the investigated categories of biomarkers had a predictive value for everolimus resistance or efficacy. However, we suggest that circulating endothelial progenitors might be surrogate biomarkers for angiogenesis activity in PanNETs during everolimus treatment, and their baseline levels might correlate with survival outcomes. These data have never been reported before for NETs.

Abstract: Background: The success of targeted therapies in the treatment of pancreatic neuroendocrine tumors has emphasized the strategy of targeting angiogenesis and the PI3K/AKT/mTOR pathway. However, the major challenge in the targeted era remains the early identification of resistant tumors especially when the efficacy is rarely associated to a clear tumor shrinkage at by imaging assessment. Methods: In this prospective study (NCT02305810) we investigated the predictive and prognostic role of soluble biomarkers of angiogenesis turnover (VEGF, bFGF, VEGFR2,

TSP-1) circulating endothelial cells and progenitors, in 43 patients with metastatic panNET receiving everolimus. Results: Among all tested biomarkers, we found a specific subpopulation of circulating cells, CD31+CD140b-, with a significantly increased tumor progression hazard for values less or equal to the first quartile. Conclusion: Our study suggested the evidence that circulating cells might be surrogate biomarkers of angiogenesis activity in patients treated with everolimus and their baseline levels can be correlated with survival. However, further studies are now needed to validate the role of these cells as surrogate markers for the selection of patients to be candidates for antiangiogenic treatments.

Keywords: pancreatic neuroendocrine tumor; everolimus; angiogenesis; circulating cells; biomarkers

1. Introduction

Pancreatic neuroendocrine tumors (PanNETs) are rare pancreatic neoplasms and represent less than 3% of primary pancreatic tumors [1]. Over the past decades, several therapies (other than somatostatin analogs), such as everolimus (EVE), sunitinib (SUN), and more recently, peptide receptor radionuclide therapy (PRRT), have been approved by the FDA and EMA for PanNETs based on pivotal trials [2–4]. Everolimus is an orally active mTOR inhibitor that has been reported to have anti-angiogenic properties distinct from vascular endothelial growth factor (VEGF) inhibitors [5]. In preclinical models, EVE has been shown to reduce the amount of mature and immature vessels, the total plasma, and VEGF in tumors without affecting blood vessel leakiness or tumor vascular permeability [5]. Some years later, this information was matched with clinical outcomes in a large biomarker analysis from the RADIANT-3 clinical trial. More in detail, Yao et al. proved that elevated baseline chromogranin A, neuron-specific enolase (NSE), placental growth factor (PlGF), and soluble VEGF receptor 1 (sVEGFR1) levels were found to be associated with a poor prognosis in patients with NETs receiving EVE [6]. Although some prognostic significance has been hypothesized, none of the components of the mTOR pathway have shown a reliable predictive value [7–9]. Moreover, the relative indolent behavior of NETs and the lack of sufficient discriminative power to monitor the effects of antivascular drugs make efficacy assessments even more challenging with the standard imaging techniques.

Therefore, in keeping with the concept that the early identification of responder patients is still an unmet clinical need in the targeted era, the role of angiogenesis as an adaptive prosurvival mechanism of tumor cells resistant to EVE deserves to be deeply investigated. Particularly, in the current study, we address the predictive and prognostic role of circulating biomarkers for angiogenesis turnover (BAT), as well as circulating cells (CCs), and we conduct a survival outcomes analysis. Hereby, we explain the rationale for the investigated biomarkers.

1.1. Biomarkers for Angiogenesis Turnover (BAT)

Angiogenesis is mediated by the balance between positive and negative regulators. Modulations in the expression of the following BAT have been proposed as direct/indirect biomarkers of anti-angiogenic drug activity:

1. VEGF is a strong growth factor that increases endothelial permeability. It can be released by cancer, stromal, and inflammatory cells, and it is stored in the platelets;
2. Basic fibroblast growth factor (bFGF) is a pro-angiogenic growth factor released by tumor, stromal, and inflammatory cells and/or by mobilization from the extracellular matrix (ECM). It acts on endothelial cells via a paracrine mode of action; however, it can also be produced endogenously by endothelial cells via autocrine, intracrine, or paracrine modes, trigging angiogenesis signaling;
3. VEGF receptor 2 (VEGFR2) is a member of the VEGFR family, and it is mainly localized in the vascular endothelium. VEGF ligands bind to VEGFR2, hence, triggering

endothelial cell proliferation, survival, migration, and vascular permeability. Lastly, it contributes to angiogenesis activation;

4. Thrombospondin (TSP1) is a family of five proteins involved in tissue remodeling associated with tumor cell proliferation and other physiological processes. It has been shown to suppress tumor growth by both inhibiting angiogenesis and activating transforming growth factor beta (TGF-β). Additionally, TSP1 exerts an anti-angiogenic effect through a direct effect on the migration of endothelial cells and the availability of VEGF.

1.2. Circulating Cells (CCs)

Circulating endothelial cells (CECs) are mature, differentiated endothelial cells shed from vessels during physiological endothelial turnover. They can be found in very small numbers within the blood of healthy individuals, and their number is indicative of and correlates with the degree of endothelial injury or dysfunction [10]. Circulating endothelial progenitors (CEPs) and pericyte progenitor cells (PPCs) are subsets of non-hematopoietic bone marrow-derived cells (BMDC) that are mobilized to complement local angiogenesis by acting as an alternative source of endothelial and mesenchymal cells [11]. In contrast to other bone BMDC types, CEPs and PPCs are thought to merge with the wall of a growing blood vessel, where they differentiate into mature endothelial and mesenchymal cells, thus, contributing to vessel growth [10,11]. Circulating mature endothelial cells (CECs) comprise: DNA (Syto16)+CD45-CD31+CD140bCD146+, including CD109+ and CD109-, and viable and apoptotic subpopulations. Circulating endothelial progenitors (CEPs) comprise: DNA (Syto16)+CD45-CD31+CD34+CD140b, including CD133+ and CD133-, and VEGFR2+ and VEGFR2- subpopulations. Circulating pericyte progenitors (PPCs) comprise: DNA (Syto16)+CD45-CD140b-, including CD31- subpopulations. To assess the blood-based biomarkers for angiogenesis that may predict the outcome of targeted therapies in cancer patients, many approaches have been tested in both preclinical and clinical studies; among these, the quantification of CECs and CEPs by flow cytometry has found wide application [12,13]. Increased plasma levels of CECs and CEPs have been reported in cancer patients. Modifications to their number and viability have shown predictive, prognostic, and dynamic biomarker value during patient selection and follow-up. Patients who responded to treatment with anti-angiogenic drugs showed clear changes in CEC and CEP levels when compared to baseline levels, while a subsequent increase predicted worse PFS [14–16]. At the time of this paper, no data regarding the predictive or prognostic role of these cells in patients with NETs were available, regardless of the therapeutic strategy.

In conclusion, EVE has been reported to have antivascular properties distinct from VEGF inhibitors. However, the role of blood-based biomarkers and circulating cells as direct or indirect indicators of angiogenesis activation and early predictors of EVE efficacy still needs to be clearly established in PanNETS.

2. Materials and Methods

This was a prospective clinical-biological study (clinicaltrials.gov: NCT02305810) including patients with well or moderately differentiated metastatic PanNETs (WHO, 2010 histology classification) who were treated with EVE and enrolled at the European Institute of Oncology between 2011 and 2016. This research has been approved by the local ethics committee (IEO S543/310). Patients with poorly differentiated neuroendocrine carcinoma, adenocarcinoid, goblet cell carcinoid, small cell carcinoma, and Merkel cell carcinoma were excluded from this study, as well as patients who received prior therapy with mTOR inhibitors.

2.1. Study Procedures

The written informed consent was signed and dated by the patients and investigators during the screening consultation. A clinical examination was scheduled at least monthly. Blood tests for CECs, CEPs, VEGF, bFGF, VEGFR2, and TSP1 were collected at baseline after one and three months of treatment, then at disease progression. A tissue biopsy at baseline, or optionally, at disease progression was required.

2.2. Sample Size

This is an exploratory study on the potential predictive and prognostic value of blood-based biomarkers (as direct or indirect indicators of angiogenesis activation) in patients with metastatic PanNETs treated with EVE. The two-tailed log-rank test ((α = 0.05, 1-β = 0.20) null hypothesis of HR = 0.30 (HR = Hazard Ratio), at three months from the start of treatment, for blood-based biomarkers values above the baseline median required 43 patients. The sample size was calculated to for the compensate the power loss of the log-rank test, assuming an average non-informative drop-out rate of 10%.

2.3. Statistical Analysis

The patients' categorical variables were summarized by the count and percentage by mean and standard deviation (SD). BATs and CCs were summarized by the mean and interquartile range (IQR), and changes from the baseline were analyzed using repeated measures ANOVA. The time and the subjects' ID entered the analysis as fixed and random factors, respectively. Patients whose time of visit did not fall within the range of ± 10 days around the expected time, at 1 and 3 months after treatment started, were excluded from the analysis. Means comparison tests, with respect to the baseline, were adjusted for multiplicity using a simulation approach. Progression-free survival (PFS) and overall survival (OS) were defined as the time from EVE start to progression or death and the time from EVE start to death, respectively. OS and PFS risks, by the median cut-off value of the angiogenetic factors and CTC, were estimated using the Cox model; the resulting HRs were tabulated alongside 95% confidence intervals (CI). The median OS and PFS were estimated using the Kaplan–Meier method.

3. Results

Forty-three patients with histological diagnosis of well/moderately differentiated metastatic PanNETs were eligible and signed the informed consent for the study. The data analysis included 38 patients. Two were excluded due to screening failure (one due to a fast clinical deterioration and one due to thrombocytopenia); one patient was excluded due to an extreme irregularity of EVE assumption and, therefore, an unreliable correlation with the biological parameters; two patients were excluded due to an internal pathology review which did not confirm a well-differentiated tumor morphology. The mean age at diagnosis was 50 years (26–66). The median duration of treatment was 10.1 months. One-third of the patients had synchronous metastases. The complete baseline of the patient/tumor's characteristics is summarized in Table 1.

Serum concentrations of BAT (VEGF, bFGF, VEGFR2, and TSP1) at the time from EVE start and their mean comparisons with the baselines at 1 and 3 months are shown in Figure 1. A number of significant changes were observed, except for in VEGF, for which the mean was significantly higher at 1 month (612 pg/mL vs. 448 pg/mL, p = 0.02) compared to the baseline, and VEGFR2, which showed a significant decreasing trend from the baseline (Table S1).

The serum levels of CCs (CECs and CEPs) measured by the time from EVE start are shown in Table 2 (graphically represented in Figure S1). Among CECs, CD146+, vital CD146+, apoptotic CECs, and CD109+ subpopulations all significantly decreased for up to 3 months after the treatment started. Additionally, CD146+ (p = 0.01) and apoptotic CECs (p = 0.02) levels remained significantly lower than the baseline even at the progression timeline. Among pericyte precursors (progenitor perivascular cells, PPCs) and CEPs, the CD31-CD140b+ and Syto16+CD45dimCD34+ subpopulations mean counts were significantly lower at 1 and 3 months compared to the baseline, without any apparent trend. A significant lower mean compared to the baseline was observed for Syto16+CD45dimCD133+CD34+ at

3 months ($p = 0.04$) and for Syto16+CD45dimVEGFR2+ at 1 month ($p = 0.007$). Figure S2 shows the CCs' evaluation by flow cytometry.

Table 1. Patient's characteristics and clinical course, $N = 38$.

Characteristic	Statistics [1]
Age (years) at	
Diagnosis	50.0 (10.1) [2]
Everolimus start	54.4 (10.2)
Metastases	
Synchronous	29 (76.3)
Metachronous	9 (23.7)
Ki 67 (%)	
(<3)	1 (2.7)
(3–20)	31 (81.5)
(21–55)	5 (13.1)
missing	1 (2.7)
Sex	
Male	19 (50.0)
Female	19 (50.0)
Baseline ^{68}Ga-PET/CT	32 (84.2)
Previous Treatments [3]	
Liver-directed treatments	10 (26.3)
Chemotherapy	11 (29.0)
Peptide Receptor Radionuclide Therapy (PRRT)	20 (52.6)
Somatostatin Analogs (SSA)	30 (78.9)
Sunitinib	5 (13.1)
Surgery	
primary site	14 (36.8)
metastatic site	2 (5.3)
primary and metastatic site	9 (23.7)
none	13 (34.2)
Functionally active tumors	
Yes	5 (13.2)
No	33 (86.8)

[1] Statistics are: Mean (SD) for Age, [2] (min = 26, max = 66), N (%) otherwise, [3] Not mutually exclusive treatments; SD = Standard Deviation.

Survival Analysis

Median PFS and OS were 14.9 months (95% CI: (10.3–27.7) and 33.6 months (95% CI: (28.5—upper limit not estimable)), respectively. Kaplan–Meier curves for PFS and OS are shown in Figure 2. According to the BAT median cut-off at the baseline, no statistically significant hazard ratio (HR) was found for either PFS or OS, except for TPS1, which had a borderline significant ($p = 0.04$) OS risk reduction (HR = 0.33, 95% CI: 0.12–0.95) for TPS1 > 144 ng/mL (Table 3). Progression-free survival risk estimates according to the first (Q1), second (median), and third (Q3) quartiles of the baseline CCs are summarized as Hazard Ratios (HR) in Table S2. After adjusting for multiple comparisons, only the PPC CD31-CD140b+ showed a significantly increased in PFS hazard for values less than or equal to the first quartile [Q1 = 51.4 counts/mL, HR = 3.78, 95% CI: (1.53–9.33), adjusted $p = 0.01$]. However, both the number of events and the subjects at risk were as few as eight and nine, respectively. No significant HRs were found for any other CCs, with the least significant hazard being for Syto16+CD45dim, CD133+CD34+ [Q1 = 87.4 counts/mL, HR = 2.70, 95% CI: (1.07–6.79), adjusted $p = 0.06$]. The Kaplan–Meier PFS curve, according to the baseline of the first quartile, for PPC CD31-CD140b+ is shown in Figure 3.

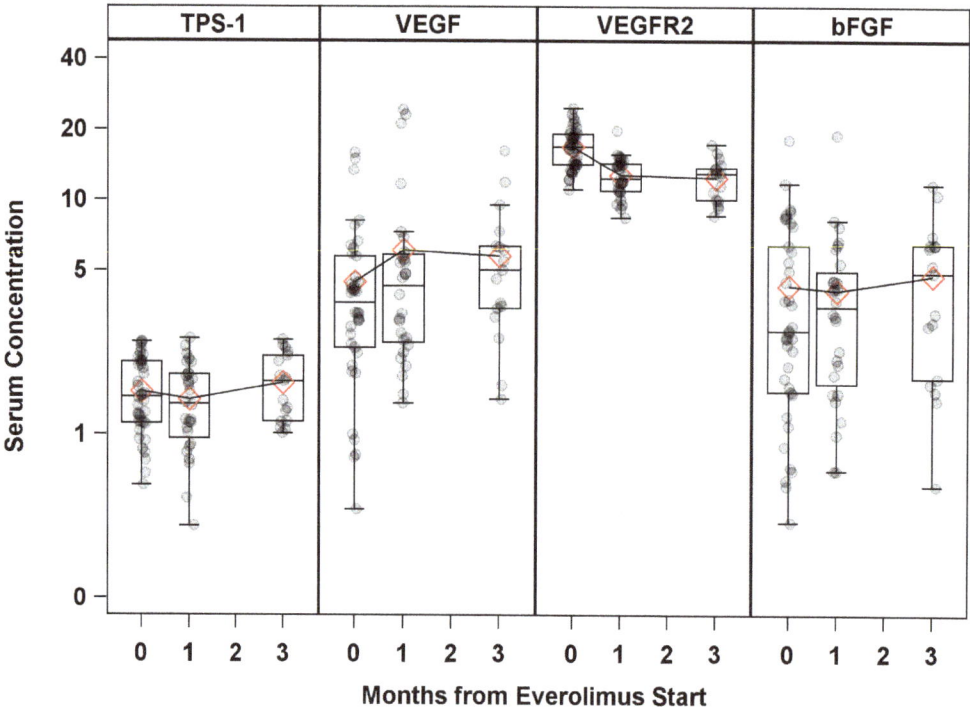

Figure 1. Serum BAT concentration by time from Everolimus start. Serum concentration units: TPS1 (ng/mL) × 100; VEGF (pg/mL) × 100; VEGFR2 (pg/mL) × 100; bFGF (pg/mL).

Table 2. Summary Statistics of CCs by time from everolimus start.

	Time	N	Mean (IQR) [1]	Adj p-Value [2]
CEC CD146+	Baseline	36	119 (67.7–163)	-
	Month 1	37	64.6 (31.9–73.7)	<0.001
	Month 3	34	54.8 (23.4–66.0)	<0.001
	at PD	13	52.4 (22.8–66.5)	0.01
CEC, Apo (%)	Baseline	36	51.3 (39.0–68.0)	-
	Month 1	37	59.5 (38.0–80.0)	0.34
	Month 3	34	57.6 (42.0–70.0)	0.59
	at PD	13	52.9 (46.0–67.0)	1.00
CEC CD146+ Vital	Baseline	36	61.0 (24.5–84.3)	-
	Month 1	37	31.4 (6.3–36.7)	0.01
	Month 3	34	26.9 (7.3–30.6)	0.003
	at PD	13	23.3 (11.4–33.4)	0.05
Apoptotic CEC	Baseline	35	59.6 (28.3–68.0)	-
	Month 1	36	33.7 (16.4–42.8)	0.002
	Month 3	33	28.6 (13.6–38.9)	<0.001
	at PD	13	29.2 (11.4–33.3))	0.02
CD140b+ pericytes	Baseline	36	22.4 (7.6–30.8)	-
	Month 1	37	15.6 (0.0–16.2)	0.50
	Month 3	33	13.2 (2.5–14.7)	0.25
	at PD	13	11.4 (3.6–16.5)	0.36

Table 2. Cont.

	Time	N	Mean (IQR)[1]	Adj p-Value[2]
CEC CD109+	Baseline	34	111 (50.4–160)	-
	Month 1	37	51.5 (21.6–71.3)	0.003
	Month 3	34	51.3 (21.0–54.1)	0.004
	at PD	13	50.9 (19.6–75.0)	0.05
PPC CD31-CD140b+	Baseline	36	107 (51.4–153)	-
	Month 1	37	49.9 (27.3.61.8)	0.001
	Month 3	33	62.0 (26.8–73.5)	0.02
	at PD	13	53.1 (24.9–75.6)	0.04
Syto16+CD45dimCD34+	Baseline	36	729 (401–909)	-
	Month 1	37	481 (226–601)	0.002
	Month 3	33	534 (256–711)	0.01
	at PD	12	537 (186–611)	0.33
Syto16+CD45-CD34+	Baseline	36	52.3 (27.8–67.2)	-
	Month 1	37	36.7 (23.5–44.8)	0.56
	Month 3	33	55.2 (25.057.6)	0.99
	at PD	12	56.8 (37.5–63.7)	0.99
Syto16+CD45dimCD133+(	Baseline	36	213 (87.4–269)	-
	Month 1	37	164 (62.3–234)	0.46
	Month 3	33	126 (67.6–160)	0.04
	at PD	12	157 (46.2–295)	0.66
Syto16+CD45dimVEGFR2+	Baseline	36	6.57 (0.00–9.25)	-
	Month 1	37	1.90 (0.00–2.50)	0.007
	Month 3	32	2.84 (0.00–4.78)	0.06
	at PD	11	2.11 (0.00–3.55)	0.14

[1] IQR = Interquartile Range; [2] Repeated Measures Adjusted p-values for Multiple comparisons vs. Baseline.

Table 3. Progression-free survival and overall survival risk estimates according to BAT median cut-off values at baseline.

		Cut-Off (Median)	No. Failures /at Risk	Hazard Ratio (95% CI)	Adj p-Value
PFS	VEGF (pg/mL)	≤365	12/19	Ref	
		>365	13/19	1.06 (0.48–2.33)	0.88
	VEGF R (pg/mL)	≤1689	12/19	Ref	
		>1689	13/19	1.30 (0.59–2.85)	0.52
	BFGF (pg/mL)	≤2.8	15/19	Ref	
		>2.8	10/19	0.50 (0.22–1.12)	0.09
	TPS1 (ng/mL)	≤144	14/19	Ref	
		>144	11/19	0.65 (0.29–1.44)	0.29
OS	VEGF (pg/mL)	≤365	8/19	Ref	
		>365	8/19	1.05 (0.39–2.79)	0.93
	VEGF R (pg/mL)	≤1689	9/19	Ref	
		>1689	7/19	0.61 (0.23–1.66)	0.33
	BFGF (pg/mL)	≤2.8	8/19	Ref	
		>2.8	8/19	0.60 (0.22–1.62)	0.31
	TPS1 (ng/mL)	≤144	10/19	Ref	
		>144	6/19	0.33 (0.12–0.95)	0.04

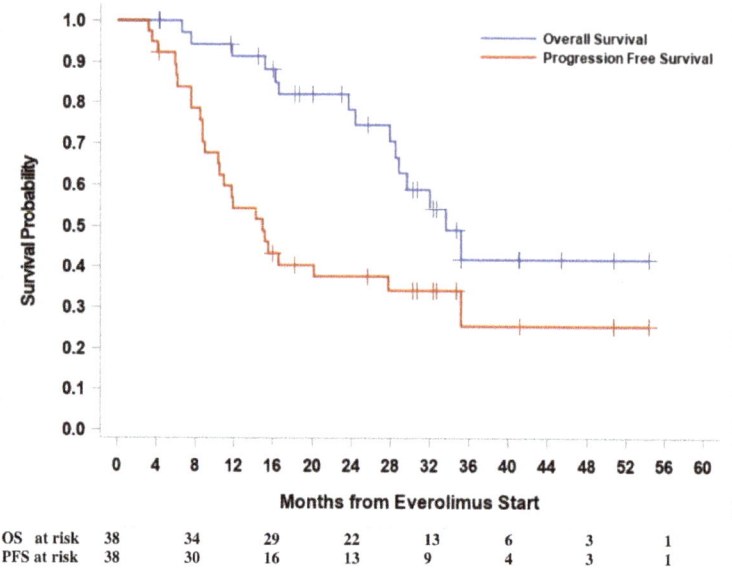

Figure 2. Survival outcomes.

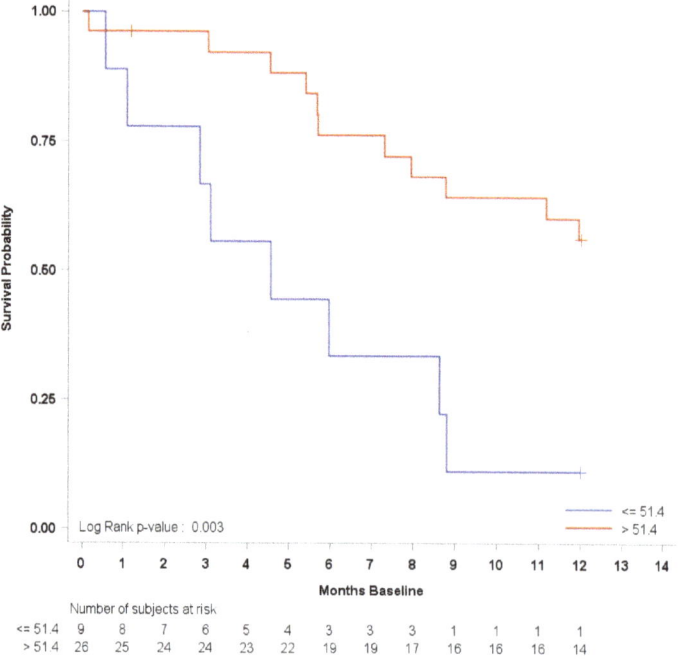

Figure 3. Progression-free survival Kaplan–Meier curve by first quartile of baseline PPC CD31-CD140b+.

4. Discussion

In our study, neither soluble BAT, CECs, nor CEPs showed any predictive value for EVE efficacy. However, a specific subpopulation of circulating progenitors, CD31-CD140b+ (pericytes), was associated with a significantly shorter PFS when its values were less than or equal to the values in the first quartile.

Regarding BAT assessment, our study did not prove any prognostic nor predictive role, with the only exception being VEGFR2, which showed a significant decreasing trend over time. Similarly, TPS1, presented a borderline significant ($p = 0.04$) OS risk reduction. Conflicting results were previously reported regarding the implication of angiogenesis biomarker measurement (mainly focused on this discussion on VEGF and VEGFR2-3 values) in clinical practice, along with a more uncertain interpretation of their modulation over time [17–20]. Some robust data about the prognostic and clinico-pathological role of the tissue markers of angiogenesis were collected by Pinato et al. [21]. In their work, the clinical and follow-up information of 88 patients who underwent surgical treatment for gastro-entero-pancreatic neuroendocrine tumors (GEPNETs) were matched with histopathological features, such as vascular invasion and necrosis. Despite the identification that VEGFA expression correlated with the presence of liver metastases in the PanNet cohort, there was not any association demonstrated between VEGFA and OS. Furthermore, the majority of tumors displayed evidence of VEGFA expression, in line with the concept that GEPNETs are highly vascular tumors, and VEGFA expression and microvascular count seem to paradoxically reduce with progressive tumor de-differentiation in PanNETs [22]. Nonetheless, soluble biomarkers are likely more reliable predictive or prognostic drivers of angiogenesis turnover.

Surprisingly, in our analysis, the trend of VEGF and VEGFR2 levels seemed to show an inverse correlation, meaning that VEGF levels tended to increase while VEGFR2 concentrations decreased over time after EVE treatment started (from the baseline to 1- or 3-month timepoints). Similar findings have previously emerged with the antivascular agent SUN in different cancer settings. The first-in-human trial with SUN, including an analysis of the plasma levels of VEGF and sVEGFR2 at the baseline and after 28 days of treatment, showed a progressive increase in VEGF and a decrease in sVEGFR2 concentrations, demonstrating the on-target effects of the drug [23]. DePrimo et al. observed similar trends in metastatic renal cell carcinoma (mRCC) by the end of the first 4 weeks of SUN treatment, whereas the concentrations of soluble biomarkers tended to return close to baseline levels at the end of the first 2-week-off period. [24]. Consistent with the results observed in mRCC, Zurita found that high pre-treatment levels of sVEGFR2 were associated with longer OS in 107 patients with PanNETs and carcinoids, with higher sVEGFR2 concentrations in PanNETs compared to carcinoids. Patients with PanNETs also showed a trend toward higher baseline VEGF levels. Notably, at the end of the first cycle of sunitinib treatment (considering a 4-week schedule), an increase in VEGF levels and a decrease in sVEGFR2 and sVEGFR3 concentrations were observed [25].

Overall, these data demonstrate how far we are from interpreting any prognostic nor predictive role of baseline BAT in NETs, which may constitutively overexpress an angiogenic signature. Conversely, the modulation of soluble biomarkers of angiogenesis over time might be a surrogate endpoint of response to antivascular compounds. In our analysis, the inverse trends of soluble VEGF and VEGFR2 during EVE treatment might be consistent with a drug-related inhibitory effect on angiogenesis in patients with metastatic PanNETs.

Regarding the circulating cells (CCs), we found a specific subpopulation of circulating progenitors, CD31-CD140b+ (pericytes), with a significantly shorter PFS for values less than or equal to the first quartile. Conversely, none of the other CCs showed a significant predictive value for EVE activity. Despite the absence of any significant predictability, we found that the number of CCs (CECs and CEPs) decreased during EVE treatment, hence, corroborating the role of EVE in targeting angiogenesis. Former evidence suggested that pericytes could play an important part in tumor angiogenesis due to their ability to trigger the formation of abnormal microvessel networks embedding the tumor cells [26]. A long-standing in-home experience on the potential predictive or prognostic role of CCs has been reported by Bertolini et al., demonstrating that CECs, CEPs, and PPCs significantly increased in untreated cancer patients compared to healthy controls [10,13]. Additionally, they reached similar conclusions in a cohort of advanced breast cancer patients treated with metronomic chemotherapy, alone or in association with antivascular drugs, where the baseline CEC count was an indicator of efficacy [14–16]. Other results found in clear-cell RCC, which were reported by Cao et al., showed that an increased pericyte-generated microvessel formation conferred an anti-angiogenic resistance to treatments [26]. Paradoxically, a lowered pericyte population not only damaged the tumor vascular network, hence impairing tumor growth, but also increased the likelihood of metastatic dissemination [27,28]. In this sense, our analysis is in line with the above-mentioned data, suggesting that variations in the number and viability of PPCs (or committed pericytes) could provide relevant prognostic, but less likely predictive, information. No prior data about the correlation between CEP levels and EVE efficacy are available, except for a single preclinical study, where median values of CEPs were reduced by EVE monotherapy in severe human gastric cancer and a combined immunodeficient (SCID) mouse xenograft model. Despite the high variability in measurements, the decreasing trend of CEP levels under EVE monotherapy might always reflect the inhibitory effect on angiogenesis [29].

These data are also consistent with a previous experience gathered in gastro-enteropancreatic (GEPNET) during SUN treatment, whereas expected, the number of CECs significantly decreased during the first 4 weeks of treatment as a consequence of an angiogenesis blockade. Conversely, no changes in CEPs were observed in the same study [25].

Our findings show that modulation of CEC, CEP, and PPC levels over time might represent an indirect measurement of the endothelial and pericyte turnover during EVE exposure, even though no predictive role can be established based on our analysis.

Our study presents several limitations. Firstly, although at the time of conceptualization it appeared timely, our study has been negatively affected by the long duration and high heterogeneity of the assessment, which invalidated a number of tests. Secondly, the timing of the sample collection was not strictly observed due to administrative delays and low compliance, as often happens in real-world evidence (RWE) studies. Therefore, this flexible management might have conditioned the reliability of statistical analyses.

On the other hand, a possible strength of our study is that a subpopulation of CCs (CD31-CD140b+) correlated with a significantly increased tumor progression hazard for values that were less than or equal to the first quartile, thus, demonstrating a prognostic value for CCs in PanNETs for the first time. Furthermore, the study population was quite homogeneous for types of treatment (EVE) and primary sites (PanNETs).

Finally, although other drugs with preponderant antivascular effects could have been more suitable for our study, the initial hypothesis that angiogenesis might be ascribed as a mechanism for resistance to EVE treatment remains original and innovative, and it deserves to be rigorously investigated, as already addressed in a previous literature review [30]. EVE has been shown to exert anti-angiogenic activity by both direct effects on vascular cell proliferation and indirect effects on growth factor production, with in vitro evidence in colon, breast, renal, melanoma, cervical, and glioma cell lines. However, reports on the activity of EVE during the early stages of in vitro vasculogenesis and angiogenesis in NETs need to be further addressed [31].

5. Conclusions

In conclusion, our study did not provide conclusive results about the predictive role of EVE resistance or the efficacy of biomarkers for angiogenic turnover/activity. However, we reported that the baseline count of CCs (CEP) might represent an indirect measure of endothelial and pericyte turnover and, consequently, can be advocated as a surrogate biomarker of angiogenesis activation. Intriguingly, the hypothesis generated by our study needs to be further investigated in other homogenous populations (e.g., extrapancreatic NENs) treated with EVE.

Supplementary Materials: The following supporting information can be downloaded at: https://www.mdpi.com/article/10.3390/cancers14184471/s1, Figure S1: CCs (CECS and CEPs) by time from Everolimus start; Figure S2: CCs evaluation by flow cytometry; Table S1: Summary Statistics of serum BAT by time from EVE start; Table S2: Progression Free Survival according to the first (Q1), the median and the third quartile (Q3) of the CCs at baseline.

Author Contributions: For this research article, the following contributions were provided: Conceptualization, N.F., C.A.C., F.S., F.B., M.B., D.R., A.L., M.R., P.M., L.F., S.P., L.Z., L.G., E.P., G.P. and A.C.; Methodology, N.F., C.A.C., F.S., F.B., A.B., M.B., D.R., A.L., M.R., P.M., L.F., S.P., L.Z., L.G., E.P., G.P. and A.C.; Software, D.R., L.F., G.P. and M.B.; Formal analysis, D.R.; Investigation, N.F., C.A.C. and F.S.; Resources, N.F.; Data curation, N.F., C.A.C., F.S., F.B., M.B., D.R., A.L., M.R., P.M., L.F., S.P., L.Z., L.G., E.P., G.P. and A.C.; Writing—original draft preparation, N.F. and C.A.C.; Writing—review and editing, N.F., C.A.C., A.B., F.S., F.B., M.B., D.R., A.L., M.R., P.M., L.F., S.P., L.Z., L.G., E.P., G.P. and A.C.; Visualization, N.F., C.A.C., A.B., F.S., F.B., M.B., D.R., A.L., M.R., P.M., L.F., S.P., L.Z., L.G., E.P., G.P. and A.C.; Supervision, N.F., C.A.C., A.B., F.S., F.B., M.B., D.R., A.L., M.R., P.M., L.F., S.P., L.Z., L.G., E.P., G.P. and A.C.; Project administration, N.F. and C.A.C. All authors have read and agreed to the published version of the manuscript.

Funding: This research received no external funding.

Institutional Review Board Statement: The study was conducted in accordance with the Declaration of Helsinki and approved by the Institutional Ethics Committee of European Institute of Oncology (protocol code IEOS543/310;date of approval 9 November 2010).

Informed Consent Statement: Informed consent was obtained from all subjects involved in the study.

Data Availability Statement: This study did not report any data.

Acknowledgments: We acknowledge the AIRC and Italian Ministry of Health for covering the expenses for the circulating cells analysis. We acknowledge Darina Tamayo and Sabrina Boselli for their administrative and technical support.

Conflicts of Interest: C.A.C. reports personal fees from BMS and Leo Pharma, and a research grant from IPSEN (institutional). F.S. received personal fees from Ipsen, Novartis, Pfizer, Advanced Accelerator Applications, and Merck; F.S. also has institutional financial interest in GETNE, Incyte, and MSD. A.B. received fees from Novartis-AAA, Amgen, Bayer, Ipsen, Janssen, and Astellas for an advisory board and public speech. N.F. received personal fees from AAA, Hutchinson MediPharma, Merck, and Novartis; has a financial interest in 4SC, Astellas, Beigene, FIBROGEN, Incyte, IPSEN, MSD, and NUCANA; and has received research grant form IPSEN (institutional).

References

1. Halfdanarson, T.R.; Rabe, K.G.; Rubin, J.; Petersen, G.M. Pancreatic neuroendocrine tumors (PNETs): Incidence, prognosis and recent trend toward improved survival. *Ann. Oncol.* **2008**, *19*, 1727–1733. [CrossRef] [PubMed]
2. Yao, J.C.; Shah, M.H.; Ito, T.; Bohas, C.L.; Wolin, E.M.; Van Cutsem, E.; Hobday, T.J.; Okusaka, T.; Capdevila, J.; de Vries, E.G.; et al. Everolimus for Advanced Pancreatic Neuroendocrine Tumors. *N. Engl. J. Med.* **2011**, *364*, 514–523. [CrossRef] [PubMed]
3. Raymond, E.; Dahan, L.; Raoul, J.-L.; Bang, Y.-J.; Borbath, I.; Lombard-Bohas, C.; Valle, J.; Metrakos, P.; Smith, D.; Vinik, A.; et al. Sunitinib Malate for the Treatment of Pancreatic Neuroendocrine Tumors. *N. Engl. J. Med.* **2011**, *364*, 501–513. [CrossRef] [PubMed]
4. Strosberg, J.; El-Haddad, G.; Wolin, E.; Hendifar, A.; Yao, J.; Chasen, B.; Mittra, E.; Kunz, P.L.; Kulke, M.H.; Jacene, H.; et al. Phase 3 Trial of ^{177}Lu-Dotatate for Midgut Neuroendocrine Tumors. *N. Engl. J. Med.* **2017**, *376*, 125–135. [CrossRef] [PubMed]
5. Lane, H.A.; Wood, J.M.; McSheehy, P.M.; Allegrini, P.R.; Boulay, A.; Brueggen, J.; Littlewood-Evans, A.; Maira, S.; Martiny-Baron, G.; Schnell, C.R.; et al. mTOR inhibitor RAD001 (everolimus) has antiangiogenic/vascular properties dis-tinct from a VEGFR tyrosine kinase inhibitor. *Clin. Cancer Res.* **2009**, *15*, 1612–1622. [CrossRef]
6. Yao, J.C.; Pavel, M.; Lombard-Bohas, C.; Van Cutsem, E.; Voi, M.; Brandt, U.; He, W.; Chen, D.; Capdevila, J.; De Vries, E.G.E.; et al. Everolimus for the Treatment of Advanced Pancreatic Neuroendocrine Tumors: Overall Survival and Circulating Biomarkers From the Randomized, Phase III RADIANT-3 Study. *J. Clin. Oncol.* **2016**, *34*, 3906–3913. [CrossRef]

7. Qian, Z.R.; Ter-Minassian, M.; Chan, J.A.; Imamura, Y.; Hooshmand, S.M.; Kuchiba, A.; Morikawa, T.; Brais, L.K.; Daskalova, A.; Heafield, R.; et al. Prognostic Significance of MTOR Pathway Component Expression in Neuroendocrine Tumors. *J. Clin. Oncol.* **2013**, *31*, 3418–3425. [CrossRef] [PubMed]
8. Missiaglia, E.; Dalai, I.; Barbi, S.; Beghelli, S.; Falconi, M.; della Peruta, M.; Piemonti, L.; Capurso, G.; Florio, A.D.; delle Fave, G.; et al. Pancreatic endocrine tumors: Expression profiling evidences a role for AKT-mTOR pathway. *J. Clin. Oncol.* **2010**, *28*, 245–255. [CrossRef]
9. O'Reilly, K.E.; Rojo, F.; She, Q.-B.; Solit, D.; Mills, G.B.; Smith, D.; Lane, H.; Hofmann, F.; Hicklin, D.J.; Ludwig, D.L.; et al. mTOR Inhibition Induces Upstream Receptor Tyrosine Kinase Signaling and Activates Akt. *Cancer Res.* **2006**, *66*, 1500–1508. [CrossRef]
10. Bertolini, F.; Shaked, Y.; Mancuso, P.; Kerbel, R.S. The multifaceted circulating endothelial cell in cancer: Towards marker and target identification. *Nat. Cancer* **2006**, *6*, 835–845. [CrossRef]
11. Mancuso, P.; Martin-Padura, I.; Calleri, A.; Marighetti, P.; Quarna, J.; Rabascio, C.; Braidotti, P.; Bertolini, F. Circulating perivascular progenitos: A target of PDGFR inhibition. *Int. J. Cancer.* **2011**, *129*, 1344–1350. [CrossRef] [PubMed]
12. Mancuso, P.; Antoniotti, P.; Quarna, J.; Calleri, A.; Rabascio, C.; Tacchetti, C.; Braidotti, P.; Wu, H.-K.; Zurita, A.J.; Saronni, L.; et al. Validation of a Standardized Method for Enumerating Circulating Endothelial Cells and Progenitors: Flow Cytometry and Molecular and Ultrastructural Analyses. *Clin. Cancer Res.* **2008**, *15*, 267–273. [CrossRef] [PubMed]
13. Baig, M.H.; Sudhakar, D.R.; Kalaiarasan, P.; Subbarao, N.; Wadhawa, G.; Lohani, M.; Khan, M.K.A.; Khan, A.U. Insight into the Effect of Inhibitor Resistant S130G Mutant on Physico-Chemical Properties of SHV Type BetaLactamase: A Molecular Dynamics Study. *PLoS ONE* **2014**, *9*, e112456. [CrossRef] [PubMed]
14. Mancuso, P.; Colleoni, M.; Calleri, A.; Orlando, L.; Maisonneuve, P.; Pruneri, G.; Agliano, A.; Goldhirsch, A.; Shaked, Y.; Kerbel, R.S.; et al. Circulating endothelial-cell kinetics and viability predict survival in breast cancer patients receiving metronomic chemotherapy. *Blood* **2006**, *108*, 452–459. [CrossRef] [PubMed]
15. Calleri, A.; Bono, A.; Bagnardi, V.; Quarna, J.; Mancuso, P.; Rabascio, C.; Dellapasqua, S.; Campagnoli, E.; Shaked, Y.; Goldhirsch, A.; et al. Predictive Potential of Angiogenic Growth Factors and Circulating Endothelial Cells in Breast Cancer Patients Receiving Metronomic Chemotherapy Plus Bevacizumab. *Clin. Cancer Res.* **2009**, *15*, 7652–7657. [CrossRef] [PubMed]
16. Dellapasqua, S.; Bertolini, F.; Bagnardi, V.; Campagnoli, E.; Scarano, E.; Torrisi, R.; Shaked, Y.; Mancuso, P.; Goldhirsch, A.; Rocca, A.; et al. Metronomic Cyclophosphamide and Capecitabine Combined With Bevacizumab in Advanced Breast Cancer. *J. Clin. Oncol.* **2008**, *26*, 4899–4905. [CrossRef]
17. Bello, C.; DePrimo, S.E.; Friece, C.; Smeraglia, J.; Sherman, L.; Tye, L.; Baum, C.; Meropol, N.J.; Lenz, H.; Kulke, M.H. Analysis of circulating biomarkers of sunitinib malate in patients with unresectable neuroendocrine tumors (NET): VEGF, IL-8, and soluble VEGF receptors 2 and 3. *J. Clin. Oncol.* **2006**, *24*, 4045. [CrossRef]
18. Zhang, J.; Jia, Z.; Li, Q.; Wang, L.W.; Rashid, A.; Zhu, Z.G.; Evans, D.B.; Vauthey, J.N.; Xie, K.P.; Yao, J.C. Elevated expression of vascular endothelial growth factor correlates with increased angiogenesis and decreased progression-free survival among patients with low-grade neuroendocrine tumors. *Cancer* **2007**, *109*, 1478–1486. [CrossRef]
19. Takahashi, Y.; Akishima-Fukasawa, Y.; Kobayashi, N.; Sano, T.; Kosuge, T.; Nimura, Y.; Kanai, Y.; Hiraoka, N. Prognostic value of tumor architecture, tumor-associated vascular characteristics, and expression of angiogenic molecules in pancreatic en-docrine tumors. *Clin. Cancer Res.* **2007**, *13*, 187–196. [CrossRef]
20. Fazio, N.; Martini, J.-F.; E Croitoru, A.; Schenker, M.; Li, S.; Rosbrook, B.; Fernandez, K.; Tomasek, J.; Thiis-Evensen, E.; Kulke, M.; et al. Pharmacogenomic analyses of sunitinib in patients with pancreatic neuroendocrine tumors. *Future Oncol.* **2019**, *15*, 1997–2007. [CrossRef]
21. Pinato, D.J.; Tan, T.M.; Toussi, S.T.K.; Ramachandran, R.; Martin, N.; Meeran, K.; Ngo, N.; Dina, R.; Sharma, R. An expression signature of the angiogenic response in gastrointestinal neuroendocrine tumours: Correlation with tumour phenotype and survival outcomes. *Br. J. Cancer* **2013**, *110*, 115–122. [CrossRef] [PubMed]
22. Scoazec, J.Y. Angiogenesis in neuroendocrine tumors: Therapeutic applications. *Neuroendocrinology* **2012**, *97*, 45–56. [CrossRef] [PubMed]
23. Faivre, S.; Delbaldo, C.; Vera, K.; Robert, C.; Lozahic, S.; Lassau, N.; Bello, C.; Deprimo, S.; Brega, N.; Massimini, G.; et al. Safety, pharmacokinetic, and antitumor activity of SU11248, a novel oral multitarget ty-rosine kinase inhibitor, in patients with cancer. *J. Clin. Oncol.* **2006**, *24*, 25–35. [CrossRef] [PubMed]
24. E DePrimo, S.; Bello, C.L.; Smeraglia, J.; Baum, C.M.; Spinella, D.; I Rini, B.; Michaelson, M.D.; Motzer, R.J. Circulating protein biomarkers of pharmacodynamic activity of sunitinib in patients with metastatic renal cell carcinoma: Modulation of VEGF and VEGF-related proteins. *J. Transl. Med.* **2007**, *5*, 32. [CrossRef] [PubMed]
25. Zurita, A.J.; Khajavi, M.; Wu, H.-K.; Tye, L.; Huang, X.; Kulke, M.H.; Lenz, H.-J.; Meropol, N.J.; Carley, W.; E DePrimo, S.; et al. Circulating cytokines and monocyte subpopulations as biomarkers of outcome and biological activity in sunitinib-treated patients with advanced neuroendocrine tumours. *Br. J. Cancer* **2015**, *112*, 1199–1205. [CrossRef] [PubMed]
26. Sims, D.E. The pericyte—A review. *Tissue Cell.* **1986**, *18*, 153–174. [CrossRef] [PubMed]
27. Cao, Y.; Zhang, Z.-L.; Zhou, M.; Elson, P.; Rini, B.; Aydin, H.; Feenstra, K.; Tan, M.-H.; Berghuis, B.; Tabbey, R.; et al. Pericyte coverage of differentiated vessels inside tumor vasculature is an independent unfavorable prognostic factor for patients with clear cell renal cell carcinoma. *Cancer* **2012**, *119*, 313–324. [CrossRef]

28. Cooke, V.G.; LeBleu, V.S.; Keskin, D.; Khan, Z.; O'Connell, J.T.; Teng, Y.; Duncan, M.B.; Xie, L.; Maeda, G.; Vong, S.; et al. Pericyte Depletion Results in Hypoxia-Associated Epithelial-to-Mesenchymal Transition and Metastasis Mediated by Met Signaling Pathway. *Cancer Cell.* **2012**, *21*, 66–81. [CrossRef]
29. Cejka, D.; Preusser, M.; Fuereder, T.; Sieghart, W.; Werzowa, J.; Strommer, S.; Wacheck, V. mTOR inhibition sensitizes gastric cancer to alkylating chemotherapy in vivo. *Anticancer Res.* **2009**, *28*, 3801–3808.
30. Martins, D.; Spada, F.; Lambrescu, I.; Rubino, M.; Cella, C.; Gibelli, B.; Grana, C.; Ribero, D.; Bertani, E.; Ravizza, D.; et al. Predictive Markers of Response to Everolimus and Sunitinib in Neuroendocrine Tumors. *Target. Oncol.* **2017**, *12*, 611–622. [CrossRef]
31. Ceausu, R.A.; Cimpean, A.M.; Dimova, I.; Hlushchuk, R.; Djonov, V.; Gaje, P.N.; Raica, M. Everolimus dual effects of an area vas-culosa angiogenesis and lymphangiogenesis. *In Vivo* **2013**, *27*, 61–66. [PubMed]

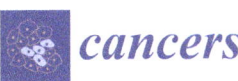

Article

Clinical Management of Neuroendocrine Neoplasms in Clinical Practice: A Formal Consensus Exercise

Mirco Bartolomei [1], Alfredo Berruti [2,*], Massimo Falconi [3], Nicola Fazio [4], Diego Ferone [5], Secondo Lastoria [6], Giovanni Pappagallo [7], Ettore Seregni [8] and Annibale Versari [9]

1. Azienda Ospedaliero-Universitaria di Ferrara, Presidio Ospedaliero Arcispedale Sant'Anna di Cona, 44124 Ferrara, Italy; mirco.bartolomei@unife.it
2. Department of Medical and Surgical Specialties, Radiological Sciences, and Public Health, Medical Oncology, University of Brescia, ASST Spedali Civili di Brescia, 25123 Brescia, Italy
3. Pancreas Surgical Unit, ENETS Center of Excellence, San Raffaele Hospital IRCCS, Vita Salute University, 20132 Milan, Italy; falconi.massimo@hsr.it
4. Division of Gastrointestinal Medical Oncologya and Neuroendocrine Tumors, European Institute of Oncology, 20132 Milan, Italy; nicola.fazio@ieo.it
5. Endocrinology Unit, Department of Internal Medicine and Medical Specialties, IRCCS, Ospedale Policlinico San Martino, Università di Genova, 16132 Genova, Italy; ferone@unige.it
6. Nuclear Medicine Unit, Istituto Nazionale Tumori, Fondazione G. Pascale, 80131 Naples, Italy; s.lastoria@istitutotumori.na.it
7. School of Clinical Methodology IRCCS "Sacred Heart–Don Calabria" Hospital; 37024 Negrar di Valpolicella, Italy; giovanni.pappagallo@gmail.com
8. Nuclear Medicine Unit, Fondazione IRCCS Istituto Nazionale dei Tumori, 20132 Milano, Italy; ettore.seregni@istitutotumori.mi.it
9. Nuclear Medicine Unit, Azienda Unità Sanitaria Locale-IRCCS of Reggio Emilia, 42100 Reggio Emilia, Italy; annibale.versari@ausl.re.it
* Correspondence: alfredo.berruti@gmail.com

Citation: Bartolomei, M.; Berruti, A.; Falconi, M.; Fazio, N.; Ferone, D.; Lastoria, S.; Pappagallo, G.; Seregni, E.; Versari, A. Clinical Management of Neuroendocrine Neoplasms in Clinical Practice: A Formal Consensus Exercise. *Cancers* 2022, 14, 2501. https://doi.org/10.3390/cancers14102501

Academic Editor: David Wong

Received: 3 May 2022
Accepted: 16 May 2022
Published: 19 May 2022

Publisher's Note: MDPI stays neutral with regard to jurisdictional claims in published maps and institutional affiliations.

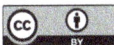

Copyright: © 2022 by the authors. Licensee MDPI, Basel, Switzerland. This article is an open access article distributed under the terms and conditions of the Creative Commons Attribution (CC BY) license (https://creativecommons.org/licenses/by/4.0/).

Simple Summary: Well-structured international guidelines are currently available regarding the management of patients with neuroendocrine neoplasms (NENs). However, in relation to the multiplicity of treatments and the relative rarity and heterogeneity of NENs, there are many controversial issues in which clinical evidence is insufficient and for which expert opinion can be of help. A group of experts selected 14 relevant topics and formulated relative statements concerning controversial issues in several areas on diagnosis, prognosis, therapeutic strategies, and patient follow-up. Specific statements have also been formulated regarding patient management on radioligand therapy (RLT), as well as in the presence of co-morbidities or bone metastases. All the statements were drafted, discussed, modified, and then approved. The Nominal Group Technique (NGT) method was used to obtain consensus. The results of this paper can facilitate the clinical approach of patients with NENs in daily practice in areas where there is scarcity or absence of clinical evidence.

Abstract: Many treatment approaches are now available for neuroendocrine neoplasms (NENs). While several societies have issued guidelines for diagnosis and treatment of NENs, there are still areas of controversy for which there is limited guidance. Expert opinion can thus be of support where firm recommendations are lacking. A group of experts met to formulate 14 statements relative to diagnosis and treatment of NENs and presented herein. The nominal group and estimate-talk-estimate techniques were used. The statements covered a broad range of topics from tools for diagnosis to follow-up, evaluation of response, treatment efficacy, therapeutic sequence, and watchful waiting. Initial prognostic characterization should be based on clinical information as well as histopathological analysis and morphological and functional imaging. It is also crucial to optimize RLT for patients with a NEN starting from accurate characterization of the patient and disease. Follow-up should be patient/tumor tailored with a shared plan about timing and type of imaging procedures to use to avoid safety issues. It is also stressed that patient-reported outcomes should receive greater attention, and that a multidisciplinary approach should be mandatory. Due to the clinical heterogeneity and relative lack of definitive evidence for NENs, personalization of diagnostic–therapeutic work-up is crucial.

Keywords: neuroendocrine neoplasms; management; Delphi; consensus

1. Introduction

Neuroendocrine neoplasms (NENs) are a heterogeneous group of neoplasms that arise from the neuroendocrine cell system [1]. While NENs occur within the gastroenteropancreatic (GEP) system in most cases, they may also arise from other systems. Considering data from a large population-based study, the overall incidence of low/intermediate grade NENs is 25 per 1,000,000 and they appear to be more frequent in patients ≥65 years in whom the incidence reaches 40 per 1,000,000 per year [2]. In addition, there is speculation that the incidence of NENs is increasing, although this may be related to use of more sensitive diagnostic methods and increased awareness among clinicians [1]. The classification system from the International Agency for Research on Cancer (IARC) and World Health Organization (WHO) considers the anatomic location, category, family history, type, and grade of tumor [3]. While well-differentiated NENs are called neuroendocrine tumors (NETs) poorly differentiated NENs are referred to as neuroendocrine carcinomas (NEC). Neuroendocrine neoplasms are clinically classified as functioning or non-functioning, depending on whether the tumor has the ability to secrete biogenic amines or peptide hormones that give rise to clinical symptoms.

A wide range of treatment approaches are now available for NENs, which broadly comprise surgical and ablative treatment, and use of somatostatin analogs (SSAs), targeted agents, chemotherapy, and peptide receptor radionuclide therapy (PRRT)/radioligand therapy (RLT), in addition to watchful waiting in very selected patients [4]. Several societies have issued guidelines for diagnosis and treatment of NENs, including the National Comprehensive Cancer Network (NCCN), European Society for Medical Oncology (ESMO), and European Neuroendocrine Tumor Society (ENETS) [5–7]. Notwithstanding, there are still several areas of controversy for which there is limited guidance, and diagnostic and therapeutic protocols may vary significantly among centers according to their expertise and geographic location.

The scope of this paper is to provide a valuable source of guidance where firm recommendations are lacking, made by a group of experts, who discussed current issues and formulated a series of statements relative to diagnosis and treatment, in order to facilitate daily practice in the management of patients with NENs.

2. Materials and Methods

The Nominal Group Technique (NGT) is a formal method of obtaining consensus that was developed to overcome a portion of the negative aspects of group dynamics and help ensure that a group decision is made used to obtain consensus [8,9]. The NGT is especially well-suited for obtaining consensus in smaller groups, where extensive face-to-face discussion and exchange of ideas can take place. The NGT is a structured group interaction, and allows participants to express their opinions and have their opinions considered by the other participants, thus overcoming a portion of the negative aspects of group dynamics and help ensure that a group decision is made [8,9]. A maximum of 7 participants is recommended, which is the number of members who took part in the present consensus meeting. The NGT used herein was composed of facilitated and structured steps, in broad agreement with current recommendations [8,9]. The members of the board initially agreed on areas of interest (ideas) through an NGT session held on 16 July 2020.

The overall process was divided into the following steps. First, each member of the board independently produced ideas, expressed in short sentences, which were deemed to be of interest. At this stage there is no limit to the ideas that each participant can indicate. A list of 46 statements was then produced with no discussion. A senior epidemiologist (GP), trained in gaining consensus among stakeholders (facilitator), then reorganized and categorized the ideas, which were then discussed on voted upon independently and a priority was assigned. Based on priority, a list of 14 topics were chosen.

Afterward, finalized topics were used by board members to draft one statement for each idea individually through an Estimate–Talk–Estimate (E–T–E) approach [10,11]. This process resulted in a certain number of statements, which were then harmonized by the facilitator. The E–T–E, similarly to NGT combines a nominal group activity restricting verbal interaction with face-to-face interaction processes [12]. In the second face-to-face meeting, the board members and the facilitator reviewed and further discussed the harmonized statements, reaching a final version. The overall process is summarized in Figure 1.

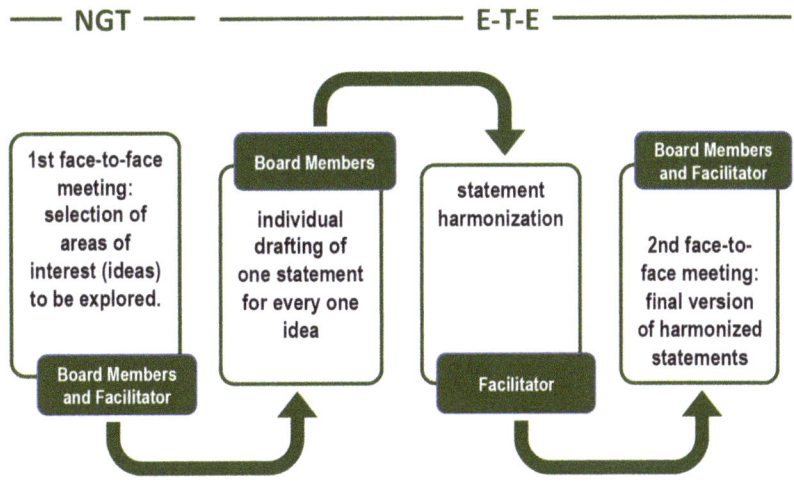

NGT: Nominal Group Technique; **E-T-E**: Estimate-Talk-Estimate

Figure 1. Overall process used to obtain consensus.

3. Results

A total of 14 statements were drafted, discussed, modified, and approved by the board of experts (Table 1). Each of the statements is commented upon below along with the main supporting evidence.

Table 1. Statements on diagnosis and management of NENs.

	Statement
1. Multidisciplinary discussion	A network among "tumor boards" working on NEN patients is advisable NEN-dedicated multidisciplinary teams should adopt the same main criteria independently of local experience.
2. Initial prognostic characterization	Initial prognostic characterization should be based on clinical information (functioning/non-functioning, performance status, comorbidity), histopathology (differentiation and grading), and morphological and functional imaging. There is no recommended definition of disease at high risk after radical surgery across NEN primary diseases.
3. Watchful waiting	A watchful waiting strategy is generally not recommended in locally advanced/metastatic patients.

Table 1. Cont.

	Statement
4. Follow-up of radically resected NENs	Follow-up should be patient-tailored in patients with NEN after radical surgery and should include a panel of conventional tests, including circulating markers, plus a list of optional instrumental tests, chosen based on the characteristics of the tumor and patient. A patient-tailored long term follow-up strategy is still lacking and needs to be defined. The timing should be modulated on the basis of prognostic parameters, while strongly taking into account safety issues related to potentially invasive exams.
5. Therapeutic strategies	There is poor evidence regarding a specific sequence or integration of various treatments in NENs. The therapeutic strategy with sequence and type of treatments should be decided in a tumor board considering the characteristics of the patient, literature data, and regulatory aspects.
6. Informed consent for RLT	A standard informed consent form for RLT should be used. Informed consent should include specific information about the purpose, mode of execution, risk-benefit balance, and potential for early and late side effects, allowing optimization of communication about the risks, benefits, and possible alternative options, to provide the same level of information within all institutions.
7. Dosimetry of RLT (for therapy)	Dosimetry evaluation should be recommended to prevent potential risks to bone marrow and kidney function to provide data to clinicians, especially in patients with long survival expectancy.
8. Management of patients with comorbidities	Comorbidities not representing an absolute contraindication to RLT (i.e., severe hypertension, brittle diabetes, functioning tumors, concomitant meningioma, etc.) should require specific protocols.
9. Management of therapy with SSA during RLT	SSA therapy should be continued during the entire course of RLT. Dosage may be adjusted in case of functioning tumors.
10. Evaluation of response (morphological vs. functional and clinical) after RLT	Assessment of tumor response after RLT should carefully consider both morphological and functional imaging. However, the timing of imaging should be correlated with characteristics of the individual tumor.
11. Follow-up after RLT	Follow-up should be patient-tailored and include morphological (CT and/or MRI) and/or functional (PET/CT with radiolabeled somatostatin analogs and/or FDG) imaging and biomarkers, chosen based on the characteristics of the tumor. The timing should be modulated based on prognostic parameters, while strongly considering safety issues. It is suggested to intercalate morphological and functional imaging to reduce the patient's irradiation dose given the very long follow-up.
12. Off-label use of RLT	Alternative schedules, means of administration, indications other than approved, and rechallenge should be limited to specific clinical studies.
13. Approach to patients with bone metastases	Bone involvement with appropriate imaging techniques must be carefully assessed in patients with a metastatic NEN to identify those at risk of skeletal-related events.
14. Role of PROs in management	Patient-reported outcomes (PROs) should be considered as a critical endpoint of benefit. Thus, guidelines should consider PROs, pointing out that their lack may have a bearing on the ultimate recommendation.

3.1. Multidisciplinary Management

Multidisciplinary care of patients with NENs at referral centers has been associated with improvements in diagnosis, planning of treatment, and overall survival, as well as greater satisfaction by both the patient and clinician [13]. The role of a multidisciplinary team (MDT), which plays a pivotal function in the care of patients with NENs, should be always promoted in order to share common indications, optimize therapeutic strategies and allow integration of treatments, also between different centers. Considering these aspects, the participants agreed and strongly suggested that a network among "tumor boards" (dedicated to patients with NENs) is advisable. Adopting a similar approach independently of local experience, the harmonization of diagnostic and therapeutic pathways may be obtained everywhere. In addition, patients treated at two or more institutions can become part of an integrated therapeutic program generated from the cooperation among specialists from the different centers involved.

3.2. Baseline Prognostic Characterization

The panel agreed that initial prognostic characterization should be based on clinical information as well as histopathological analysis and morphological and functional imaging. In advanced disease, for all NETs somatostatin receptor (SSTR) imaging with ^{68}Ga-SSAs PET/CT has a main role in this context, and can combine prognostic, staging, and predictive information [14–17] (Figure 2A,B).

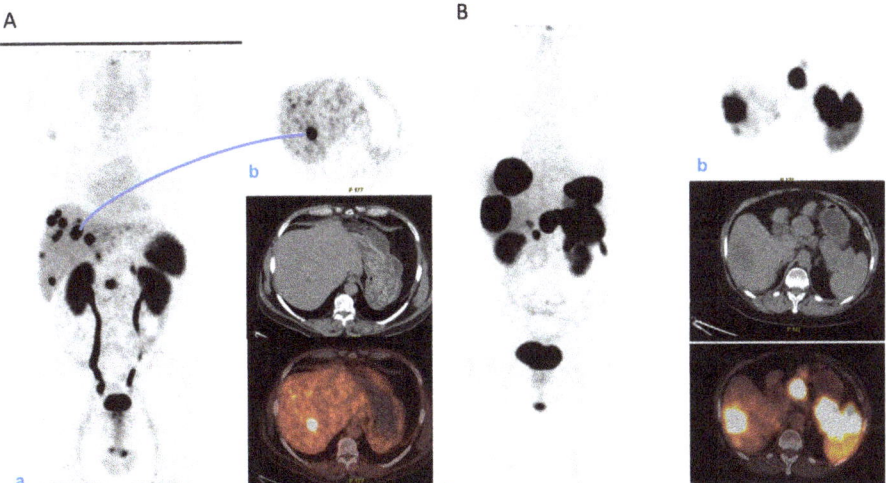

Figure 2. (**A**) PET/CT initial staging in metastatic pNET. (a) Male, 62 years old, pNEN, G1, initial staging. PET/CT ^{68}Ga-DOTATOC MIP: depicts the intense uptake within primary pancreatic NEN (SUVmax 16.6) and in multiple liver metastases (SUVmax range: 6.6-62). (b) Axial image of the hottest liver metastasis along with corresponding CT and fused slice. (**B**) Female, 68 years old, pNEN, G3, staging during therapy with SSA and FOLFIRI. PET/CT ^{68}Ga-DOTATOC MIP: (a) depicts the intense uptake within primary pancreatic NEN (SUVmax 38.6) and in large liver metastases (SUVmax range: 3-92). (b) Axial image of the primary pancreatic NEN, mesenteric lymph node, and largest liver metastasis.

Moreover, the sensitivity and specificity of ^{68}Ga-SSAs PET/CT for most NETs is high (>90%), except for insulinomas, which express SSTRs less frequently [18]. ^{68}Ga-SSAs PET/CT can be useful in guiding the therapeutic strategy, as patients with a high and homogeneous expression of SSTRs are selected for radiolabeled SSAs [19]. ^{18}F-FDG PET can be useful for NECs and NETs with high Ki-67, but also for NETs with low or inhomogeneous expression of SSTRs. Elevated ^{18}F-FDG uptake, is a negative prognostic factor [20,21]. There is insufficient evidence for the use of circulating chromogranin A as a routine prognostic marker [22].

For resected NENs, a number of pathological factors have been associated with prognosis, such as tumor stage (pTNM), tumor grade, tumor size, and vascular/lymphatic/perineural invasion, and there are several nomograms that can be used to classify the patient's risk of disease recurrence or progression [23–25].

Tumor tissue samples, preferably histological, should be always obtained (by percutaneous biopsy or surgery) for diagnosis and classification before starting medical anti-cancer treatment [26]. Endoscopic ultrasound-guided fine-needle biopsy (EUS-FNB) is crucial for the evaluation of pancreatic neuroendocrine tumors [27]. In addition to tumor differentiation (well, moderately, and poorly), the grade should be determined using the Ki-67 and mitotic index. The Ki-67 proliferative index is the most commonly used prognostic factor [28,29] and should be requested to pathologists, if not present in the initial report.

3.3. Watchful Waiting

A watchful waiting strategy means clinical observation to assess the spontaneous clinical history of the tumor in the absence of anti-tumor therapy [30]. Furthermore, its application in clinical practice can differ in terms of type and timing of imaging or other exams utilized [30]. In locally advanced/metastatic NENs, the experts did not recommend a watchful waiting strategy. Although watchful waiting has been reported in several guidelines and recommendations, it has never been validated, nor has it been specifically investigated or standardized. In patients with metastatic NENs, watchful waiting does not seem to have a role, on the basis of the results from the PROMID and CLARINET trials [31,32]. Watchful waiting to delay first-line therapy for a short period may be justified in asymptomatic patients with good performance status and a low-grade NET with the aim to better characterize the disease and define the optimal therapeutic strategy [14,33,34]. However, in metastatic disease a *watchful waiting* to definitively avoid treatment is not justified, as even NENs with very favorable biological characteristics tend to grow [30].

3.4. Follow-Up of Radically Resected NENs

Follow-up has been recommended in virtually all patients after radical resection of local or locally advanced and metastatic NENs [35,36]. Generally, guidelines and recommendations suggest that following complete resection morphological imaging is recommended every 3–6 months for 5 years and then every 12–24 months for up to 10 years [35,37]. The expert panel of this consensus suggests that, considering the long-term nature of follow-up, magnetic resonance imaging (MRI) with diffusion-weighted (DW) sequences should progressively substitute and has to be preferred over computed tomography (CT) with the aim of reducing exposure of the entire body to ionizing radiation and renal exposure to iodinated contrast media. Nevertheless, the choice of the morphologic modality has to be based on its accuracy in the visualization of the target lesions. Of note, periodic functional imaging (namely ^{68}Ga-SSAs PET/CT) has not been demonstrated to have clinical utility in radically resected NETs, and is recommended only in patients with suspected recurrence of disease at morphological imaging or in those presenting new, suspicious, clinical signs and/or symptoms [14,15,33,35]. In general, considering that NENs are remarkably heterogeneous and this heterogeneity greatly influences the risk of relapse or progression and patient prognosis, the expert panel agreed that a fixed follow-up schedule might be inadequate in many cases. Current guidelines do not mention the possibility of risk-adapted individual follow-up. The experts agreed that follow-up for radically resected NEN should be patient/tumor tailored; the timing should be based on individual prognostic parameters, with a balanced analysis of risks and benefits. Stratification by risk of recurrence can help the clinician in avoiding unnecessary examinations in low-risk patients (e.g., reduction of exposure to radiation). In this regard, there is some evidence to suggest that the frequency of follow-up investigations can be based on tumor features, such as tumor differentiation, Ki-67 index, presence of metastases, and tumor size, even if no formal consensus has been reached in this regard [23,25]. Due to the well-known heterogeneity of NENs, it is clear that follow-up cannot be standardized on the basis of the primary site or pathology classification only, e.g., the WHO. It should be contextualized based on the specific characteristics of the disease in the individual patient and discussed within the NEN-dedicated multidisciplinary team. In other words, follow-up should be personalized.

3.5. Therapeutic Strategies

The expert panel recognized that there is little consensus on the optimal sequence of treatments for patients with NENs [7]. Patients with G1- and low G2 NETs that are not amenable to surgery often receive SSAs as first-line therapy [6,14,35], as recommended by international guidelines [7,38], in order to control tumor growth and/or associated clinical syndromes. For patients who show tumor progression after first-line treatment with SSAs, the selection of second-line therapy may be difficult due to the lack of an absolute standard. The sequence SSAs followed by PRRT/RLT upon progression has become a common/standard approach in G1-G2 SI-NEN patients, thanks to the results of the NETTER-1 trial [39]. The panel agreed with a previous suggestion that comorbidities and goal of treatment can help to drive the therapeutic choice [14]. For example, if the goal of therapy is to achieve tumor shrinkage, then various treatments, mainly chemotherapy and PRRT, may be considered according to the evidence, to be discussed within the NEN-dedicated MDT [40]. In a selected patient population and after a careful multidisciplinary discussion, a cytoreductive surgery on primary malignancy could be considered, due to the potential positive relationship of this approach with patient survival in retrospective case series [41,42].

If, however, effective long-term control of the endocrine clinical syndrome is the priority, then the most appropriate targeted therapy must be chosen. Patients with a malignant pancreatic insulinoma, for example, can gain long-term blood glucose control with everolimus, which would thus be preferred to control clinical progression vs. a SSA. Everolimus could even be continued in order to control the syndrome even in case of further progression, in association with subsequent tanti-tumor therapies (e.g., chemotherapy or PRRT), at least for a short period [43]. Conversely, based on its effects on glucose metabolism, sunitinib could have detrimental effects in patients with an insulinoma [44], and might be preferentially indicated in patients with a glucagonoma.

Systemic therapies can be suitably integrated with loco-regional therapies when clinically indicated and following multidisciplinary discussion. Liver-directed treatments (LDTs) such as trans-arterial chemoembolization (TACE), trans-arterial embolization (TAE), and thermo-ablation (TA), in fact, are usually considered for selected patients with liver metastases from NETs [6,45]. Finally, when deciding the sequence of treatments, additional toxicities should be taken into consideration as well as their impact on the patient's quality of life.

3.6. Informed Consent for RLT

The expert panel agreed that specific and detailed, oral and written information should be given to the patients before obtaining the signed consent form before starting treatment. The information provided should include notes about the purpose, procedure, and risk-benefit balance deriving from radiation use in RLT. Moreover, the potential for early and late side effects (reversible hematological toxicity, nephrotoxicity), and the rare but severe long-term complications (myelodysplastic syndromes (MDS) and leukemia) have to be exhaustively and comprehensively discussed with the patient [43,46]. A relevant item concerns the information for patients (of both sexes) about the period of abstention from procreation.

3.7. Dosimetry of RLT

Dosimetric evaluation is currently not recommended during standard RLT, since the NETTER 1 trial demonstrated that four fixed doses of ^{177}Lu- Lutathera® (Basel, Switzerland, Novartis)(7.4 GBq) in most patients are characterized by a favorable toxicity profile and are effective [47]. Dosimetry should optimize the efficacy of therapy and minimize potential side effects to the organs at risk, namely red bone marrow and kidney. The use of individual dosimetry during RLT has the potential to tailor treatment after the standard four cycles [46], possibly receiving additional cycles (up to 10) before reaching dose-limiting toxicity levels [48,49].

In a prospective study with dosimetric assessment, patients who had, after the 4 cycles, an absorbed dose to the kidneys ≥23 Gy showed significantly better survival outcomes than those who did not reach such a preset dose [50]. Thus, using a predetermined cut-off of four cycles of 7.4 GBq ^{177}Lu-DOTATATE, some patients would benefit from additional therapy, further highlighting the value of dosimetric evaluation. The panelists suggest that dosimetry should be performed in trials or for re-treatment. In this setting, the development of more accurate, simplified, and standardized methods will enable routine use of dosimetry in a clinical setting.

3.8. Management of Patients with Comorbidities

Comorbidities and safety of medical therapies must be always considered when choosing the most appropriate treatment. Comorbidities not representing an absolute contraindication to RLT (i.e., severe hypertension, brittle diabetes, functioning tumors, concomitant meningioma, etc.) should require specific protocols. Eligibility for RLT requires the absence of a significant impairment of renal function (creatinine clearance <30 mL/min). Given that some comorbidities are related with a higher risk of adverse reactions [51], patients with the certain characteristics should be more strictly monitored during treatment and considered for dose reduction or postponement of therapy. These include morphological abnormalities in the kidney/urinary tract, incontinence, creatinine clearance 30–50 mL/min, prior chemotherapy, diabetes mellitus, hypertension, heart failure, pre-existing hematologic toxicity (other than lymphopenia) ≥ grade 2 prior to therapy, and widespread bone metastases, as well as previous radiometabolic therapies, (including radioiodine therapy previously performed for thyroid cancer) and extended external bean radiation modalities.

In terms of medical therapies, sunitinib should be preferred over everolimus for patients with a pre-existing diabetes mellitus or underlying pulmonary disease, whereas everolimus should be preferred over sunitinib in patients with cardiovascular diseases, arterial hypertension, or bleeding diathesis [14]. In patients with mild and moderate hepatic impairment (Child-Pugh A-B), the dose of everolimus should be reduced down to 5 mg/day, respectively [6].

3.9. Management of Therapy with SSA during RLT

The association of SSAs and RLT has been suggested to play a role in tumor growth control [52]. A recent retrospective study reported better survival for patients with advanced NENs receiving combined treatment with SSAs and RLT vs. RLT alone [52]. While the type of SSA and its formulation and dose are yet to be standardized, the experts held that SSA therapy should be continued during the entire course of RLT, with dose adjustment in patients with functioning tumors.

In the NETTER-1 study, the combination of ^{177}Lu-DOTATATE and octreotide LAR 30 mg every 4 weeks was reported to be safe with longer progression-free survival (PFS) and higher overall response rate (ORR) compared to high-dose octreotide LAR alone [47]. The PRELUDE study further demonstrated that the combination of lanreotide and ^{177}Lu-DOTATOC/DOTATATE was effective and safe in patients with metastatic or locally advanced NENs [53]. Thus, the available evidence appears to suggest that the association of either octreotide or lanreotide with RLT is both safe and feasible, even if further studies are advisable.

3.10. Evaluation of Tumor Response (Morphological vs. Functional and Clinical) after RLT

The expert panel held that tumor response assessment after RLT should carefully consider both morphological and functional imaging, and that the timing of imaging should be correlated with characteristics of the individual tumor based on histopathological, morphological, functional, and clinical parameters. Evaluation of morphological tumor response (with CT-scan and/or MRI) is mandatory in all patients undergoing medical therapies of a NEN and is usually based on RECIST 1.1 criteria [35,37]. Moreover, radiological tumor response assessment should be made comparing the same technique (e.g., CT-scan or MRI). The preferred imaging modality should be chosen initially on an individualized basis depending on how well it allows visualization of the parameter tumor lesions at baseline [14,35,54]. In this sense, PET with FDG could also be useful in evaluating the response (Figure 3).

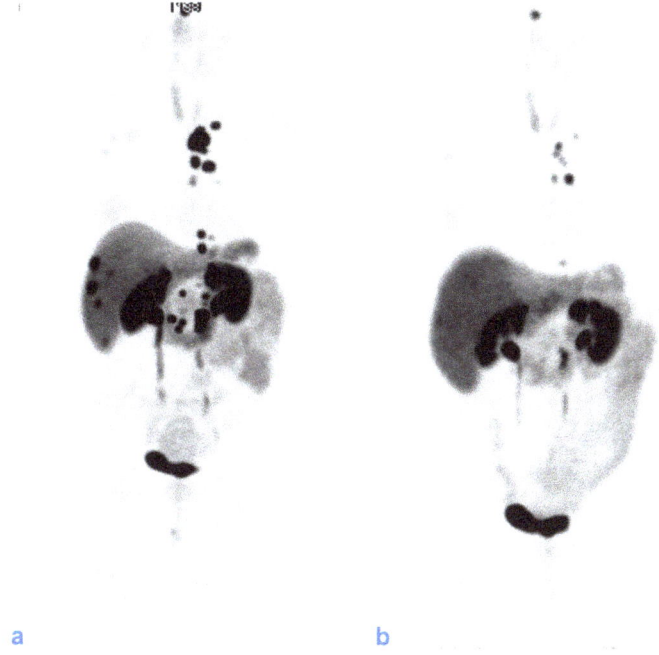

Figure 3. Monitoring response to RLT with PET/CT ^{68}Ga-DOTATOC. Female, 58 years old, pNEN, G2, surgically removed in 2016. Staging before and after RLT with ^{177}Lu-Lutathera. PET/CT 68Ga-DOTATOC MIP (**a**) depicts the extent metastatic disease (thoracic, axillary and abdominal LNs, liver metastases) before RLT. (**b**) MIP after RLT with no evidence of liver metastases and abdominal lymph nodes along with a significant reduction in the radioligand uptake of thoracic lymph nodes, which is suggestive for a partial response.

Functional imaging also plays a role in evaluation of response to RLT. Appearance of new uptake lesions and/or disappearance of previous uptake areas at ^{68}Ga DOTA-peptide PET/CT may mean tumor progression or regression [54,55]. A decrease in uptake at ^{68}Ga DOTA-peptide PET/CT after RLT may be a predictor of longer PFS and improvement of symptoms [56]. Conversely, loss of SSTR expression at ^{68}Ga DOTA-peptide PET/CT and the appearance of 18F-FDG uptake on the same or different lesions may be associated with rapid tumor progression and poor prognosis [57,58].

3.11. Follow-Up after RLT

As with the prior statement, follow-up should be patient-tailored and include both morphological (CT and/or MRI) and/or functional (PET/CT with radiolabeled somatostatin analogs and/or ^{18}F-FDG) imaging and biomarkers chosen based on the characteristics of the tumor. The timing should be based on the prognosis, avoiding unnecessary use. Additional use of imaging modalities is justified when discordant results are obtained by CT (i.e., stable lesions) and PET/CT (increased uptake or greater number of detected lesions); the suggestion might be to repeat the PET/CT in 2 or 3 months to verify the extent of the disease. The most appropriate use of morphological and functional imaging modalities should also be guided to minimize the doses of ionizing radiations to patients considering the prospect of long-term follow-up. Following RLT with ^{177}Lu-DOTA-SSAs, clinicians should be aware of previously-identified predictors of poor outcomes which can help to stratify patients by risk [59]. These include high hepatic tumor load and skeletal metastases, elevated blood chromogranin A, metastases at uncommon sites, and ascites [59].

3.12. Off-Label Use of RLT

While acknowledging that off-label use of RLT is possible, it was held that alternative schedules, types of administration, indications other than those approved, and rechallenge should be limited to specific clinical studies.

A standard course of ^{177}Lu-DOTATATE RLT consists of four cycles administered every 6–8 weeks [57]. It is believed that optimal results are achieved when the dose absorbed is close to, but not exceeding, the maximum acceptable dose for radiosensitive organs [50]. Given this, by relying on individual dosimetry, a substantial proportion of patients could possibly receive additional cycles of RLT before reaching dose-limiting toxicity for the kidneys and bone marrow [49]. However, it should be considered that the relationships between the dose absorbed and the clinical effects depends on unknown factors such as dose rate, intracellular distribution of the radionuclide, and radiosensitivity of the tumor. Additional data are needed to clarify the precise role of RLT beyond a standard course.

While the combination of ^{90}Y-DOTATOC and ^{177}Lu-DOTATATE has been advocated by several groups [60,61], and some studies have documented a higher ORR and survival advantages using the combination [62,63], in the opinion of the expert panelists these regimens cannot yet be recommended in routine clinical practice in the absence of additional information about their safety and efficacy.

In selected patients who initially respond to RLT, but subsequently progress, retreatment with RLT might be considered up to a lifetime maximum of around eight cycles [64–66]. Indeed, salvage therapy with ^{177}Lu-DOTATATE has been documented to be both safe and effective even in patients who underwent prior, extensive multimodal treatments [67–69]. In a phase II trial investigating retreatment with low-dosage ^{177}Lu-DOTATATE in 26 patients who progressed after ≥12 months following ^{90}Y-DOTATOC reported a disease control rate of 85%, indicating that in some patients retreatment with RLT may be a valid therapeutic option for progressive disease [70]. Data on the efficacy of RLT retreatment in patients with advanced NET are depicted in Table 2 [67–72].

Table 2. Efficacy of radioligand therapy re-treatment in patients with advanced NET.

Study	Number of Patients	Initial RLT	Re-Treatment RLT	PFS (Months)	95% CI
Sabet et al., 2014 [72]	33	^{177}Lu-DOTATATE	^{177}Lu-DOTATATE	13.0	9.0–18.0
Severi et al., 2015 [70]	26	^{90}Y-DOTATOC	^{177}Lu-DOTATATE	9.0	5.0–17.0
Vaughan et al., 2018 [69]	47	^{177}Lu-DOTATATE or 90Y-DOTATOC	^{177}Lu-DOTATATE or 90Y-DOTATOC	17.5	11.0–23.8
Baum et al. [71]	470	^{177}Lu-DOTATATE or ^{90}Y-DOTATOC	^{177}Lu-DOTATATE or ^{90}Y-DOTATOC	11.0	9.4–12.5
Van der Zwal et al., 2019 [68]	168	^{177}Lu-DOTATATE	^{177}Lu-DOTATATE	14.6	12.4–19.6
Rudisile S et al., 2019 [67]	32	^{177}Lu-DOTATATE	^{177}Lu-DOTATATE	6.0	0.0–16.00

Since RLT is often associated with good responses and is generally well tolerated, this has stimulated its use beyond the indicated recommendations. Such a situation includes G3 NENs with a Ki-67 index between 20% and 30% [7,73,74]. Since high ^{18}F-FDG uptake is generally observed in these patients, combined chemo-RLT may be a reasonable therapeutic option [75].

There is some encouraging evidence suggesting that RLT efficacy could be improved by the concomitant administration of several antineoplastic therapies (Figure 4).

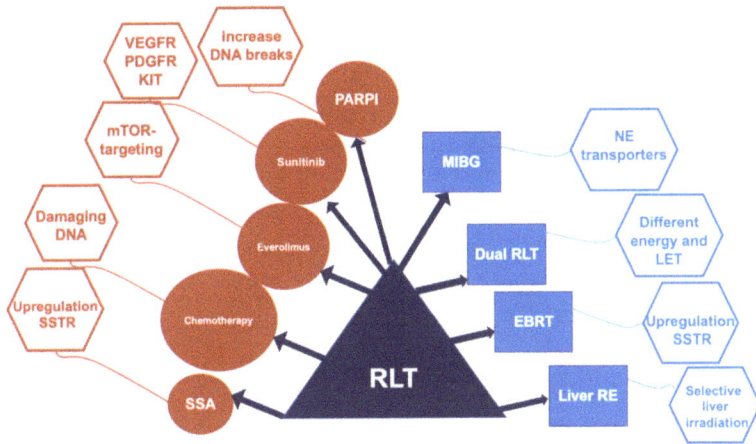

Figure 4. Current therapies proposed in combination with RLT.

Treatment with SSAs can upregulate SSTR. The overexpression of the tumor targets SSTR2 in NETs can increase the effectiveness of RLT without increasing the toxicity profile. More than one-third of patients with progressive NETs in the multicenter retrospective trial PRELUDE, treated with SSA lanreotide combined with RLT, had an objective response, and 95% were, at the last follow-up visit 1 year post-treatment, still progression-free [53].

In patients with NETs characterized by heterogeneous grading, with lesions simultaneously showing high and low Ki-67 values, the combined use of RLT and chemotherapeutic regimen with capecitabine and temozolomide (CAPTEM) has been reported to be effective. However, such a combination is suggested to be adopted in dedicated protocols taking into account the potential toxicity of CAPTEM in combination with RLT [76–78].

Clinical experience with the combined treatment of everolimus and RLT is extremely limited. In a phase I study, patients received escalating doses of everolimus: 5 to 10 mg/d for 24 weeks, and RLT, the maximum tolerated dose of everolimus in combination with RLT was 7.5 mg/d [79].

An ongoing randomized phase II study is aiming to compare the efficacy of sunitinib and RLT in advanced metastatic pancreatic NETs (NCT02230176). The focus is to determine the results of the cross-over groups, since sunitinib seems to be a potential radiosensitizer that might improve the effects of RLT. However, to date, there are no substantial clinical data on the combined use of RLT and sunitinib.

Combination of the anti-PD-1 checkpoint inhibitor nivolumab with increasing doses of RLT has been tested in a phase I/II trial including nine patients with small cell lung cancer (NCT03325816). Low-level activity RLT (3.7 GBq LUTATHERA) every 8 weeks and nivolumab every 2 weeks for a period of 6 months showed no dose limiting toxicity. More intense RLT (7.4 GBq LUTATHERA) led, in the six patients with measurable disease, to one partial response and two stable disease, with a single case of a grade 3 rash [80].

Another promising partner of RLT might be poly (ADP-ribose) polymerase-1 inhibitors (PARPi). In preclinical studies, PARPi combined with PRRT increased DNA double-strand tumor breaks and increased survival compared to PRRT as a monotherapy [81].

A recent sub-analysis of the NETTER-1-study showed that PFS in NET patients with large tumor lesions (>3 cm in diameter) was significantly shorter ($p = 0.022$) than in patients with small lesions [82]. A possible explanation for the failure in large liver lesions is due to the maximum tissue penetration of ^{177}Lu, which is limited to 2–4 mm. In a comparative analysis, patients treated with radioembolization plus RLT showed a superior OS (87% vs. 67%) than those receiving radioembolization alone (68 months vs. 35 months) [83]. Radioembolization after initial RLT is feasible, with objective responses of 16% after ^{90}Y and 43% after ^{166}Ho radioembolization. Such combined therapies should be verified in larger cohorts of patients with prevalent liver spreading of NETs, also focusing on the related hepatotoxicity, which may lead, besides the radionuclide, used to death [83,84].

Tandem RLT (using ^{177}Lu- and ^{90}Y-DOTA-SSA), in published series, shows a better overall survival than RLT with 90Y-DOTA-SSA alone (5.51 y vs. 3.96 y) along with a higher response rate and similar related toxicity [85,86]. At present, the off-label use of RLT should be limited to specific clinical circumstances and should always be discussed within the NEN-dedicated MDT. These studies are summarized in Table 3.

Table 3. Efficacy and safety of combination treatment with RLT.

Combination Partner	ORR (%)	OS (Months)	PFS (Months)	SAE (%)	Reference
SSA	37	NR	48	3% hepatotoxicity	[52,53,65]
Capecitabine	24–30	NR	31	15% hematotoxicity	[87,88]
CAPTEM	53–70	NR	22–48	6% hematotoxicity	[76–78]
5-FU	25	NR	-	-	[89]
Everolimus	44	NR	63 at 2 years	100% hematotoxicity	[79]
EBRT	0	NR	108	-	[90]
Liver Embolization					
(^{90}Y)	16	42–68	-	50% liver enzyme elevation	[83,84,91]
(^{166}Ho)	43			10% abdominal pain	
Dual RLT (^{177}Lu/^{90}Y)	42	66–127	-	2% MDS	[63,85,86]
(^{177}Lu/^{225}Ac)			-	7% hematotoxicity	
MIBG (^{131}I)	0		-	33% thrombocytopenia	[92]

3.13. Approach to Patients with Bone Metastases

In this statement, the experts recommended that bone involvement detected by appropriate imaging techniques must be carefully assessed in patients with a metastatic NEN to identify patients at risk of skeletal-related events (SREs). Bone metastases are detectable in 10–20% of patients with NENs and associated with poor prognosis [93]. Bone metastases are usually identified using appropriately sensitive functional imaging techniques, such as ^{68}Ga-DOTA-peptide PET/CT [94,95]. Bone MRI can also be performed to assess suspicious lesions [7,35]. At present, it remains uncertain if identification of micro-metastases (<5 mm) to bone should prompt to changes in management [35]. Palliative radiotherapy should be considered for patients with painful bone metastases that are difficult to control with medical therapy and for bone lesions at sites with a high risk of clinical complications [93,96]. Relief of pain has been described in the majority of patients treated with external beam radiotherapy [96]. In a prophylactic setting, radiotherapy may be beneficial in avoiding bone fractures [97]. Surgical therapy for neuroendocrine bone metastases is rarely indicated and mostly for mechanical reasons or isolated lesions [93]. Although there is little practical guidance, bisphosphonates or rank ligand inhibitors can be administered [97,98].

When required for disease control, symptomatic patients with bone metastases generally require systemic chemotherapy [93]. However, the optimal regimens are still debated and are likely to depend on the site of the primary tumor. RLT may be effective in some patients with bone metastases, who demonstrated high expression of SSTRs. In fact, two retrospective series have shown that RLT appears to be associated with ORR in bone lesions in around half of patients with NENs and bone metastases, although there is a potentially increased risk of myelotoxicity [99,100]. However, additional studies are warranted to confirm this data.

3.14. Role of Patient-Reported Outcomes in Management

Increasing importance is being given to patient-reported outcomes (PROs) in many fields of oncology, which are used to evaluate the health and quality of life of patients. The FDA defined PROs as "any report of the status of a patient's health condition that comes directly from the patient, without interpretation of the patient's response by a clinician or anyone else" [101]. Even in clinical trials, the use of PROs has become common in patients with NENs [102–104]. PROs allow for integration of clinical outcomes with the patient's opinion of their own health [105]. This is important since NENs pose considerable burden for patients [105]. PROs should be incorporated in oncology to guarantee optimal delivery of patient-centered care. Furthermore, the routine evaluation of PROs will allow clinicians to better recognize and understand the unmet needs of patients with NENs. PROs can be evaluated using validated tools such as the EORTC QOL-C30 questionnaire and, in the opinion of the experts, should receive greater consideration by management guidelines in the future, which is at the basis of this statement.

4. Conclusions

Herein, consensus on a series of statements regarding diagnosis and clinical management of patients with NENs was reached by a panel of experts. The statements covered a broad range of topics from tools for diagnosis to follow-up, evaluation of response, treatment efficacy, therapeutic sequence, and watchful waiting. Most of these topics are not addressed directly in treatment guidelines, and in the opinion of the board members additional guidance would thus be helpful in daily practice. The experts tried to define indications and suggestions, taken from the existing literature and their own experience.

At present, RLT is both effective and safe for a large proportion of patients. Therefore, it is crucial to optimize RLT for NET patients starting from accurate characterization of the patient and his/her disease. This initial characterization must be based on clinical information as well as histopathological analysis, morphological and functional imaging useful in guiding the therapeutic strategy. Somatostatin receptor imaging with ^{68}Ga-SSAs PET/CT has a main role for selecting patients who can be treated with radiolabeled SSAs. In our opinion, the future challenges for RLT involve not only the optimal therapeutic advantage by focusing on more precise dosimetric protocols, but also in greater understanding of the genotypic and phenotypic characteristics that differentiate the various subpopulations of NET patients [106]. Only in this way will it be possible to identify and stratify the potentially "responsive" and "non-responsive" forms to RLT [107]. The result will be the earlier and more accurate selection of patients, who can avoid ineffective treatments with unnecessary toxicity and benefit from the most appropriate line of therapy, with increased expectations and quality of life. This methodological approach can also bring about the definition of shared guidelines and standardized therapeutic algorithms that can aid in unravelling the biological, clinical, and prognostic uncertainties that still surround NENs. RLT with ^{177}Lu-DOTATATE is a well-established second-line treatment, after SSA, of SI-NENs G1 and G2, approved by EMA and FDA [47]. For pancreatic NENs, there is no similar evidence, lacking head-to-head comparisons with everolimus or sunitinib. However, RLT may have greater efficacy with better safety compared to the two targeted therapies. The experts did not exclude the opportunity to consider RLT as second line therapy in all GEP NETs (G1 and G2) with a strong and homogeneous expression of SSTR at ^{68}Ga-PET/CT, always considering comorbidities, goals of treatment, and treatment-related adverse events as well as the patient's QoL. Radioligand therapy may also be effective (ORR) in some patients with bone metastases with high expression of SSTRs.

Follow-up should be patient/tumor tailored with a shared plan about timing and type of imaging procedures to use in order to avoid safety issues. Stratification of patients, by risk of recurrence based on individual prognostic parameters and tumor features, can help clinicians in avoiding unnecessary and potentially invasive examinations. Dosimetry evaluation is recommended to optimize the efficacy of RLT and to minimize dose limits exceeding for the organs at risk. The use of dosimetry during RLT has also the potential to safely administrate supplementary cycles that may be associated with better survival outcomes indicating that in some patients' retreatment may be a valid therapeutic option for progressive disease.

The experts also stressed that PROs should receive greater attention during treatment and follow-up, given that they provide important insights to treating physicians about the patient's perspective. Another important aspect is the role that the NEN-dedicated MDT should have in NEN patient care. A multidisciplinary approach should be mandatory, and whenever feasible within the context of a NEN-referral center. The MDT should be dedicated to NEN, in the sense that each specialist should have particular expertise in NEN field and routinely interact with colleagues from different specialists deeply involved in NEN. In this regard, and in order to achieve greater harmonization in treatment and facilitate comparison among centers and therapies, a series of quality indicators have been recommended for care of patients with NENs, which include the use of a detailed pathology report and tumor board review was also included among the performance indicators [108]. In considering harmonization of care, the therapeutic benefits of RLT should be considered while at the same time minimizing the use of off-label RLT and watchful waiting unless carried out within part of a dedicated clinical study. While several aspects in the treatment of NENs undoubtedly warrant additional study before specific recommendations can be made, clinicians should obviously use evidence-based best judgment according to the individual characteristics of the patient and tumor, as well as regulatory aspects. Due to the clinical heterogeneity and the relative lack of absolute evidence in NENs, personalization of the diagnostic–therapeutic work-up is crucial, more than in other fields of oncology.

Author Contributions: Writing—Review and Editing, M.B., A.B., M.F., N.F., D.F., S.L., G.P., E.S. and A.V. All authors have read and agreed to the published version of the manuscript.

Funding: The funders had no role in the design of the study; in the collection, analyses, or interpretation of data; in the writing of the manuscript, or in the decision to publish the results. Mirco Bartolomei: participation to Advisory Board funded by Novartis and AAA; Alfredo Berruti: participates on the advisory board funded by Novartis and AAA; Massimo Falconi: participates on the advisory board funded by Novartis and AAA; Nicola Fazio: participates on the advisory board funded by Novartis and AAA; Diego Ferone: participates on the advisory board funded by Novartis and AAA; Secondo Lastoria: participates on the advisory board funded by Novartis and AAA; Giovanni Pappagallo: participates on the advisory board funded by Novartis and AAA; Ettore Seregni: participates on the advisory board funded by Novartis and AAA; Annibale Versari: participates on the advisory board funded by Novartis and AAA.

Acknowledgments: We thank Patrick Moore., an independent medical writer, who provided English-language editing and journal styling prior to submission on behalf of Prex Srl. The manuscript writing and open access fees for publication were funded by AAA, a Novartis company.

Conflicts of Interest: A.V.: GE Healthcare (webinar speaker), the other authors declare no conflict of interest a part the participation to an advisory board funded by Novartis AAA as previously stated.

References

1. Dasari, A.; Shen, C.; Halperin, D.; Zhao, B.; Zhou, S.; Xu, Y.; Shih, T.; Yao, J.C. Trends in the Incidence, Prevalence, and Survival Outcomes in Patients with Neuroendocrine Tumors in the United States. *JAMA Oncol.* **2017**, *3*, 1335–1342. [CrossRef] [PubMed]
2. Xu, Z.; Wang, L.; Dai, S.; Chen, M.; Li, F.; Sun, J.; Luo, F. Epidemiologic Trends of and Factors Associated With Overall Survival for Patients With Gastroenteropancreatic Neuroendocrine Tumors in the United States. *JAMA Netw. Open* **2021**, *4*, e2124750. [CrossRef] [PubMed]
3. Rindi, G.; Klimstra, D.S.; Abedi-Ardekani, B.; Asa, S.L.; Bosman, F.T.; Brambilla, E.; Busam, K.J.; De Krijger, R.R.; Dietel, M.; El-Naggar, A.K.; et al. A common classification framework for neuroendocrine neoplasms: An International Agency for Research

on Cancer (IARC) and World Health Organization (WHO) expert consensus proposal. *Mod. Pathol.* **2018**, *31*, 1770–1786. [CrossRef] [PubMed]
4. Kaderli, R.M.; Spanjol, M.; Kollar, A.; Butikofer, L.; Gloy, V.; Dumont, R.A.; Seiler, C.A.; Christ, E.R.; Radojewski, P.; Briel, M.; et al. Therapeutic Options for Neuroendocrine Tumors: A Systematic Review and Network Meta-analysis. *JAMA Oncol.* **2019**, *5*, 480–489. [CrossRef]
5. NCCN. Available online: https://www.nccn.org/professionals/physician_gls/pdf/neuroendocrine.pdf (accessed on 15 February 2022).
6. Pavel, M.; O'Toole, D.; Costa, F.; Capdevila, J.; Gross, D.; Kianmanesh, R.; Krenning, E.; Knigge, U.; Salazar, R.; Pape, U.F.; et al. ENETS Consensus Guidelines Update for the Management of Distant Metastatic Disease of Intestinal, Pancreatic, Bronchial Neuroendocrine Neoplasms (NEN) and NEN of Unknown Primary Site. *Neuroendocrinology* **2016**, *103*, 172–185. [CrossRef]
7. Pavel, M.; Oberg, K.; Falconi, M.; Krenning, E.P.; Sundin, A.; Perren, A.; Berruti, A. Gastroenteropancreatic neuroendocrine neoplasms: ESMO Clinical Practice Guidelines for diagnosis, treatment and follow-up. *Ann. Oncol.* **2020**, *31*, 844–860. [CrossRef]
8. Delbecq, A.L.; Van de Ven, A.H. A Group Process Model for Problem Identification and Program Planning. *J. Appl. Behav. Sci.* **1971**, *7*, 466–492. [CrossRef]
9. Rohrbaugh, J. Improving the quality of group judgment: Social judgment analysis and the nominal group technique. *Organ. Behav. Hum. Perform.* **1981**, *28*, 272–288. [CrossRef]
10. Rowe Wright, G. Expert opinions in forecasting: Role of the Delphi technique. In *Principles of Forecasting*; Armstrong, J.S., Ed.; Kluwer Academic Press: Norwell, MA, USA, 2001.
11. Gustafson, D.H.; Shukla, R.K.; Delbecq, A.; Walster, G.W. A comparative study of differences in subjective likelihood estimates made by individuals, interacting groups, Delphi groups, and nominal groups. *Organ. Behav. Hum. Perform.* **1973**, *9*, 280–291. [CrossRef]
12. Gallego, D.; Bueno, S. Exploring the application of the Delphi method as a forecasting tool in Information Systems and Technologies research. *Technol. Anal. Strateg. Manag.* **2014**, *26*, 987–999. [CrossRef]
13. Singh, S.; Law, C. Multidisciplinary reference centers: The care of neuroendocrine tumors. *J. Oncol. Pract.* **2010**, *6*, e11–e16. [CrossRef]
14. Falconi, M.; Eriksson, B.; Kaltsas, G.; Bartsch, D.K.; Capdevila, J.; Caplin, M.; Kos-Kudla, B.; Kwekkeboom, D.; Rindi, G.; Kloppel, G.; et al. ENETS Consensus Guidelines Update for the Management of Patients with Functional Pancreatic Neuroendocrine Tumors and Non-Functional Pancreatic Neuroendocrine Tumors. *Neuroendocrinology* **2016**, *103*, 153–171. [CrossRef]
15. Halfdanarson, T.R.; Strosberg, J.R.; Tang, L.; Bellizzi, A.M.; Bergsland, E.K.; O'Dorisio, T.M.; Halperin, D.M.; Fishbein, L.; Eads, J.; Hope, T.A.; et al. The North American Neuroendocrine Tumor Society Consensus Guidelines for Surveillance and Medical Management of Pancreatic Neuroendocrine Tumors. *Pancreas* **2020**, *49*, 863–881. [CrossRef]
16. Ramage, J.K.; De Herder, W.W.; Delle Fave, G.; Ferolla, P.; Ferone, D.; Ito, T.; Ruszniewski, P.; Sundin, A.; Weber, W.; Zheng-Pei, Z.; et al. ENETS Consensus Guidelines Update for Colorectal Neuroendocrine Neoplasms. *Neuroendocrinology* **2016**, *103*, 139–143. [CrossRef]
17. Ramage, J.K.; Punia, P.; Faluyi, O.; Frilling, A.; Meyer, T.; Saharan, R.; Valle, J.W. Observational Study to Assess Quality of Life in Patients with Pancreatic Neuroendocrine Tumors Receiving Treatment with Everolimus: The OBLIQUE Study (UK Phase IV Trial). *Neuroendocrinology* **2019**, *108*, 317–327. [CrossRef]
18. Nockel, P.; Babic, B.; Millo, C.; Herscovitch, P.; Patel, D.; Nilubol, N.; Sadowski, S.M.; Cochran, C.; Gorden, P.; Kebebew, E. Localization of Insulinoma Using 68Ga-DOTATATE PET/CT Scan. *J. Clin. Endocrinol. Metab.* **2017**, *102*, 195–199. [CrossRef]
19. Crown, A.; Rocha, F.G.; Raghu, P.; Lin, B.; Funk, G.; Alseidi, A.; Hubka, M.; Rosales, J.; Lee, M.; Kennecke, H. Impact of initial imaging with gallium-68 dotatate PET/CT on diagnosis and management of patients with neuroendocrine tumors. *J. Surg. Oncol.* **2020**, *121*, 480–485. [CrossRef]
20. Ezziddin, S.; Adler, L.; Sabet, A.; Poppel, T.D.; Grabellus, F.; Yuce, A.; Fischer, H.P.; Simon, B.; Holler, T.; Biersack, H.J.; et al. Prognostic stratification of metastatic gastroenteropancreatic neuroendocrine neoplasms by 18F-FDG PET: Feasibility of a metabolic grading system. *J. Nucl. Med.* **2014**, *55*, 1260–1266. [CrossRef]
21. Rinzivillo, M.; Partelli, S.; Prosperi, D.; Capurso, G.; Pizzichini, P.; Iannicelli, E.; Merola, E.; Muffatti, F.; Scopinaro, F.; Schillaci, O.; et al. Clinical Usefulness of (18)F-Fluorodeoxyglucose Positron Emission Tomography in the Diagnostic Algorithm of Advanced Entero-Pancreatic Neuroendocrine Neoplasms. *Oncologist* **2018**, *23*, 186–192. [CrossRef]
22. Pulvirenti, A.; Rao, D.; McIntyre, C.A.; Gonen, M.; Tang, L.H.; Klimstra, D.S.; Fleisher, M.; Ramanathan, L.V.; Reidy-Lagunes, D.; Allen, P.J. Limited role of Chromogranin A as clinical biomarker for pancreatic neuroendocrine tumors. *HPB* **2019**, *21*, 612–618. [CrossRef]
23. Genc, C.G.; Jilesen, A.P.; Partelli, S.; Falconi, M.; Muffatti, F.; van Kemenade, F.J.; van Eeden, S.; Verheij, J.; Van Dieren, S.; Van Eijck, C.H.J.; et al. A New Scoring System to Predict Recurrent Disease in Grade 1 and 2 Nonfunctional Pancreatic Neuroendocrine Tumors. *Ann. Surg.* **2018**, *267*, 1148–1154. [CrossRef]
24. Pulvirenti, A.; Javed, A.A.; Landoni, L.; Jamieson, N.B.; Chou, J.F.; Miotto, M.; He, J.; Gonen, M.; Pea, A.; Tang, L.H.; et al. Multi-institutional Development and External Validation of a Nomogram to Predict Recurrence After Curative Resection of Pancreatic Neuroendocrine Tumors. *Ann. Surg.* **2019**, *274*, 1051–1057. [CrossRef]

25. Zaidi, M.Y.; Lopez-Aguiar, A.G.; Switchenko, J.M.; Lipscomb, J.; Andreasi, V.; Partelli, S.; Gamboa, A.C.; Lee, R.M.; Poultsides, G.A.; Dillhoff, M.; et al. A Novel Validated Recurrence Risk Score to Guide a Pragmatic Surveillance Strategy After Resection of Pancreatic Neuroendocrine Tumors: An International Study of 1006 Patients. *Ann. Surg.* **2019**, *270*, 422–433. [CrossRef]
26. Lloyd, R.V.; Osamura, R.Y.; Klöppel, G.; Rosai, J. Neoplasms of the neuroendocrine pancreas. In *WHO Classification of Tumours of Endocrine Organs*, 4th ed.; WHO/IARC Classification of Tumours; WHO: Geneva, Switzerland, 2017; Volume 10, pp. 209–239.
27. Crino, S.F.; Ammendola, S.; Meneghetti, A.; Bernardoni, L.; Conti Bellocchi, M.C.; Gabbrielli, A.; Landoni, L.; Paiella, S.; Pin, F.; Parisi, A.; et al. Comparison between EUS-guided fine-needle aspiration cytology and EUS-guided fine-needle biopsy histology for the evaluation of pancreatic neuroendocrine tumors. *Pancreatology* **2021**, *21*, 443–450. [CrossRef]
28. Genc, C.G.; Falconi, M.; Partelli, S.; Muffatti, F.; van Eeden, S.; Doglioni, C.; Klumpen, H.J.; Van Eijck, C.H.J.; Nieveen van Dijkum, E.J.M. Recurrence of Pancreatic Neuroendocrine Tumors and Survival Predicted by Ki67. *Ann. Surg. Oncol.* **2018**, *25*, 2467–2474. [CrossRef]
29. Wu, Z.; Wang, Z.; Zheng, Z.; Bi, J.; Wang, X.; Feng, Q. Risk Factors for Lymph Node Metastasis and Survival Outcomes in Colorectal Neuroendocrine Tumors. *Cancer Manag. Res.* **2020**, *12*, 7151–7164. [CrossRef]
30. Fazio, N. Watch and wait policy in advanced neuroendocrine tumors: What does it mean? *World J. Clin. Oncol.* **2017**, *8*, 96–99. [CrossRef]
31. Caplin, M.E.; Pavel, M.; Cwikla, J.B.; Phan, A.T.; Raderer, M.; Sedlackova, E.; Cadiot, G.; Wolin, E.M.; Capdevila, J.; Wall, L.; et al. Lanreotide in metastatic enteropancreatic neuroendocrine tumors. *N. Engl. J. Med.* **2014**, *371*, 224–233. [CrossRef]
32. Rinke, A.; Wittenberg, M.; Schade-Brittinger, C.; Aminossadati, B.; Ronicke, E.; Gress, T.M.; Muller, H.H.; Arnold, R.; Group, P.S. Placebo-Controlled, Double-Blind, Prospective, Randomized Study on the Effect of Octreotide LAR in the Control of Tumor Growth in Patients with Metastatic Neuroendocrine Midgut Tumors (PROMID): Results of Long-Term Survival. *Neuroendocrinology* **2017**, *104*, 26–32. [CrossRef]
33. Howe, J.R.; Merchant, N.B.; Conrad, C.; Keutgen, X.M.; Hallet, J.; Drebin, J.A.; Minter, R.M.; Lairmore, T.C.; Tseng, J.F.; Zeh, H.J.; et al. The North American Neuroendocrine Tumor Society Consensus Paper on the Surgical Management of Pancreatic Neuroendocrine Tumors. *Pancreas* **2020**, *49*, 1–33. [CrossRef]
34. Partelli, S.; Bartsch, D.K.; Capdevila, J.; Chen, J.; Knigge, U.; Niederle, B.; Nieveen van Dijkum, E.J.M.; Pape, U.F.; Pascher, A.; Ramage, J.; et al. ENETS Consensus Guidelines for Standard of Care in Neuroendocrine Tumours: Surgery for Small Intestinal and Pancreatic Neuroendocrine Tumours. *Neuroendocrinology* **2017**, *105*, 255–265. [CrossRef] [PubMed]
35. De Mestier, L.; Lepage, C.; Baudin, E.; Coriat, R.; Courbon, F.; Couvelard, A.; Do Cao, C.; Frampas, E.; Gaujoux, S.; Gincul, R.; et al. Digestive Neuroendocrine Neoplasms (NEN): French Intergroup clinical practice guidelines for diagnosis, treatment and follow-up (SNFGE, GTE, RENATEN, TENPATH, FFCD, GERCOR, UNICANCER, SFCD, SFED, SFRO, SFR). *Dig. Liver Dis.* **2020**, *52*, 473–492. [CrossRef] [PubMed]
36. Knigge, U.; Capdevila, J.; Bartsch, D.K.; Baudin, E.; Falkerby, J.; Kianmanesh, R.; Kos-Kudla, B.; Niederle, B.; Nieveen van Dijkum, E.; O'Toole, D.; et al. ENETS Consensus Recommendations for the Standards of Care in Neuroendocrine Neoplasms: Follow-Up and Documentation. *Neuroendocrinology* **2017**, *105*, 310–319. [CrossRef] [PubMed]
37. Singh, S.; Moody, L.; Chan, D.L.; Metz, D.C.; Strosberg, J.; Asmis, T.; Bailey, D.L.; Bergsland, E.; Brendtro, K.; Carroll, R.; et al. Follow-up Recommendations for Completely Resected Gastroenteropancreatic Neuroendocrine Tumors. *JAMA Oncol.* **2018**, *4*, 1597–1604. [CrossRef] [PubMed]
38. Baudin, E.; Caplin, M.; Garcia-Carbonero, R.; Fazio, N.; Ferolla, P.; Filosso, P.L.; Frilling, A.; de Herder, W.W.; Horsch, D.; Knigge, U.; et al. Lung and thymic carcinoids: ESMO Clinical Practice Guidelines for diagnosis, treatment and follow-up. *Ann. Oncol.* **2021**, *32*, 439–451. [CrossRef] [PubMed]
39. Strosberg, J.R.; Caplin, M.E.; Kunz, P.L.; Ruszniewski, P.B.; Bodei, L.; Hendifar, A.; Mittra, E.; Wolin, E.M.; Yao, J.C.; Pavel, M.E.; et al. (177)Lu-Dotatate plus long-acting octreotide versus highdose long-acting octreotide in patients with midgut neuroendocrine tumours (NETTER-1): Final overall survival and long-term safety results from an open-label, randomised, controlled, phase 3 trial. *Lancet Oncol.* **2021**, *22*, 1752–1763. [CrossRef]
40. Pozzari, M.; Maisonneuve, P.; Spada, F.; Berruti, A.; Amoroso, V.; Cella, C.A.; Laffi, A.; Pellicori, S.; Bertani, E.; Fazio, N. Systemic therapies in patients with advanced well-differentiated pancreatic neuroendocrine tumors (PanNETs): When cytoreduction is the aim. A critical review with meta-analysis. *Cancer Treat. Rev.* **2018**, *71*, 39–46. [CrossRef]
41. Citterio, D.; Pusceddu, S.; Facciorusso, A.; Coppa, J.; Milione, M.; Buzzoni, R.; Bongini, M.; deBraud, F.; Mazzaferro, V. Primary tumour resection may improve survival in functional well-differentiated neuroendocrine tumours metastatic to the liver. *Eur. J. Surg. Oncol.* **2017**, *43*, 380–387. [CrossRef]
42. Partelli, S.; Cirocchi, R.; Rancoita, P.M.V.; Muffatti, F.; Andreasi, V.; Crippa, S.; Tamburrino, D.; Falconi, M. A Systematic review and meta-analysis on the role of palliative primary resection for pancreatic neuroendocrine neoplasm with liver metastases. *HPB* **2018**, *20*, 197–203. [CrossRef]
43. Tovazzi, V.; Ferrari, V.D.; Dalla Volta, A.; Consoli, F.; Amoroso, V.; Berruti, A. Should everolimus be stopped after radiological progression in metastatic insulinoma? A "cons" point of view. *Endocrine* **2020**, *69*, 481–484. [CrossRef]
44. Berruti, A.; Pia, A.; Terzolo, M. Advances in pancreatic neuroendocrine tumor treatment. *N. Engl. J. Med.* **2011**, *364*, 1871–1872.
45. Kennedy, A.; Bester, L.; Salem, R.; Sharma, R.A.; Parks, R.W.; Ruszniewski, P. Role of hepatic intra-arterial therapies in metastatic neuroendocrine tumours (NET): Guidelines from the NET-Liver-Metastases Consensus Conference. *HPB* **2015**, *17*, 29–37. [CrossRef]

46. Hicks, R.J.; Kwekkeboom, D.J.; Krenning, E.; Bodei, L.; Grozinsky-Glasberg, S.; Arnold, R.; Borbath, I.; Cwikla, J.; Toumpanakis, C.; Kaltsas, G.; et al. ENETS Consensus Guidelines for the Standards of Care in Neuroendocrine Neoplasia: Peptide Receptor Radionuclide Therapy with Radiolabeled Somatostatin Analogues. *Neuroendocrinology* **2017**, *105*, 295–309. [CrossRef]
47. Strosberg, J.; El-Haddad, G.; Wolin, E.; Hendifar, A.; Yao, J.; Chasen, B.; Mittra, E.; Kunz, P.L.; Kulke, M.H.; Jacene, H.; et al. Phase 3 Trial of 177Lu-Dotatate for Midgut Neuroendocrine Tumors. *N. Engl. J. Med.* **2017**, *376*, 125–135. [CrossRef]
48. Bison, S.M.; Konijnenberg, M.W.; Melis, M.; Pool, S.E.; Bernsen, M.R.; Teunissen, J.J.; Kwekkeboom, D.J.; De Jong, M. Peptide receptor radionuclide therapy using radiolabeled somatostatin analogs: Focus on future developments. *Clin. Transl. Imaging* **2014**, *2*, 55–66. [CrossRef]
49. Sandstrom, M.; Garske-Roman, U.; Granberg, D.; Johansson, S.; Widstrom, C.; Eriksson, B.; Sundin, A.; Lundqvist, H.; Lubberink, M. Individualized dosimetry of kidney and bone marrow in patients undergoing 177Lu-DOTA-octreotate treatment. *J. Nucl. Med.* **2013**, *54*, 33–41. [CrossRef]
50. Garske-Roman, U.; Sandstrom, M.; Fross Baron, K.; Lundin, L.; Hellman, P.; Welin, S.; Johansson, S.; Khan, T.; Lundqvist, H.; Eriksson, B.; et al. Prospective observational study of (177)Lu-DOTA-octreotate therapy in 200 patients with advanced metastasized neuroendocrine tumours (NETs): Feasibility and impact of a dosimetry-guided study protocol on outcome and toxicity. *Eur. J. Nucl. Med. Mol. Imaging* **2018**, *45*, 970–988. [CrossRef]
51. Bodei, L.; Cremonesi, M.; Ferrari, M.; Pacifici, M.; Grana, C.M.; Bartolomei, M.; Baio, S.M.; Sansovini, M.; Paganelli, G. Long-term evaluation of renal toxicity after peptide receptor radionuclide therapy with 90Y-DOTATOC and 177Lu-DOTATATE: The role of associated risk factors. *Eur. J. Nucl. Med. Mol. Imaging* **2008**, *35*, 1847–1856. [CrossRef]
52. Yordanova, A.; Wicharz, M.M.; Mayer, K.; Brossart, P.; Gonzalez-Carmona, M.A.; Strassburg, C.P.; Fimmers, R.; Essler, M.; Ahmadzadehfar, H. The Role of Adding Somatostatin Analogues to Peptide Receptor Radionuclide Therapy as a Combination and Maintenance Therapy. *Clin. Cancer Res.* **2018**, *24*, 4672–4679. [CrossRef]
53. Prasad, V.; Srirajaskanthan, R.; Toumpanakis, C.; Grana, C.M.; Baldari, S.; Shah, T.; Lamarca, A.; Courbon, F.; Scheidhauer, K.; Baudin, E.; et al. Lessons from a multicentre retrospective study of peptide receptor radionuclide therapy combined with lanreotide for neuroendocrine tumours: A need for standardised practice. *Eur. J. Nucl. Med. Mol. Imaging* **2020**, *47*, 2358–2371. [CrossRef]
54. Garcia-Carbonero, R.; Garcia-Figueiras, R.; Carmona-Bayonas, A.; Sevilla, I.; Teule, A.; Quindos, M.; Grande, E.; Capdevila, J.; Aller, J.; Arbizu, J.; et al. Imaging approaches to assess the therapeutic response of gastroenteropancreatic neuroendocrine tumors (GEP-NETs): Current perspectives and future trends of an exciting field in development. *Cancer Metastasis Rev.* **2015**, *34*, 823–842. [CrossRef]
55. Huizing, D.M.V.; Aalbersberg, E.A.; Versleijen, M.W.J.; Tesselaar, M.E.T.; Walraven, I.; Lahaye, M.J.; De Wit-van der Veen, B.J.; Stokkel, M.P.M. Early response assessment and prediction of overall survival after peptide receptor radionuclide therapy. *Cancer Imaging* **2020**, *20*, 57. [CrossRef]
56. Haug, A.R.; Auernhammer, C.J.; Wangler, B.; Schmidt, G.P.; Uebleis, C.; Goke, B.; Cumming, P.; Bartenstein, P.; Tiling, R.; Hacker, M. 68Ga-DOTATATE PET/CT for the early prediction of response to somatostatin receptor-mediated radionuclide therapy in patients with well-differentiated neuroendocrine tumours. *J. Nucl. Med.* **2010**, *51*, 1349–1356. [CrossRef]
57. Ramage, J.; Naraev, B.G.; Halfdanarson, T.R. Peptide receptor radionuclide therapy for patients with advanced pancreatic neuroendocrine tumors. *Semin. Oncol.* **2018**, *45*, 236–248. [CrossRef]
58. Sansovini, M.; Severi, S.; Ianniello, A.; Nicolini, S.; Fantini, L.; Mezzenga, E.; Ferroni, F.; Scarpi, E.; Monti, M.; Bongiovanni, A.; et al. Long-term follow-up and role of FDG PET in advanced pancreatic neuroendocrine patients treated with (177)Lu-D OTATATE. *Eur. J. Nucl. Med. Mol. Imaging* **2017**, *44*, 490–499. [CrossRef]
59. Swiha, M.M.; Sutherland, D.E.K.; Sistani, G.; Khatami, A.; Abazid, R.M.; Mujoomdar, A.; Wiseman, D.P.; Romsa, J.G.; Reid, R.H.; Laidley, D.T. Survival predictors of (177)Lu-Dotatate peptide receptor radionuclide therapy (PRRT) in patients with progressive well-differentiated neuroendocrine tumors (NETS). *J. Cancer Res. Clin. Oncol.* **2021**, *148*, 225–236. [CrossRef]
60. Baum, R.P.; Kulkarni, H.R.; Carreras, C. Peptides and receptors in image-guided therapy: Theranostics for neuroendocrine neoplasms. *Semin. Nucl. Med.* **2012**, *42*, 190–207. [CrossRef]
61. Cives, M.; Strosberg, J. Radionuclide Therapy for Neuroendocrine Tumors. *Curr. Oncol. Rep.* **2017**, *19*, 9. [CrossRef]
62. Kunikowska, J.; Krolicki, L.; Hubalewska-Dydejczyk, A.; Mikolajczak, R.; Sowa-Staszczak, A.; Pawlak, D. Clinical results of radionuclide therapy of neuroendocrine tumours with 90Y-DOTATATE and tandem 90Y/177Lu-DOTATATE: Which is a better therapy option? *Eur. J. Nucl. Med. Mol. Imaging* **2011**, *38*, 1788–1797. [CrossRef]
63. Villard, L.; Romer, A.; Marincek, N.; Brunner, P.; Koller, M.T.; Schindler, C.; Ng, Q.K.; Macke, H.R.; Muller-Brand, J.; Rochlitz, C.; et al. Cohort study of somatostatin-based radiopeptide therapy with [(90)Y-DOTA]-TOC versus [(90)Y-DOTA]-TOC plus [(177)Lu-DOTA]-TOC in neuroendocrine cancers. *J. Clin. Oncol.* **2012**, *30*, 1100–1106. [CrossRef]
64. Cives, M.; Strosberg, J.R. Gastroenteropancreatic Neuroendocrine Tumors. *CA Cancer J. Clin.* **2018**, *68*, 471–487. [CrossRef] [PubMed]
65. Van Essen, M.; Krenning, E.P.; Kam, B.L.; De Herder, W.W.; Feelders, R.A.; Kwekkeboom, D.J. Salvage therapy with (177)Lu-octreotate in patients with bronchial and gastroenteropancreatic neuroendocrine tumors. *J. Nucl. Med.* **2010**, *51*, 383–390. [CrossRef] [PubMed]
66. Strosberg, J.; Leeuwenkamp, O.; Siddiqui, M.K. Peptide receptor radiotherapy re-treatment in patients with progressive neuroendocrine tumors: A systematic review and meta-analysis. *Cancer Treat. Rev.* **2021**, *93*, 102141. [CrossRef] [PubMed]

67. Rudisile, S.; Gosewisch, A.; Wenter, V.; Unterrainer, M.; Boning, G.; Gildehaus, F.J.; Fendler, W.P.; Auernhammer, C.J.; Spitzweg, C.; Bartenstein, P.; et al. Salvage PRRT with (177)Lu-DOTA-octreotate in extensively pretreated patients with metastatic neuroendocrine tumor (NET): Dosimetry, toxicity, efficacy, and survival. *BMC Cancer* **2019**, *19*, 788. [CrossRef]
68. Van der Zwan, W.A.; Brabander, T.; Kam, B.L.R.; Teunissen, J.J.M.; Feelders, R.A.; Hofland, J.; Krenning, E.P.; De Herder, W.W. Salvage peptide receptor radionuclide therapy with [(177)Lu-DOTA,Tyr(3)]octreotate in patients with bronchial and gastroenteropancreatic neuroendocrine tumours. *Eur. J. Nucl. Med. Mol. Imaging* **2019**, *46*, 704–717. [CrossRef]
69. Vaughan, E.; Machta, J.; Walker, M.; Toumpanakis, C.; Caplin, M.; Navalkissoor, S. Retreatment with peptide receptor radionuclide therapy in patients with progressing neuroendocrine tumours: Efficacy and prognostic factors for response. *Br. J. Radiol.* **2018**, *91*, 20180041. [CrossRef]
70. Severi, S.; Sansovini, M.; Ianniello, A.; Bodei, L.; Nicolini, S.; Ibrahim, T.; Di Iorio, V.; D'Errico, V.; Caroli, P.; Monti, M.; et al. Feasibility and utility of re-treatment with (177)Lu-DOTATATE in GEP-NENs relapsed after treatment with (90)Y-DOTATOC. *Eur. J. Nucl. Med. Mol. Imaging* **2015**, *42*, 1955–1963. [CrossRef]
71. Baum, R.P.; Kulkarni, H.R.; Singh, A.; Kaemmerer, D.; Mueller, D.; Prasad, V.; Hommann, M.; Robiller, F.C.; Niepsch, K.; Franz, H.; et al. Results and adverse events of personalized peptide receptor radionuclide therapy with (90)Yttrium and (177)Lutetium in 1048 patients with neuroendocrine neoplasms. *Oncotarget* **2018**, *9*, 16932–16950. [CrossRef]
72. Sabet, A.; Haslerud, T.; Pape, U.F.; Sabet, A.; Ahmadzadehfar, H.; Grunwald, F.; Guhlke, S.; Biersack, H.J.; Ezziddin, S. Outcome and toxicity of salvage therapy with 177Lu-octreotate in patients with metastatic gastroenteropancreatic neuroendocrine tumours. *Eur. J. Nucl. Med. Mol. Imaging* **2014**, *41*, 205–210. [CrossRef]
73. Sorbye, H.; Kong, G.; Grozinsky-Glasberg, S. PRRT in high-grade gastroenteropancreatic neuroendocrine neoplasms (WHO G3). *Endocr. Relat. Cancer* **2020**, *27*, R67–R77. [CrossRef]
74. Thang, S.P.; Lung, M.S.; Kong, G.; Hofman, M.S.; Callahan, J.; Michael, M.; Hicks, R.J. Peptide receptor radionuclide therapy (PRRT) in European Neuroendocrine Tumour Society (ENETS) grade 3 (G3) neuroendocrine neoplasia (NEN)—A single-institution retrospective analysis. *Eur. J. Nucl. Med. Mol. Imaging* **2018**, *45*, 262–277. [CrossRef]
75. Kashyap, R.; Hofman, M.S.; Michael, M.; Kong, G.; Akhurst, T.; Eu, P.; Zannino, D.; Hicks, R.J. Favourable outcomes of (177)Lu-octreotate peptide receptor chemoradionuclide therapy in patients with FDG-avid neuroendocrine tumours. *Eur. J. Nucl. Med. Mol. Imaging* **2015**, *42*, 176–185. [CrossRef]
76. Claringbold, P.G.; Price, R.A.; Turner, J.H. Phase I-II study of radiopeptide 177Lu-octreotate in combination with capecitabine and temozolomide in advanced low-grade neuroendocrine tumors. *Cancer Biother. Radiopharm.* **2012**, *27*, 561–569. [CrossRef]
77. Claringbold, P.G.; Turner, J.H. Pancreatic Neuroendocrine Tumor Control: Durable Objective Response to Combination 177Lu-Octreotate-Capecitabine-Temozolomide Radiopeptide Chemotherapy. *Neuroendocrinology* **2016**, *103*, 432–439. [CrossRef]
78. Ostwal, V.; Basu, S.; Bhargava, P.; Shah, M.; Parghane, R.V.; Srinivas, S.; Chaudhari, V.; Bhandare, M.S.; Shrikhande, S.V.; Ramaswamy, A. Capecitabine-Temozolomide in Advanced Grade 2 and Grade 3 Neuroendocrine Neoplasms: Benefits of Chemotherapy in Neuroendocrine Neoplasms with Significant 18FDG Uptake. *Neuroendocrinology* **2021**, *111*, 998–1004. [CrossRef]
79. Claringbold, P.G.; Turner, J.H. NeuroEndocrine Tumor Therapy with Lutetium-177-octreotate and Everolimus (NETTLE): A Phase I Study. *Cancer Biother. Radiopharm.* **2015**, *30*, 261–269. [CrossRef]
80. Kim, C.; Liu, S.V.; Subramaniam, D.S.; Torres, T.; Loda, M.; Esposito, G.; Giaccone, G. Phase I study of the (177)Lu-DOTA(0)-Tyr(3)-Octreotate (lutathera) in combination with nivolumab in patients with neuroendocrine tumors of the lung. *J. Immunother. Cancer* **2020**, *8*, e000980. [CrossRef]
81. Cullinane, C.; Waldeck, K.; Kirby, L.; Rogers, B.E.; Eu, P.; Tothill, R.W.; Hicks, R.J. Enhancing the anti-tumour activity of (177)Lu-DOTA-octreotate radionuclide therapy in somatostatin receptor-2 expressing tumour models by targeting PARP. *Sci. Rep.* **2020**, *10*, 10196. [CrossRef]
82. Strosberg, J.; Kunz, P.L.; Hendifar, A.; Yao, J.; Bushnell, D.; Kulke, M.H.; Baum, R.P.; Caplin, M.; Ruszniewski, P.; Delpassand, E.; et al. Impact of liver tumour burden, alkaline phosphatase elevation, and target lesion size on treatment outcomes with (177)Lu-Dotatate: An analysis of the NETTER-1 study. *Eur. J. Nucl. Med. Mol. Imaging* **2020**, *47*, 2372–2382. [CrossRef]
83. Yilmaz, E.; Engin, M.N.; Ozkan, Z.G.; Kovan, B.; Buyukkaya, F.; Poyanli, A.; Saglam, S.; Basaran, M.; Turkmen, C. Y90 selective internal radiation therapy and peptide receptor radionuclide therapy for the treatment of metastatic neuroendocrine tumors: Combination or not? *Nucl. Med. Commun.* **2020**, *41*, 1242–1249. [CrossRef]
84. Braat, A.; Bruijnen, R.C.G.; van Rooij, R.; Braat, M.; Wessels, F.J.; van Leeuwaarde, R.S.; van Treijen, M.J.C.; de Herder, W.W.; Hofland, J.; Tesselaar, M.E.T.; et al. Additional holmium-166 radioembolisation after lutetium-177-dotatate in patients with neuroendocrine tumour liver metastases (HEPAR PLuS): A single-centre, single-arm, open-label, phase 2 study. *Lancet Oncol.* **2020**, *21*, 561–570. [CrossRef]
85. Kunikowska, J.; Pawlak, D.; Bak, M.I.; Kos-Kudla, B.; Mikolajczak, R.; Krolicki, L. Long-term results and tolerability of tandem peptide receptor radionuclide therapy with (90)Y/(177)Lu-DOTATATE in neuroendocrine tumors with respect to the primary location: A 10-year study. *Ann. Nucl. Med.* **2017**, *31*, 347–356. [CrossRef]
86. Seregni, E.; Maccauro, M.; Chiesa, C.; Mariani, L.; Pascali, C.; Mazzaferro, V.; De Braud, F.; Buzzoni, R.; Milione, M.; Lorenzoni, A.; et al. Treatment with tandem [90Y]DOTA-TATE and [177Lu]DOTA-TATE of neuroendocrine tumours refractory to conventional therapy. *Eur. J. Nucl. Med. Mol. Imaging* **2014**, *41*, 223–230. [CrossRef]

87. Claringbold, P.G.; Brayshaw, P.A.; Price, R.A.; Turner, J.H. Phase II study of radiopeptide 177Lu-octreotate and capecitabine therapy of progressive disseminated neuroendocrine tumours. *Eur. J. Nucl. Med. Mol. Imaging* **2011**, *38*, 302–311. [CrossRef]
88. Nicolini, S.; Bodei, L.; Bongiovanni, A.; Sansovini, M.; Grassi, I.; Ibrahim, T.; Monti, M.; Caroli, P.; Sarnelli, A.; Diano, D.; et al. Combined use of 177Lu-DOTATATE and metronomic capecitabine (Lu-X) in FDG-positive gastro-entero-pancreatic neuroendocrine tumors. *Eur. J. Nucl. Med. Mol. Imaging* **2021**, *48*, 3260–3267. [CrossRef]
89. Kong, G.; Thompson, M.; Collins, M.; Herschtal, A.; Hofman, M.S.; Johnston, V.; Eu, P.; Michael, M.; Hicks, R.J. Assessment of predictors of response and long-term survival of patients with neuroendocrine tumour treated with peptide receptor chemoradionuclide therapy (PRCRT). *Eur. J. Nucl. Med. Mol. Imaging* **2014**, *41*, 1831–1844. [CrossRef]
90. Hartrampf, P.E.; Hanscheid, H.; Kertels, O.; Schirbel, A.; Kreissl, M.C.; Flentje, M.; Sweeney, R.A.; Buck, A.K.; Polat, B.; Lapa, C. Long-term results of multimodal peptide receptor radionuclide therapy and fractionated external beam radiotherapy for treatment of advanced symptomatic meningioma. *Clin. Transl. Radiat. Oncol.* **2020**, *22*, 29–32. [CrossRef]
91. Braat, A.; Ahmadzadehfar, H.; Kappadath, S.C.; Stothers, C.L.; Frilling, A.; Deroose, C.M.; Flamen, P.; Brown, D.B.; Sze, D.Y.; Mahvash, A.; et al. Radioembolization with (90)Y Resin Microspheres of Neuroendocrine Liver Metastases After Initial Peptide Receptor Radionuclide Therapy. *Cardiovasc. Interv. Radiol.* **2020**, *43*, 246–253. [CrossRef]
92. Bushnell, D.L.; Bodeker, K.L.; O'Dorisio, T.M.; Madsen, M.T.; Menda, Y.; Graves, S.; Zamba, G.K.D.; O'Dorisio, M.S. Addition of (131)I-MIBG to PRRT ((90)Y-DOTATOC) for Personalized Treatment of Selected Patients with Neuroendocrine Tumors. *J. Nucl. Med.* **2021**, *62*, 1274–1277. [CrossRef]
93. Kos-Kudla, B.; O'Toole, D.; Falconi, M.; Gross, D.; Kloppel, G.; Sundin, A.; Ramage, J.; Oberg, K.; Wiedenmann, B.; Komminoth, P.; et al. ENETS consensus guidelines for the management of bone and lung metastases from neuroendocrine tumors. *Neuroendocrinology* **2010**, *91*, 341–350. [CrossRef]
94. Putzer, D.; Gabriel, M.; Henninger, B.; Kendler, D.; Uprimny, C.; Dobrozemsky, G.; Decristoforo, C.; Bale, R.J.; Jaschke, W.; Virgolini, I.J. Bone metastases in patients with neuroendocrine tumor: 68Ga-DOTA-Tyr3-octreotide PET in comparison to CT and bone scintigraphy. *J. Nucl. Med.* **2009**, *50*, 1214–1221. [CrossRef] [PubMed]
95. Sadowski, S.M.; Neychev, V.; Millo, C.; Shih, J.; Nilubol, N.; Herscovitch, P.; Pacak, K.; Marx, S.J.; Kebebew, E. Prospective Study of 68Ga-DOTATATE Positron Emission Tomography/Computed Tomography for Detecting Gastro-Entero-Pancreatic Neuroendocrine Tumors and Unknown Primary Sites. *J. Clin. Oncol.* **2016**, *34*, 588–596. [CrossRef] [PubMed]
96. Guan, M.; He, I.; Luu, M.; David, J.; Gong, J.; Placencio-Hickok, V.R.; Reznik, R.S.; Tuli, R.; Hendifar, A.E. Palliative Radiation Therapy for Bone Metastases in Neuroendocrine Neoplasms. *Adv. Radiat. Oncol.* **2019**, *4*, 513–519. [CrossRef] [PubMed]
97. Cives, M.; Pelle, E.; Rinzivillo, M.; Prosperi, D.; Tucci, M.; Silvestris, F.; Panzuto, F. Bone Metastases in Neuroendocrine Tumors: Molecular Pathogenesis and Implications in Clinical Practice. *Neuroendocrinology* **2021**, *111*, 207–216. [CrossRef]
98. Costa, L.; Major, P.P. Effect of bisphosphonates on pain and quality of life in patients with bone metastases. *Nat. Clin. Pract. Oncol.* **2009**, *6*, 163–174. [CrossRef]
99. Ezzidin, S.; Sabet, A.; Heinemann, F.; Yong-Hing, C.J.; Ahmadzadehfar, H.; Guhlke, S.; Holler, T.; Willinek, W.; Boy, C.; Biersack, H.J. Response and long-term control of bone metastases after peptide receptor radionuclide therapy with (177)Lu-octreotate. *J. Nucl. Med.* **2011**, *52*, 1197–1203. [CrossRef]
100. Sabet, A.; Khalaf, F.; Haslerud, T.; Al-Zreiqat, A.; Sabet, A.; Simon, B.; Poppel, T.D.; Biersack, H.J.; Ezzidin, S. Bone metastases in GEP-NET: Response and long-term outcome after PRRT from a follow-up analysis. *Am. J. Nucl. Med. Mol. Imaging* **2013**, *3*, 437–445.
101. Newman, C.B.; Melmed, S.; Snyder, P.J.; Young, W.F.; Boyajy, L.D.; Levy, R.; Stewart, W.N.; Klibanski, A.; Molitch, M.E.; Gagel, R.F. Safety and efficacy of long-term octreotide therapy of acromegaly: Results of a multicenter trial in 103 patients—A clinical research center study. *J. Clin. Endocrinol. Metab.* **1995**, *80*, 2768–2775. [CrossRef]
102. Ruszniewski, P.; Valle, J.W.; Lombard-Bohas, C.; Cuthbertson, D.J.; Perros, P.; Holubec, L.; Delle Fave, G.; Smith, D.; Niccoli, P.; Maisonobe, P.; et al. Patient-reported outcomes with lanreotide Autogel/Depot for carcinoid syndrome: An international observational study. *Dig. Liver Dis.* **2016**, *48*, 552–558. [CrossRef]
103. Singh, S.; Granberg, D.; Wolin, E.; Warner, R.; Sissons, M.; Kolarova, T.; Goldstein, G.; Pavel, M.; Oberg, K.; Leyden, J. Patient-Reported Burden of a Neuroendocrine Tumor (NET) Diagnosis: Results From the First Global Survey of Patients With NETs. *J. Glob. Oncol.* **2017**, *3*, 43–53. [CrossRef]
104. Wolin, E.M.; Leyden, J.; Goldstein, G.; Kolarova, T.; Hollander, R.; Warner, R.R.P. Patient-Reported Experience of Diagnosis, Management, and Burden of Neuroendocrine Tumors: Results From a Large Patient Survey in the United States. *Pancreas* **2017**, *46*, 639–647. [CrossRef]
105. Snyder, C.F.; Aaronson, N.K. Use of patient-reported outcomes in clinical practice. *Lancet* **2009**, *374*, 369–370. [CrossRef]
106. Bodei, L.; Kidd, M.S.; Singh, A.; van der Zwan, W.A.; Severi, S.; Drozdov, I.A.; Malczewska, A.; Baum, R.P.; Kwekkeboom, D.J.; Paganelli, G.; et al. PRRT neuroendocrine tumor response monitored using circulating transcript analysis: The NETest. *Eur. J. Nucl. Med. Mol. Imaging* **2020**, *47*, 895–906. [CrossRef]

107. Roll, W.; Weckesser, M.; Seifert, R.; Bodei, L.; Rahbar, K. Imaging and liquid biopsy in the prediction and evaluation of response to PRRT in neuroendocrine tumors: Implications for patient management. *Eur. J. Nucl. Med. Mol. Imaging* **2021**, *48*, 4016–4027. [CrossRef]
108. Woodhouse, B.; Pattison, S.; Segelov, E.; Singh, S.; Parker, K.; Kong, G.; Macdonald, W.; Wyld, D.; Meyer-Rochow, G.; Pavlakis, N.; et al. Consensus-Derived Quality Performance Indicators for Neuroendocrine Tumour Care. *J. Clin. Med.* **2019**, *8*, 1455. [CrossRef]

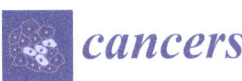

Article

Establishment of Novel Neuroendocrine Carcinoma Patient-Derived Xenograft Models for Receptor Peptide-Targeted Therapy

Catherine G. Tran [1,†], Luis C. Borbon [1,†], Jacqueline L. Mudd [2], Ellen Abusada [3], Solmaz AghaAmiri [4], Sukhen C. Ghosh [4], Servando Hernandez Vargas [4], Guiying Li [1], Gabriella V. Beyer [1], Mary McDonough [1], Rachel Li [1], Carlos H.F. Chan [1], Susan A. Walsh [5], Thaddeus J. Wadas [5], Thomas O'Dorisio [6], M Sue O'Dorisio [7], Ramaswamy Govindan [8], Paul F. Cliften [9], Ali Azhdarinia [4], Andrew M. Bellizzi [3], Ryan C. Fields [2], James R. Howe [1,*] and Po Hien Ear [1,*]

1. Department of Surgery, University of Iowa Carver College of Medicine, Iowa City, IA 52242, USA; catherine-tran@uiowa.edu (C.G.T.); luis-borbon@uiowa.edu (L.C.B.); guiying-li@uiowa.edu (G.L.); gabriella-holmes@uiowa.edu (G.V.B.); marymcdonough23@gmail.com (M.M.); binrui-li@uiowa.edu (R.L.); carlos-chan@uiowa.edu (C.H.F.C.)
2. Department of Surgery, Washington University School of Medicine, St. Louis, MO 63110, USA; jmudd@wustl.edu (J.L.M.); rcfields@wustl.edu (R.C.F.)
3. Department of Pathology, University of Iowa Carver College of Medicine, Iowa City, IA 52242, USA; ellen-abusada@uiowa.edu (E.A.); andrew-bellizzi@uiowa.edu (A.M.B.)
4. The Brown Foundation Institute of Molecular Medicine, McGovern Medical School, The University of Texas Health Science Center at Houston, Houston, TX 77054, USA; solmaz.aghaamiri@uth.tmc.edu (S.A.); sukhen.ghosh@uth.tmc.edu (S.C.G.); servando.hernandezvargas@uth.tmc.edu (S.H.V.); ali.azhdarinia@uth.tmc.edu (A.A.)
5. Department of Radiology, University of Iowa Carver College of Medicine, Iowa City, IA 52242, USA; susan-walsh@uiowa.edu (S.A.W.); thaddeus-wadas@uiowa.edu (T.J.W.)
6. Department of Internal Medicine, University of Iowa Carver College of Medicine, Iowa City, IA 52242, USA; thomas-odorisio@uiowa.edu
7. Department of Pediatrics, University of Iowa Carver College of Medicine, Iowa City, IA 52242, USA; sue-odorisio@uiowa.edu
8. Department of Medicine, Washington University School of Medicine, St. Louis, MO 63110, USA; rgovindan@wustl.edu
9. Department of Genetics, Washington University School of Medicine, St. Louis, MO 63110, USA; pcliften@wustl.edu
* Correspondence: james-howe@uiowa.edu (J.R.H.); pohien-ear@uiowa.edu (P.H.E.)
† These authors contributed equally to this work.

Simple Summary: Gastroenteropancreatic neuroendocrine neoplasms (GEP NENs) are a family of rare cancers with rising incidence in recent years. GEP NEN tumor cells are difficult to propagate, and few cellular and patient-derived xenograft (PDX) models are available for testing new therapies and studying the heterogeneous nature of these cancers. Here, we described the establishment and characterization of two novel NEC cellular and PDX models (NEC913 and NEC1452). NEC913 PDX tumors express somatostatin receptor 2 (SSTR2), whereas NEC1452 PDX tumors are SSTR2 negative. As a proof-of-concept study, we demonstrated how these PDX models can be used for peptide imaging experiments targeting SSTR2 using fluorescently labelled octreotide. The NEC913 and NEC1452 PDX lines represent valuable new tools for accelerating the process of drug discovery for GEP NENs.

Abstract: Gastroenteropancreatic neuroendocrine neoplasms (GEP NENs) are rare cancers consisting of neuroendocrine carcinomas (NECs) and neuroendocrine tumors (NETs), which have been increasing in incidence in recent years. Few cell lines and pre-clinical models exist for studying GEP NECs and NETs, limiting the ability to discover novel imaging and treatment modalities. To address this gap, we isolated tumor cells from cryopreserved patient GEP NECs and NETs and injected them into the flanks of immunocompromised mice to establish patient-derived xenograft (PDX) models. Two of six mice developed tumors (NEC913 and NEC1452). Over 80% of NEC913 and NEC1452 tumor cells stained positive for Ki67. NEC913 PDX tumors expressed neuroendocrine markers such as chromogranin A (CgA), synaptophysin (SYP), and somatostatin receptor-2 (SSTR2), whereas NEC1452 PDX tumors did not express SSTR2. Exome sequencing revealed loss of *TP53* and *RB1* in both NEC tumors. To demonstrate an application of these novel NEC PDX models for SSTR2-targeted peptide imaging, the NEC913 and NEC1452 cells were bilaterally injected into mice. Near infrared-labelled octreotide was administered and the fluorescent signal was specifically observed for the NEC913 SSTR2 positive tumors. These 2 GEP NEC PDX models serve as a valuable resource for GEP NEN therapy testing.

Keywords: gastroenteropancreatic neuroendocrine neoplasms; patient-derived xenograft; tumor spheroids; somatostatin receptor-2; near infrared-labelled octreotide analog

1. Introduction

Tumors can arise within neuroendocrine cells throughout the body, and some of the most common sites that lead to human morbidity and mortality originate within the GI system, most commonly within the small bowel and pancreas, collectively known as gastroenteropancreatic neuroendocrine neoplasms (GEP NENs). The age-adjusted incidence of GEP NENs increased over sixfold in the United States between 1973 and 2012, with an annual incidence of 3.56 per 100,000 persons [1]. These tumors are typically slow growing, but over 60% of patients present with metastatic disease and survival is greatly diminished [2–4]. In addition to the stage of the disease, both tumor grade and cell morphology/degree of differentiation are also powerful predictors of survival. Based on the 2019 World Health Organization classification of neuroendocrine neoplasms, GEP NENs are comprised of well-differentiated neuroendocrine tumors (NETs) and poorly-differentiated neuroendocrine carcinomas (NECs) [5]. Grade 1, 2, and 3 NETs are all morphologically well-differentiated and have Ki-67 values of <3%, 3–20%, and >20%, respectively. NECs are poorly differentiated tumors with a Ki-67 proliferation index >20% and/or a mitotic rate of over 20 mitoses per 2 mm^2, and many NECs have Ki-67 indices >50% [5]. In addition to these distinguishing features of poor differentiation and high Ki-67, GEP NECs have frequent mutations in *TP53* and *RB1*, while mutations in NET tumors are less common, and include *MEN1*, *DAXX*, and *ATRX* for pancreatic NETs (PNETs) and *CDKN1B* and 18q loss in small bowel NETs (SBNETs) [5–7].

Clinically, NECs are very aggressive, rapidly dividing tumors. They are associated with high rates of metastatic disease at presentation and poor prognosis. The incidence of NECs is not as well-defined due to changes in the WHO classification over the past decade, but epidemiological studies estimate this to be about 0.4/100,000 person-years [1,8]. The optimal treatment for GEP NECs has not been established due in part to the rarity of these tumors and difficulty with performing randomized trials. As a result, current guidelines for treatment of GEP NEC are based on lower-level evidence (NCCN Guidelines 2021) [9]. Therapeutic strategies are largely derived from experience in management of small cell lung cancer due to the pathologic and immunohistochemical similarities between small cell lung cancer and GEP NECs [10–12]. The appropriateness of this has been called into question as small cell lung cancer differs from NECs in several ways including higher association with smoking, higher rate of brain metastases, and higher sensitivity to platinum-based chemotherapy [11–14]. Patients are generally treated with chemotherapy regimens including platinum-based alkylating agents (carboplatin) and topoisomerase inhibitors (etoposide). Despite treatment, response rates are only 30–50% and median overall survival is 9 to 20 months [13–15].

Current therapies for both NETs and NECs are limited to somatostatin analogues (SSAs), mTOR inhibitors (everolimus), tyrosine kinase inhibitors (sunitinib), limited chemotherapy regimens, and peptide receptor radionuclide therapy (PRRT) [16–18]. One of the biggest barriers to identifying additional active therapeutics has been the inability to establish GEP NEN cell lines and mouse models that can be grown robustly. Some of these tumor cells can be grown in culture as spheroids, but they grow very slowly and are difficult to propagate as xenografts [19–21]. The two widely used cell lines, BON [22] and QGP1 [23] resemble poorly differentiated NECs [24–26], and unfortunately express low levels of NEN markers such as the somatostatin receptor 2 (SSTR2) [24]. Although well-differentiated GEP NET cell lines, such as the P-STS, GOT1, and NT-3 cells, have been described [24,25,27], difficulties growing these cells in abundance have limited their distribution to other researchers. The paucity of available cell lines has been a significant hurdle towards better understanding NEN biology and to provide theranostic models, and therefore we set out to establish new models to expand these options for NEN research.

2. Methods

2.1. Patient-Derived Xenograft Models and Cell Lines

The inventory of the Washington University PDX center was searched for neuroendocrine tumors and carcinomas, which were collected under an Institutional Review Board-approved protocol (#201708051) of Washington University and cryo-preserved. All peripheral blood and patient tumor tissue were procured on the day of surgery. Peripheral blood was layered onto a Ficoll gradient, peripheral blood mononuclear cells (PBMCs) isolated, rinsed, 5×10^6/mL transferred to cryovials, and cryopreserved in FBS + 10% DMSO. Tumor tissues were kept cold, cut into multiple small pieces, 5 pieces transferred into each cryovial, and cryopreserved in FBS + 10% DMSO. All cryopreserved samples were progressively cooled in a freezing container at a controlled rate of -1 °C/min at -80 °C. Vials were subsequently transferred to liquid nitrogen for long term storage.

Six patient samples were selected for this study. Tumors were thawed, minced, digested with collagenase and DNase I, and strained to obtain a single-cell suspension [19]. One to ten thousand cells were injected subcutaneously into NOD scid gamma (NSG) mice under an Institutional Animal Care and Use Committee-approved protocol (#9051771). Once visible subcutaneous tumors developed, tumor volume was calculated by multiplying tumor length, width, and depth and expressed as mm^3. Tumors larger than 1000 mm^3 were harvested, processed, and 1 million tumor cells were injected into another generation of NSG mice, and remaining cells were placed in suspension culture. After 2 days of incubation, mouse fibroblasts from the PDX tumors were easily removed since they adhered to the plastic culture dish while the NEC cells grew in suspension. The floating NEC cells were harvested and transferred into new culture dishes. After 3 passages, the cultures consisted of only NEC cells with no fibroblast contamination was observed. NEC tumor cells can also be seeded in extracellular matrix as 3-dimensional cultures. For optimal NET marker expression, use NEC cells recently isolated from PDX tumors and avoid using cells in culture over 6 months. NEC tumor cells were grown in Dulbecco's modified Eagle's medium (DMEM)/F12 with 10% fetal bovine serum (FBS), 1% penicillin/streptomycin, 1% L-glutamine, insulin, and nicotinamide [19]. BON cells were cultured in Dulbecco's modified Eagle's medium (DMEM)/F12 with 10% fetal bovine serum (FBS), 1% penicillin/streptomycin, and 1% L-glutamine [22].

2.2. Histology and Immunohistochemistry

Patient samples from surgery were fixed in formalin, embedded in paraffin, and sectioned. Slides were deparaffinized, rehydrated, and stained with hematoxylin and eosin (H&E). Slides were immunostained using specific antibodies against chromogranin A (CgA) (Thermo Scientific, Waltham, MA, USA, #MA5-13096), synaptophysin (SYP) (Agilent Dako, Santa Clara, CA, USA, #M7315), achaete-scute family bHLH transcription factor 1 (ASCL1) (BD Pharmingen, San Diego, CA, USA, #556604), p53 (Agilent Dako, #M700101-2), retinoblastoma protein (Rb) (BD Pharmingen, #554136), somatostatin receptor 2 (SSTR2) (Abcam, Waltham, MA, USA, #ab134152), and C-X-C motif chemokine receptor 4 (CXCR4) (Abcam, #ab124824), and Ki-67 (Agilent Dako, #M724001-2). Ki-67 proliferation index was quantified by percentage of positively staining cells in ~500 tumor cells per tumor sample.

2.3. Quantitative PCR

RNA was extracted from tumors grown in mice using the RNeasy Plus Universal Kit (Qiagen, Beverly, MA, USA) and reverse transcribed to cDNA using the qScript cDNA Supermix (QuantaBio, Beverly, MA, USA). Quantitative PCR was performed with gene-specific primers and PerfeCTa SYBR Green Supermix dye (Quantabio) using the 7900HT Fast Real-Time PCR System (Applied Biosystems, Waltham, MA, USA). Primer sequences were obtained from PrimerBank (https://pga.mgh.harvard.edu/primerbank, accessed on the 8 July 2020) and were purchased from Integrated DNA Technologies (IDT). Primer sequences used for qPCR analysis are shown in Table 1.

Table 1. List of primer sequences used for qPCR experiments.

Gene Symbol	Forward	Reverse
GAPDH	GGAGCGAGATCCCTCCAAAAT	GGCTGTTGTCATACTTCTCATGG
CGA	TAAAGGGGATACCGAGGTGATG	TCGGAGTGTCTCAAAACATTCC
SYP	CTCGGCTTTGTGAAGGTGCT	CTGAGGTCACTCTCGGTCTTG
SSTR1	GCGCCATCCTGATCTCTTTCA	AACGTGGAGGTGACTAGGAAG
SSTR2	TGGCTATCCATTCCATTTGACC	AGGACTGCATTGCTTGTCAGG
SSTR3	AGAACCTGAGAATGCCTCCTC	GCCGCAGGACCACATAGATG
SSTR4	GCATGGTCGCTATCCAGTG	GCGAAGGATCACGAAGATGAC
SSTR5	GTGATCCTTCGCTACGCCAA	CACGGTGAGACAGAAGACGC
CXCR4	ACGCCACCAACAGTCAGAG	AGTCGGGAATAGTCAGCAGGA

2.4. Immunofluorescence

Cells derived from mouse tumors were fixed with 4% paraformaldehyde for 10 min, then stained with primary antibodies against SYP (Abcam, #32127) at 1:600 dilution, CgA (Invitrogen, Waltham, MA, USA, #MA5-13096) at 1:400 dilution, and SSTR2 (Sigma, St. Louis, MO, USA, #HPA007264) at 1:400 dilution overnight. Cells were washed and incubated with an FITC-conjugated secondary antibody (Jackson ImmunoResearch, West Grove, PA, USA, #115-095-062 and #711-095-152) at 1:500 dilution for 1 h. Immunofluorescent images were taken using a fluorescent microscope at 200 ms exposure time.

2.5. Genomic DNA Analyses

Genomic DNA from PDX tumors, and peripheral blood mononuclear cells (PBMCs) were extracted using a DNA extraction kit (Qiagen). Short tandem repeats (STR) analyses were performed on the DNA samples using the Cell Check9 panel of 9 human STR polymorphisms (IDEXX, Westbrook, ME, USA). Exome sequencings of PDX tumors were performed by submitting genomic DNA from NEC913 and NEC1452 PDX tumors to the Washington University Genome Technology Access Center for analyses with the IDT Exome 150X coverage. Exome sequencing data were analyzed using a DRAGEN processor and compared to the GRCh38 reference genome.

2.6. Imaging of Patient-Derived Xenograft Mouse Model with Bilateral Tumors

Five female NSG mice (Jackson Laboratory, Bar Harbor, ME, USA, Stock no: 005557) were anesthetized with 1% to 2% isoflurane at 10 weeks of age, and were subcutaneously injected with 1×10^6 SSTR2(+) cells in extracellular matrix Matrigel (Corning, Corning, NY, USA, #356235) in the left shoulder, and 1×10^6 SSTR2(−) cells in the right shoulder. When bilateral tumor size reached between 10 to 20 mm in diameter at 5 weeks post-implantation, in vivo and ex vivo near infrared (NIR) fluorescence imaging were conducted with NIR octreotide analog (NIR-TOC) as described by Hernandez-Vargas et al. [28,29] In brief, 6 nmol of NIR-TOC diluted in 100 µL PBS was administered via mouse tail-vein injection 24 h prior to imaging studies. NIR fluorescence imaging was acquired using the IVIS Lumina S5 small animal imaging station and Living Image® software (PerkinElmer, Waltham, MA, USA) with excitation and emission set to 740 and 790 nm, respectively. Images with favorable contrast-to-noise ratio were obtained using exposure time of 2 s for in vivo and 0.1 s for ex vivo imaging, with subject height of 1.50 cm, small binning and F/Stop setting of 2, and field of view setting C. After completing in vivo imaging, mice were euthanized and dissection was immediately performed for ex vivo isolation, and imaging of subcutaneous tumors as well as major intraabdominal and intrathoracic organs was performed. Quantification of NIR fluorescent signal was performed using ImageJ version 1.53 a (NIH, Bethesda, MD, USA). Statistical analyses for NIR fluorescent signal were performed using t-tests in Prism GraphPad. $p < 0.05$ was depicted with *.

3. Results

Tumor cells from six cryopreserved patient tumors (Table 2) were injected into the flank of NSG mice to generate PDX models (Figure 1A). At 3 months post-tumor cell injection, two mice harboring GEP NEC cells had developed subcutaneous tumors of approximately 1 cm in diameter (NEC913 and NEC1452; Figure 1A) while four GEP NET patient tumor cell samples injected into mice did not form tumors (Table 2). Subcutaneous injection of 1×10^6 NEC913 and NEC1452 cells grew into tumors about 1000 mm^3 and 1500 mm^3 in size, respectively, after 5 weeks in subsequent passages. The tumor formation rate was 100%. The NEC913 and NEC1452 xenograft tumors were harvested and collected for histological and biochemical analyses. A separate portion of the NEC913 and NEC1452 tumors was collected for tumor cell isolation and injection into another generation of mice for propagation of the PDX models and for establishment of cell lines. Both NEC913 and NEC1452 cells were successfully maintained in culture for months in enriched DMEM/F12 medium. Both PDX tumors stained positive for the neuroendocrine tumor markers chromogranin A (CgA) and synaptophysin (SYP), but only the NEC913 PDX tumor stained positive for somatostatin receptor 2 (SSTR2; Figure 1B). Exome sequencing of the NEC913 and NEC1452 PDX tumors were performed and mutations in *TP53* and *RB1* were confirmed (Figure 1C; Supplementary Tables S1 and S2).

Table 2. List of GEP NEN patient tumor samples used for patient-derived xenograft (PDX) development.

Patient Tumor ID Number	Classification of Tumor	WHO Terminology	Differentiation	Tumor Grade	Ki67 (%)	Establishment of PDX
PNET459	Pancreatic NET	NET Grade 2	Well differentiated	Intermediate	7	no
PNET560	Pancreatic NET	NET Grade 2	Well differentiated	Intermediate	8.4	no
PNET1164	Pancreatic NET	NET Grade 2	Well differentiated	Intermediate	13	no
SBNET1063	Small bowel NET	NET Grade 3	Well differentiated	High	80	no
NEC913	Ampullary NEC	NEC, small and large-cell types	Poorly differentiated	High	80–90	yes
NEC1452	Rectal NEC	NEC, large-cell type	Poorly differentiated	High	80–90	yes

We were able to retrieve the original patient tumor for the NEC913 sample for comparison with the PDX model. The NEC913 tumor came from a patient presenting with jaundice and upper GI bleeding. A biopsy revealed a Grade 3 NEC of the ampulla of Vater, and the patient was treated with carboplatin/etoposide chemotherapy for 4 months, then had a Whipple procedure, where a 0.3 cm primary tumor with multiple involved nodes were also removed (Figure 2A). Hematoxylin and eosin (H&E) staining showed the presence of both small and large NEC cells (Figure 2B). The NEC913 primary tumor stained positive for Ki-67 in over 80% of cells (Figure 2C). An outside pathology report indicated that the specimen was TTF-1 positive and CDX2 negative. We detected positive staining for CgA, SYP, SSTR2, and ASCL1 (Figure 2D–G). A low level of p53 was detected (Figure 2H); however, exome sequencing data identified several stopgain mutations where the first stopgain mutation is located in codon 147 of *TP53* (Figure 1C, Supplementary Table S1) suggesting that the IHC staining detect only the first 146 amino acid fragment of p53. Expression of Rb was lost (Figure 2I). Exome sequencing of the NEC913 PDX tumor revealed an *RB1* frameshift insertion (1091_1092insCG) leading to a premature stop codon

(Figure 1C, Supplementary Table S1). STR analyses confirmed that the NEC913 patient blood sample shared the same alleles with the NEC913 PDX tumor (Supplementary Table S3) and that these samples did not match any of the existing research samples in the IDEXX DSMZ STR database, meaning that they are being reported for the first time.

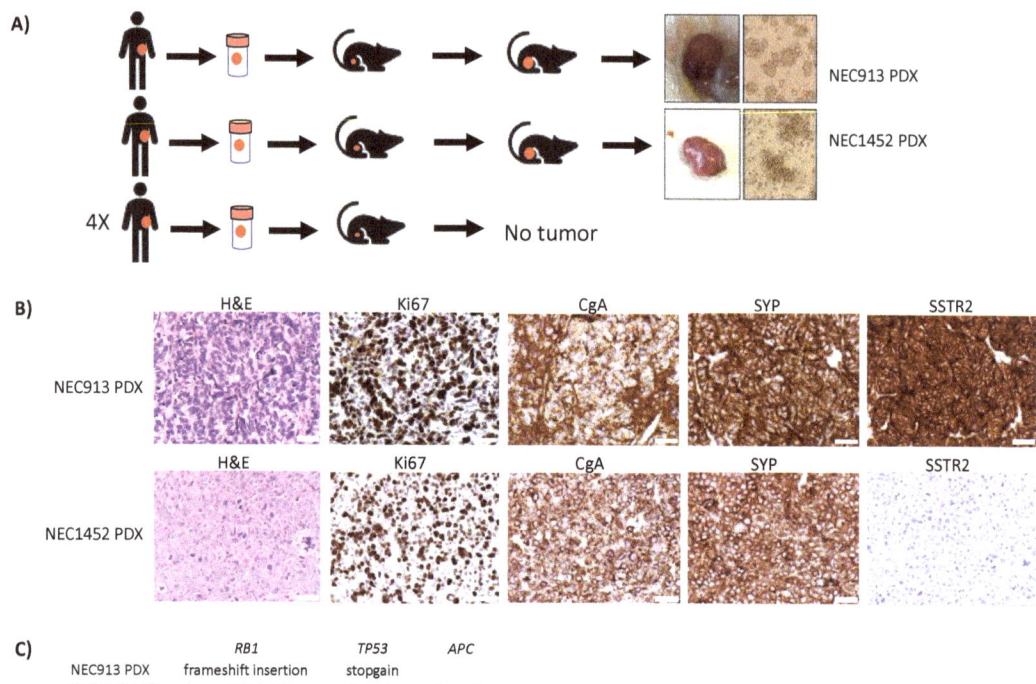

Figure 1. Establishment of neuroendocrine neoplasm (NEN) patient-derived xenograft (PDX) models: (A) Tumor samples from NEN patients were cryopreserved, thawed, and injected into the flank of immunocompromised NOD Scid Gamma (NSG) mice. Two mice developed subcutaneous tumors at three months post injection (NEC913 and NEC1452 PDX models). Both PDX models have been passaged in 6 generations of mice. (B) Formalin-fixed and paraffin-embedded tumor sections are stained with H&E and stained for Ki67 and neuroendocrine tumor markers such chromogranin A (CgA), synaptophysin (SYP), and somatostatin receptor 2 (SSTR2) by IHC. Scale bar represents 40 µm. (C) Exome sequencing of NEC913 and NEC1452 PDX tumors demonstrated mutations in *TP53* and *RB1*.

The patient giving rise to tumor NEC1452 presented with a mediastinal and supraclavicular masses, as well as liver, pancreatic, retroperitoneal, and rectal lesions that were Fluorodeoxyglucose–Positron Emission Tomography (FDG-PET) positive and only mildly DOTA-octreotate (DOTA-TATE) PET avid. A supraclavicular node biopsy showed a small cell NEC and carboplatin/etoposide were started, followed by FOLFIRI after progression, then immunotherapy. A retroperitoneal node was biopsied due to poor response, which showed large cell NEC with a Ki-67 of 80–90%, which the source of this PDX. The treating medical oncologist considered the rectum to be the primary site, because this had the highest FDG-PET avidity, with uptake in perirectal nodes, a nearly obstructing mass seen on sigmoidoscopy, and the presence of *APC* mutations in the tumor (Figure 1C, Supplementary Table S2). The NEC1452 PDX tumor sample did not match any pre-existing samples in the IDEXX DSMZ STR database (Supplementary Table S4), and exome sequencing confirmed *TP53* stopgain mutations and *RB1* frameshift mutation (Figure 1C, Supplementary Table S2).

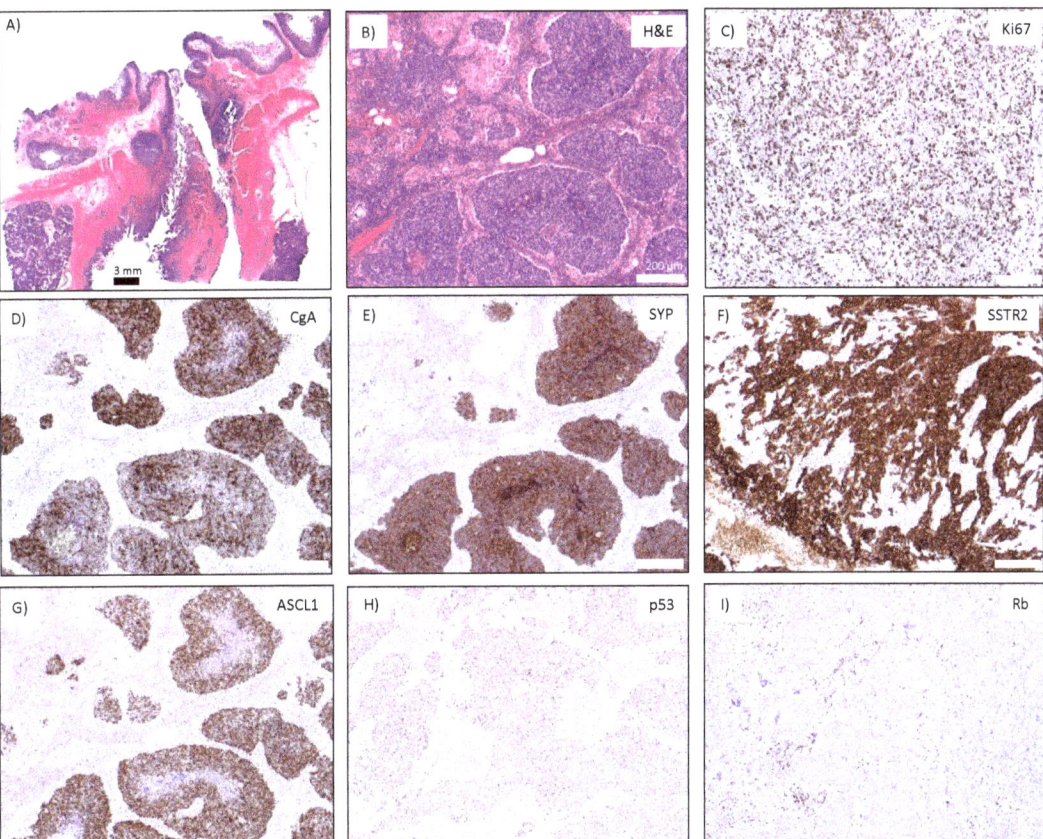

Figure 2. IHC analyses of NEC913 patient sample: (**A**) Primary NEC tumor at the ampulla of Vater. Scale bar represents 3 mm. (**B**) H&E staining of primary NEC tumor. (**C–I**) Staining for Ki67, CgA, SYP, SSTR2, ASCL1, p53, and Rb. Scale bar represents 200 μm.

Tumor cells isolated from the cryopreserved NEC913 and NEC1452 tumors yielded viable cells despite the fact that both patients had been treated with carboplatin/etoposide chemotherapy, suggesting that these NEC cells are resistant to the treatment. Both samples can be robustly passaged as PDXs and tumor cells from the xenografts grow as suspension cultures or as spheroids embedded in extracellular matrix. By immunofluorescent staining, we confirmed the expression of CgA and SYP in both cell lines and SSTR2 in only the NEC913 line (Figure 3A). To further characterize these novel cell lines for additional neuroendocrine cancer markers, gene expression analyses using quantitative PCR was performed (Figure 3B–H). In comparison to the established BON cells, NEC913 was found to have significantly increased *SYP* and *SSTR2* expression (Figure 3B,E). NEC1452 cells were determined to have increased *SSTR1* expression relative to BON cells (Figure 3D).

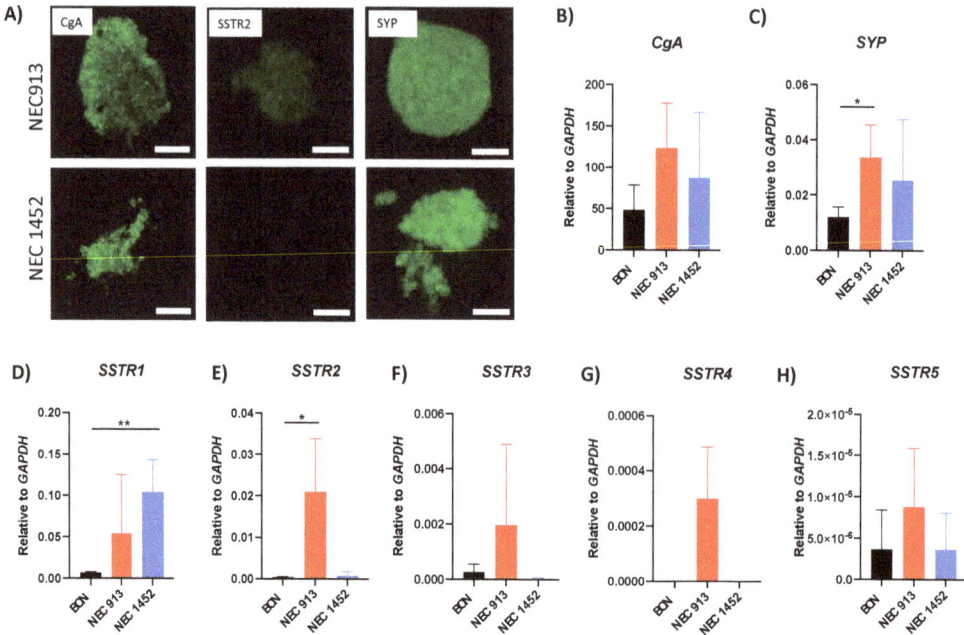

Figure 3. Characterization of NEC913 and NEC1452 cells for NET markers: (**A**) NEC913 and NEC1452 cells incubated with antibodies against CgA (1/300), SSTR2 (1/300), and SYP (1/600) overnight and with secondary antibodies coupled to FITC (1/500) for 1 h at room temperature. Microscopy pictures are taken using 200 ms exposure time. Scale bar represents 100 μm. (**B–H**) Gene expression analyses of NET markers in NEC913 and NEC1452 cells compared to BON cells. Gene expression levels were normalized to the control gene *GAPDH* to determine the relative fold change. Statistical analyses of gene expression changes were performed using T-tests in Prism GraphPad. $p < 0.05$ was depicted with *. $p < 0.01$ was depicted with **.

To demonstrate the utility of NEC PDX models as a potential tool for testing receptor-targeted theranostics, we conducted a proof-of-concept study whereby we established a mouse model with tumor implantations using the NEC913 (SSTR2+) and NEC1452 (SSTR2−) cells in opposite shoulders for SSTR2-targeted imaging (Figure 4A). We then injected these mice with a NIR-TOC, which previously was demonstrated to specifically detects SSTR2 on NEN cells, and imaged them using NIR fluorescence imaging [28,30]. Image analysis revealed that the NIR-fluorescence signal was localized only in the NEC913(SSTR2+) tumor (Figure 4B). To confirm the localization of the NIR fluorescence signal on the NEC tumors, ex vivo NIR fluorescence imaging was performed on both tumors after they were removed from the animals. The NIR fluorescence signal was detected in the NEC913 tumor but not NEC1452 (Figure 4C), corroborating the in vivo imaging results (Figure 4B). Qualitative assessment of SSTR2-mediated uptake was supported by semi-quantitative image analyses, which revealed an approximately twofold increase and a threefold increase in fluorescent signal intensity of NEC913 compared to NEC1452 tumors in the in vivo and ex vivo experiments, respectively (Figure 4D,E).

Further characterization of the NEC913 PDX tumor by IHC showed low expression of p53, which could be due to the specificity of the antibody for the truncated form of p53, and no expression of Rb (Figure 5A), which is similar to the expression pattern observed in original patient tumor IHC analyses (Figure 2H,I). The expression of ASCL1 was lower in the NEC913 PDX tumor (Figure 5A) when compared to the original tumor (Figure 2G). In addition, the NEC913 PDX tumor expressed CXCR4 (Figure 5A). The *CXCR4* expression was also detected in NEC913 spheroids by quantitative PCR and IHC using a specific antibody against CXCR4 (Figure 5B,C).

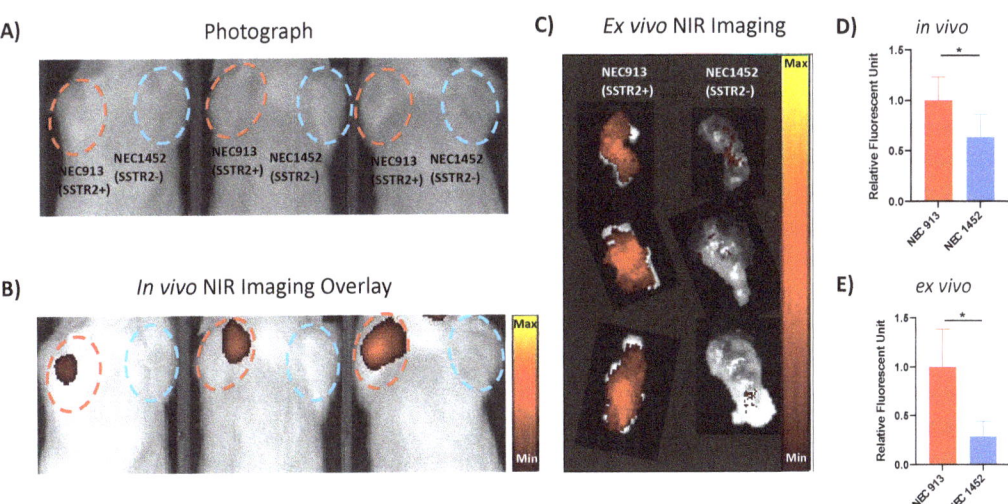

Figure 4. Application of NEC PDX models for SSTR2-targeted imaging: (**A**) Representative photograph of mice harboring NEC913 and NEC1452 tumors ranging from 1.0 to 2.0 cm in diameter 5 weeks post tumor cell injections from an $n = 5$ mice experiment. (**B**) Representative Near infrared (NIR) fluorescence imaging of mice harboring NEC913 and NEC1452 tumors using exposure time of 2 s and excitation and emission wavelengths set at 740 and 790 nm, respectively. NEC913 tumors are circled in red and NEC1452 tumors are circled in blue. (**C**) Representative ex vivo NIR fluorescence imaging of dissected NEC913 and NEC1452 tumors from an $n = 5$ mice experiment. (**D,E**) Quantifications of in vivo and ex vivo NIR fluorescence signal in NEC913 and NEC1452 tumors. T-tests were performed using Prism GraphPad. $p < 0.05$ was depicted with *.

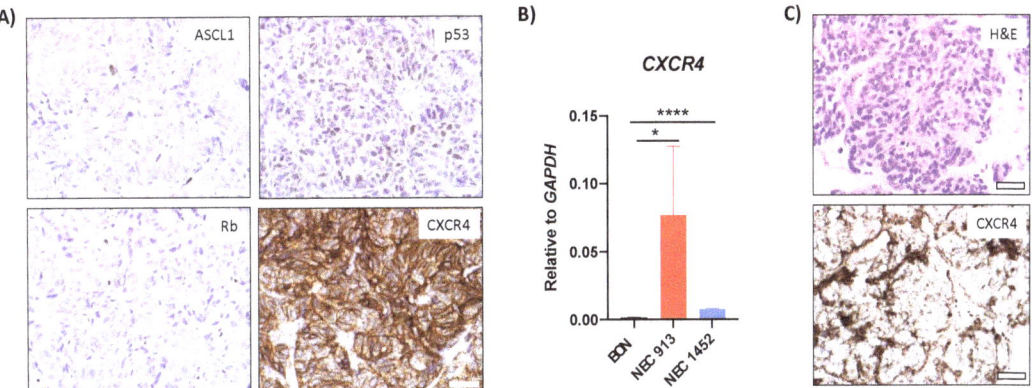

Figure 5. Additional characterization of NEC913 PDX model: (**A**) IHC analyses of NEC913 PDX tumors for NEC markers such as Rb, p53, ASCL1, and CXCR4. (**B**) Comparison of the gene expression levels of *CXCR4* in BON, NEC913, and NEC1452 cells by quantitative PCR normalized to the control gene *GAPDH* to determine the relative fold change. Statistical analyses of gene expression changes were performed using T-tests in Prism GraphPad. $p < 0.05$ was depicted with *. $p < 0.0001$ was depicted with ****. (**C**) NEC913 spheroids H&E staining and IHC analysis of CXCR4. Scale bar represents 40 μm.

4. Discussion

GEP NETs and NECs are rare cancers with few in vitro and in vivo models available for therapeutic testing [31]. GEP NET cell lines and spheroids are difficult to propagate as they take approximately 2 to 3 weeks to divide [19,22,24,32]. A limited number of GEP NEC cell and organoid lines have been recently published, but distribution remains limited. The two currently available human GEP-NEN-derived cell lines, BON and QGP-1, divide approximately every 3 days and carry *TP53* and *RB1* mutations [25]. They are morphologically poorly differentiated, and have Ki-67 rates that exceed 90%, which define them as NEC cell lines.

Because well-differentiated NETs grow slowly, attempts to propagate them long term have not generally been successful. We have shown that these can be grown in culture for up to 9 months, remained well-differentiated, and expressed NET markers such as synaptophysin, chromogranin, and SSTR2 [19]. However, after about 2 weeks, growth remains fairly constant at a low level. In this study, we were unsuccessful at establishing all four frozen NET samples in immunocompromised mice at 3 months post injection (Table 2). Considering that a majority of GEP NETs are generally slow-growing Grade 2 tumors with a Ki-67 index less than 20%, it is possible that a period longer than 3 months is required for tumor formation. Interestingly, even the SBNET sample SBNET1063 (Table 2), which was a WHO Grade 3 tumor, did not generate a subcutaneous tumor, suggesting that a xenograft model may not be ideal for NET PDX development. There have been a few NET cell lines described such as P-STS, GOT1, NT3 [24,25,27], and a well-differentiated PNET PDX model reported by Chamberlain et al. [33]. Although these appear to be promising GEP NET models, they have not been widely distributed to many investigators. The most likely explanation for this is that they cannot be grown in a large enough quantity to share, or that over time, the cells that do survive could potentially dedifferentiate into NECs.

We established two new NEC cell lines that grow well in culture and can be passaged through several generations of immunocompromised mice. These lines significantly expand the options for study of NECs and were derived from different sites. The NEC913 was derived from an ampullary NEC and NEC1452 from a retroperitoneal node from a patient suspected to have a rectal NEC. Both NEC913 and NEC1452 PDX tumors contain *TP53* and *RB1* mutations that are commonly reported in GEP NECs [6,34,35]. Both lines expressed synaptophysin, chromogranin A, and had Ki-67 of >80%. The NEC913 line expressed SSTR2 and CXCR4 while NEC1452 did not. Tumors from these PDX models can robustly be passaged in more than six generations of mice with a 100% rate of tumor formation. NEC cells from both PDX models can be maintained in culture in media supplemented with insulin and nicotinamide as suspension cultures or spheroids embedded in extracellular matrix.

Several lung NEC lines [36,37] and colon NEC lines such as the HROC47, SS-2, and NEC-DUE1 and 2 [36,38–40] have been established, but few pancreas and rectal NEC lines have been reported [39]. Considering the rarity of GEP NEC PDX and cell models, the NEC913 and NEC1452 PDX models developed in this study could be tremendously valuable for a variety of pre-clinical experiments. Here, we showed that the NEC913 line can be useful in confirming the target specificity of NIR-TOC with fluorescence imaging in a clinically relevant model, suggesting high translational potential (Figure 4). NEC913 PDX model maintains high SSTR2 (Figure 1B) and CXCR4 (Figure 5A,B) expression after six generations of passages. The NEC913 cells grew as spheroids in suspension culture or embedded in extracellular matrix, recapitulated characteristics of the PDX tumor, and stained positive for CXCR4 (Figure 5). This cell line also shows great promise as a potential tool for future investigations involving PRRT including testing of combination therapies or highly potent alpha-emitter PRRT [41]. CXCR4 is also emerging as a valuable target in atypical lung carcinoid and small cell lung cancer, and can be targeted with the radiolabeled ligand Pentixafor and Pentixather [42,43]. Thus, NEC913 could also serve as an effective pre-clinical model for PRRT directed at CXCR4. The development and characterization of these NEC913 and NEC452 PDX lines represent valuable new tools that could overcome the significant limitations of existing preclinical models in NEN research and accelerate the process of drug discovery.

5. Conclusions

Two novel NEC PDX models (NEC913 and NEC1452) were established from cryopreserved patient tumors. Tumors from these PDX models can robustly be passaged in immunocompromised mice. The NEC913 PDX model maintained SSTR2 expression after six generations of passages and can be visualized using NIR-TOC peptide. In addition, the NEC913 PDX model expressed high level of CXCR4, which makes it potentially useful for CXCR4-targeted theranostics. NEC cells from both PDX models can be maintained in culture in media supplemented with insulin and nicotinamide. Considering the rarity of GEP NEC PDX and cell lines, the NEC913 and NEC1452 PDX models are valuable pre-clinical models for peptide imaging, drug testing experiments, and studying GEP NEC tumor biology.

Supplementary Materials: The following supporting information can be downloaded at: https://www.mdpi.com/article/10.3390/cancers14081910/s1, Table S1: List of curated mutations identified in NEC913 PDX tumors by exome sequencing. Table S2: List of curated mutations identified in NEC1452 PDX tumors by exome sequencing. Table S3: Short Tandem Repeats analyses of NEC913 PDX tumors and patient periphery blood mononuclear cells. Table S4: Short Tandem Repeats analyses of NEC1452 PDX tumors.

Author Contributions: Conceptualization, P.H.E., J.R.H., R.C.F., C.H.F.C., M.S.O., T.O., A.A. and R.G.; Methodology, C.G.T., L.C.B., J.L.M., E.A., S.A., S.C.G., S.H.V., G.L., C.H.F.C., G.V.B., M.M., R.L. and S.A.W.; Software, P.F.C., S.A., S.A.W. and T.J.W.; Formal Analysis, P.H.E., A.M.B., J.R.H., R.C.F., S.A. and P.F.C.; Resources, R.C.F., A.M.B. and A.A.; Data Curation, P.H.E.; Funding acquisition, P.H.E., R.C.F., M.S.O., R.G., J.R.H., A.M.B. and T.O.; Original Draft Preparation, P.H.E.; Writing—Review and Editing, P.H.E., J.R.H., C.G.T., L.C.B., C.H.F.C., T.J.W., S.A.W., S.A., A.A. and J.L.M.; Supervision, P.H.E.; Project Administration, P.H.E., J.R.H., R.C.F. and J.L.M. All authors have read and agreed to the published version of the manuscript.

Funding: This work was funded by the PDX Center U54CA224083 Supplement Grant awarded to P.H.E., R.C.F., M.S.O. and R.G.; NANETS BTSI Award given to P.H.E.; and by the NET SPORE P50CA174521 awarded to M.S.O., T.O., A.M.B. and J.R.H. CGT was supported by T32CA148062. The PerkinElmer Lumina S5 was purchased with the NIH S5 1S10OD026835-01 grant.

Institutional Review Board Statement: Patient tumor collection was approved by the Institutional Review Board (protocol # 201708051; Washington University PDX center). All animal experiments have been approved by the Institutional Animal Care and Use Committee (protocol # 905177; University of Iowa).

Informed Consent Statement: Not applicable.

Data Availability Statement: Please contact the corresponding authors for any additional data.

Acknowledgments: We thank Mark B. Evers and Courtney M. Townsend for providing us with the BON cell line.

Conflicts of Interest: Authors declare no conflict of interest.

References

1. Dasari, A.; Shen, C.; Halperin, D.; Zhao, B.; Zhou, S.; Xu, Y.; Shih, T.; Yao, J.C. Trends in the Incidence, Prevalence, and Survival Outcomes in Patients with Neuroendocrine Tumors in the United States. *JAMA Oncol.* **2017**, *3*, 1335–1342. [CrossRef]
2. Panzuto, F.; Boninsegna, L.; Fazio, N.; Campana, D.; Pia Brizzi, M.; Capurso, G.; Scarpa, A.; De Braud, F.; Dogliotti, L.; Tomassetti, P.; et al. Metastatic and locally advanced pancreatic endocrine carcinomas: Analysis of factors associated with disease progression. *J. Clin. Oncol.* **2011**, *29*, 2372–2377. [CrossRef] [PubMed]
3. Pavel, M.; O'Toole, D.; Costa, F.; Capdevila, J.; Gross, D.; Kianmanesh, R.; Krenning, E.; Knigge, U.; Salazar, R.; Pape, U.F.; et al. ENETS Consensus Guidelines Update for the Management of Distant Metastatic Disease of Intestinal, Pancreatic, Bronchial Neuroendocrine Neoplasms (NEN) and NEN of Unknown Primary Site. *Neuroendocrinology* **2016**, *103*, 172–185. [CrossRef] [PubMed]

4. Dasari, A.; Mehta, K.; Byers, L.A.; Sorbye, H.; Yao, J.C. Comparative study of lung and extrapulmonary poorly differentiated neuroendocrine carcinomas: A SEER database analysis of 162,983 cases. *Cancer* **2018**, *124*, 807–815. [CrossRef] [PubMed]
5. Nagtegaal, I.D.; Odze, R.D.; Klimstra, D.; Paradis, V.; Rugge, M.; Schirmacher, P.; Washington, K.M.; Carneiro, F.; Cree, I.A.; WHO Classification of Tumors Editorial Board. The 2019 WHO classification of tumours of the digestive system. *Histopathology* **2020**, *76*, 182–188. [CrossRef] [PubMed]
6. Venizelos, A.; Elvebakken, H.; Perren, A.; Nikolaienko, O.; Deng, W.; Lothe, I.M.B.; Couvelard, A.; Hjortland, G.O.; Sundlov, A.; Svensson, J.; et al. The molecular characteristics of high-grade gastroenteropancreatic neuroendocrine neoplasms. *Endocr. Relat. Cancer* **2021**, *29*, 1–14. [CrossRef] [PubMed]
7. Yachida, S.; Totoki, Y.; Noe, M.; Nakatani, Y.; Horie, M.; Kawasaki, K.; Nakamura, H.; Saito-Adachi, M.; Suzuki, M.; Takai, E.; et al. Comprehensive Genomic Profiling of Neuroendocrine Carcinomas of the Gastrointestinal System. *Cancer Discov.* **2021**, *12*, 692–711. [CrossRef]
8. Korse, C.M.; Taal, B.G.; van Velthuysen, M.L.; Visser, O. Incidence and survival of neuroendocrine tumours in the Netherlands according to histological grade: Experience of two decades of cancer registry. *Eur. J. Cancer* **2013**, *49*, 1975–1983. [CrossRef]
9. Shah, M.H.; Goldner, W.S.; Benson, A.B.; Bergsland, E.; Blaszkowsky, L.S.; Brock, P.; Chan, J.; Das, S.; Dickson, P.V.; Fanta, P.; et al. Neuroendocrine and Adrenal Tumors, Version 2.2021, NCCN Clinical Practice Guidelines in Oncology. *J. Natl. Compr. Cancer Netw.* **2021**, *19*, 839–868. [CrossRef]
10. Sorbye, H.; Strosberg, J.; Baudin, E.; Klimstra, D.S.; Yao, J.C. Gastroenteropancreatic high-grade neuroendocrine carcinoma. *Cancer* **2014**, *120*, 2814–2823. [CrossRef]
11. Walenkamp, A.M.; Sonke, G.S.; Sleijfer, D.T. Clinical and therapeutic aspects of extrapulmonary small cell carcinoma. *Cancer Treat. Rev.* **2009**, *35*, 228–236. [CrossRef] [PubMed]
12. Brennan, S.M.; Gregory, D.L.; Stillie, A.; Herschtal, A.; Mac Manus, M.; Ball, D.L. Should extrapulmonary small cell cancer be managed like small cell lung cancer? *Cancer* **2010**, *116*, 888–895. [CrossRef] [PubMed]
13. Conte, B.; George, B.; Overman, M.; Estrella, J.; Jiang, Z.Q.; Mehrvarz Sarshekeh, A.; Ferrarotto, R.; Hoff, P.M.; Rashid, A.; Yao, J.C.; et al. High-Grade Neuroendocrine Colorectal Carcinomas: A Retrospective Study of 100 Patients. *Clin. Colorectal Cancer* **2016**, *15*, e1–e7. [CrossRef] [PubMed]
14. Terashima, T.; Morizane, C.; Hiraoka, N.; Tsuda, H.; Tamura, T.; Shimada, Y.; Kaneko, S.; Kushima, R.; Ueno, H.; Kondo, S.; et al. Comparison of chemotherapeutic treatment outcomes of advanced extrapulmonary neuroendocrine carcinomas and advanced small-cell lung carcinoma. *Neuroendocrinology* **2012**, *96*, 324–332. [CrossRef]
15. Sorbye, H.; Welin, S.; Langer, S.W.; Vestermark, L.W.; Holt, N.; Osterlund, P.; Dueland, S.; Hofsli, E.; Guren, M.G.; Ohrling, K.; et al. Predictive and prognostic factors for treatment and survival in 305 patients with advanced gastrointestinal neuroendocrine carcinoma (WHO G3): The NORDIC NEC study. *Ann. Oncol.* **2013**, *24*, 152–160. [CrossRef]
16. Phan, A.T.; Kunz, P.L.; Reidy-Lagunes, D.L. New and Emerging Treatment Options for Gastroenteropancreatic Neuroendocrine Tumors. *Clin. Adv. Hematol. Oncol.* **2015**, *13*, 1–18.
17. Cives, M.; Strosberg, J. Treatment Strategies for Metastatic Neuroendocrine Tumors of the Gastrointestinal Tract. *Curr. Treat. Options Oncol.* **2017**, *18*, 14. [CrossRef]
18. Perez, K.; Chan, J. Treatment of Gastroenteropancreatic Neuroendocrine Tumors. *Surg. Pathol. Clin.* **2019**, *12*, 1045–1053. [CrossRef]
19. Ear, P.H.; Li, G.; Wu, M.; Abusada, E.; Bellizzi, A.M.; Howe, J.R. Establishment and Characterization of Small Bowel Neuroendocrine Tumor Spheroids. *J. Vis. Exp.* **2019**, *152*, e60303. [CrossRef]
20. Tillotson, L.G.; Lodestro, C.; Hocker, M.; Wiedenmann, B.; Newcomer, C.E.; Reid, L.M. Isolation, maintenance, and characterization of human pancreatic islet tumor cells expressing vasoactive intestinal peptide. *Pancreas* **2001**, *22*, 91–98. [CrossRef]
21. Fujii, M.; Shimokawa, M.; Date, S.; Takano, A.; Matano, M.; Nanki, K.; Ohta, Y.; Toshimitsu, K.; Nakazato, Y.; Kawasaki, K.; et al. A Colorectal Tumor Organoid Library Demonstrates Progressive Loss of Niche Factor Requirements during Tumorigenesis. *Cell Stem Cell* **2016**, *18*, 827–838. [CrossRef] [PubMed]
22. Evers, B.M.; Townsend, C.M., Jr.; Upp, J.R.; Allen, E.; Hurlbut, S.C.; Kim, S.W.; Rajaraman, S.; Singh, P.; Reubi, J.C.; Thompson, J.C. Establishment and characterization of a human carcinoid in nude mice and effect of various agents on tumor growth. *Gastroenterology* **1991**, *101*, 303–311. [CrossRef]
23. Iguchi, H.; Hayashi, I.; Kono, A. A somatostatin-secreting cell line established from a human pancreatic islet cell carcinoma (somatostatinoma): Release experiment and immunohistochemical study. *Cancer Res.* **1990**, *50*, 3691–3693. [PubMed]
24. Benten, D.; Behrang, Y.; Unrau, L.; Weissmann, V.; Wolters-Eisfeld, G.; Burdak-Rothkamm, S.; Stahl, F.R.; Anlauf, M.; Grabowski, P.; Mobs, M.; et al. Establishment of the First Well-differentiated Human Pancreatic Neuroendocrine Tumor Model. *Mol. Cancer Res.* **2018**, *16*, 496–507. [CrossRef] [PubMed]
25. Hofving, T.; Arvidsson, Y.; Almobarak, B.; Inge, L.; Pfragner, R.; Persson, M.; Stenman, G.; Kristiansson, E.; Johanson, V.; Nilsson, O. The neuroendocrine phenotype, genomic profile and therapeutic sensitivity of GEPNET cell lines. *Endocr. Relat. Cancer* **2018**, *25*, 367–380. [CrossRef] [PubMed]
26. Parekh, D.; Ishizuka, J.; Townsend, C.M., Jr.; Haber, B.; Beauchamp, R.D.; Karp, G.; Kim, S.W.; Rajaraman, S.; Greeley, G., Jr.; Thompson, J.C. Characterization of a human pancreatic carcinoid in vitro: Morphology, amine and peptide storage, and secretion. *Pancreas* **1994**, *9*, 83–90. [CrossRef] [PubMed]

27. Pfragner, R.; Behmel, A.; Hoger, H.; Beham, A.; Ingolic, E.; Stelzer, I.; Svejda, B.; Moser, V.A.; Obenauf, A.C.; Siegl, V.; et al. Establishment and characterization of three novel cell lines -P-STS, L-STS, H-STS- derived from a human metastatic midgut carcinoid. *Anticancer Res.* **2009**, *29*, 1951–1961.
28. Hernandez Vargas, S.; Kossatz, S.; Voss, J.; Ghosh, S.C.; Tran Cao, H.S.; Simien, J.; Reiner, T.; Dhingra, S.; Fisher, W.E.; Azhdarinia, A. Specific Targeting of Somatostatin Receptor Subtype-2 for Fluorescence-Guided Surgery. *Clin. Cancer Res.* **2019**, *25*, 4332–4342. [CrossRef]
29. Herrera-Martinez, A.D.; Feelders, R.A.; Van den Dungen, R.; Dogan-Oruc, F.; van Koetsveld, P.M.; Castano, J.P.; de Herder, W.W.; Hofland, L.J. Effect of the Tryptophan Hydroxylase Inhibitor Telotristat on Growth and Serotonin Secretion in 2D and 3D Cultured Pancreatic Neuroendocrine Tumor Cells. *Neuroendocrinology* **2020**, *110*, 351–363. [CrossRef]
30. Hernandez Vargas, S.; Lin, C.; Voss, J.; Ghosh, S.C.; Halperin, D.M.; AghaAmiri, S.; Cao, H.S.T.; Ikoma, N.; Uselmann, A.J.; Azhdarinia, A. Development of a drug-device combination for fluorescence-guided surgery in neuroendocrine tumors. *J. Biomed. Opt.* **2020**, *25*, 126002. [CrossRef]
31. Grozinsky-Glasberg, S.; Shimon, I.; Rubinfeld, H. The role of cell lines in the study of neuroendocrine tumors. *Neuroendocrinology* **2012**, *96*, 173–187. [CrossRef] [PubMed]
32. Kolby, L.; Bernhardt, P.; Ahlman, H.; Wangberg, B.; Johanson, V.; Wigander, A.; Forssell-Aronsson, E.; Karlsson, S.; Ahren, B.; Stenman, G.; et al. A transplantable human carcinoid as model for somatostatin receptor-mediated and amine transporter-mediated radionuclide uptake. *Am. J. Pathol.* **2001**, *158*, 745–755. [CrossRef]
33. Chamberlain, C.E.; German, M.S.; Yang, K.; Wang, J.; VanBrocklin, H.; Regan, M.; Shokat, K.M.; Ducker, G.S.; Kim, G.E.; Hann, B.; et al. A Patient-derived Xenograft Model of Pancreatic Neuroendocrine Tumors Identifies Sapanisertib as a Possible New Treatment for Everolimus-resistant Tumors. *Mol. Cancer Ther.* **2018**, *17*, 2702–2709. [CrossRef] [PubMed]
34. Yachida, S.; Vakiani, E.; White, C.M.; Zhong, Y.; Saunders, T.; Morgan, R.; de Wilde, R.F.; Maitra, A.; Hicks, J.; Demarzo, A.M.; et al. Small cell and large cell neuroendocrine carcinomas of the pancreas are genetically similar and distinct from well-differentiated pancreatic neuroendocrine tumors. *Am. J. Surg. Pathol.* **2012**, *36*, 173–184. [CrossRef]
35. Kawasaki, K.; Toshimitsu, K.; Matano, M.; Fujita, M.; Fujii, M.; Togasaki, K.; Ebisudani, T.; Shimokawa, M.; Takano, A.; Takahashi, S.; et al. An Organoid Biobank of Neuroendocrine Neoplasms Enables Genotype-Phenotype Mapping. *Cell* **2020**, *183*, 1420–1435.e21. [CrossRef]
36. Pettengill, O.S.; Sorenson, G.D.; Wurster-Hill, D.H.; Curphey, T.J.; Noll, W.W.; Cate, C.C.; Maurer, L.H. Isolation and growth characteristics of continuous cell lines from small-cell carcinoma of the lung. *Cancer* **1980**, *45*, 906–918. [CrossRef]
37. Baillie-Johnson, H.; Twentyman, P.R.; Fox, N.E.; Walls, G.A.; Workman, P.; Watson, J.V.; Johnson, N.; Reeve, J.G.; Bleehen, N.M. Establishment and characterisation of cell lines from patients with lung cancer (predominantly small cell carcinoma). *Br. J. Cancer* **1985**, *52*, 495–504. [CrossRef]
38. Gock, M.; Mullins, C.S.; Harnack, C.; Prall, F.; Ramer, R.; Goder, A.; Kramer, O.H.; Klar, E.; Linnebacher, M. Establishment, functional and genetic characterization of a colon derived large cell neuroendocrine carcinoma cell line. *World J. Gastroenterol.* **2018**, *24*, 3749–3759. [CrossRef]
39. Detjen, K.; Hammerich, L.; Ozdirik, B.; Demir, M.; Wiedenmann, B.; Tacke, F.; Jann, H.; Roderburg, C. Models of Gastroenteropancreatic Neuroendocrine Neoplasms: Current Status and Future Directions. *Neuroendocrinology* **2021**, *111*, 217–236. [CrossRef]
40. Krieg, A.; Mersch, S.; Boeck, I.; Dizdar, L.; Weihe, E.; Hilal, Z.; Krausch, M.; Mohlendick, B.; Topp, S.A.; Piekorz, R.P.; et al. New model for gastroenteropancreatic large-cell neuroendocrine carcinoma: Establishment of two clinically relevant cell lines. *PLoS ONE* **2014**, *9*, e88713. [CrossRef]
41. Li, M.; Sagastume, E.A.; Lee, D.; McAlister, D.; DeGraffenreid, A.J.; Olewine, K.R.; Graves, S.; Copping, R.; Mirzadeh, S.; Zimmerman, B.E.; et al. (203/212)Pb Theranostic Radiopharmaceuticals for Image-guided Radionuclide Therapy for Cancer. *Curr. Med. Chem.* **2020**, *27*, 7003–7031. [CrossRef] [PubMed]
42. Kaemmerer, D.; Reimann, C.; Specht, E.; Wirtz, R.M.; Sayeg, M.; Baum, R.P.; Schulz, S.; Lupp, A. Differential expression and prognostic value of the chemokine receptor CXCR4 in bronchopulmonary neuroendocrine neoplasms. *Oncotarget* **2015**, *6*, 3346–3358. [CrossRef] [PubMed]
43. Werner, R.A.; Kircher, S.; Higuchi, T.; Kircher, M.; Schirbel, A.; Wester, H.J.; Buck, A.K.; Pomper, M.G.; Rowe, S.P.; Lapa, C. CXCR4-Directed Imaging in Solid Tumors. *Front. Oncol.* **2019**, *9*, 770. [CrossRef] [PubMed]

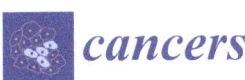

Article

Molecular Profiling of Well-Differentiated Neuroendocrine Tumours: The Role of ctDNA in Real-World Practice

Angela Lamarca [1,2,*], Melissa Frizziero [1,2], Jorge Barriuso [1,2], Zainul Kapacee [1], Wasat Mansoor [1], Mairéad G. McNamara [1,2], Richard A. Hubner [1,2] and Juan W. Valle [1,2]

[1] Department of Medical Oncology, The Christie NHS Foundation Trust, Manchester M20 4BX, UK; melissa.frizziero@cruk.manchester.ac.uk (M.F.); jorge.barriuso@manchester.ac.uk (J.B.); zainul.kapacee@nhs.net (Z.K.); was.mansoor@nhs.net (W.M.); mairead.mcnamara@nhs.net (M.G.M.); richard.hubner@nhs.net (R.A.H.); juan.valle@nhs.net (J.W.V.)

[2] Division of Cancer Sciences, Faculty of Biology, Medicine and Health, University of Manchester, Manchester M13 9PL, UK

* Correspondence: angela.lamarca@nhs.net

Citation: Lamarca, A.; Frizziero, M.; Barriuso, J.; Kapacee, Z.; Mansoor, W.; McNamara, M.G.; Hubner, R.A.; Valle, J.W. Molecular Profiling of Well-Differentiated Neuroendocrine Tumours: The Role of ctDNA in Real-World Practice. *Cancers* 2022, 14, 1017. https://doi.org/10.3390/cancers14041017

Academic Editors: Adam E. Frampton and Girish Shah

Received: 13 December 2021
Accepted: 16 February 2022
Published: 17 February 2022

Publisher's Note: MDPI stays neutral with regard to jurisdictional claims in published maps and institutional affiliations.

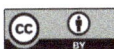

Copyright: © 2022 by the authors. Licensee MDPI, Basel, Switzerland. This article is an open access article distributed under the terms and conditions of the Creative Commons Attribution (CC BY) license (https://creativecommons.org/licenses/by/4.0/).

Simple Summary: The analysis of circulating tumour DNA (ctDNA) can help to identify genetic alterations present in cancer cells without the need to access tumour tissue, which can be an invasive approach. This study explored the feasibility of analysing ctDNA in patients with advanced well-differentiated neuroendocrine tumours (WdNETs). A total of 45 patients (15 with WdNETs) were included. Although feasible (with a non-evaluable sample rate of 27.8%), mutation-based ctDNA analysis was of limited clinical utility for patients with advanced WdNETs. While patients with WdNETs could still be offered genomic profiling (if available and reimbursed), it is important to manage patients' expectations regarding the likelihood of the results impacting their treatment.

Abstract: *Background*: The role of tumour genomic profiling in the clinical management of well-differentiated neuroendocrine tumours (WdNETs) is unclear. Circulating tumour DNA (ctDNA) may be a useful surrogate for tumour tissue when the latter is insufficient for analysis. *Methods*: Patients diagnosed with WdNETs underwent ctDNA genomic profiling (FoundationLiquid®); non-WdNETs (paraganglioma, goblet cell or poorly-differentiated neuroendocrine carcinoma) were used for comparison. The aim was to determine the rate of: test failure (primary end-point), "pathological alterations" (PAs) (secondary end-point) and patients for whom ctDNA analysis impacted management (secondary end-point). *Results*: Forty-five patients were included. A total of 15 patients with WdNETs (18 ctDNA samples) were eligible: 8 females (53.3%), median age 63.2 years (range 23.5–86.8). Primary: small bowel (8; 53.3%), pancreas (5; 33.3%), gastric (1; 6.7%) and unknown primary (1; 6.7%); grade (G)1 (n = 5; 33.3%), G2 (9; 60.0%) and G3 (1; 6.7%); median Ki-67: 5% (range 1–30). A total of 30 patients with non-WdNETs (34 ctDNA samples) were included. Five WdNETs samples (27.78%) failed analysis (vs. 17.65% in non-WdNETs; p-value 0.395). Of the 13 WdNET samples with successful ctDNA analyses, PAs were detected in 6 (46.15%) (vs. 82.14% in non-WdNETs; p-value 0.018). In WdNETs, the PA rate was independent of concomitant administration anti-cancer systemic therapies (2/7; 28.57% vs. 4/6; 66.67%; p-value 0.286) at the time of the ctDNA analysis: four, one and one samples had one, two and three PAs, respectively. These were: *CDKN2A* mutation (mut) (one sample), *CHEK2*mut (one), *TP53*mut (one), *FGFR2* amplification (one), *IDH2*mut (one), *CTNNB1*mut (one), *NF1*mut (one) and *PALB2*mut (one). None were targetable (0%) or impacted clinical management (0%). There was a lower maximum mutant allele frequency (mMAF) in WdNETs (mean 0.33 vs. non-WdNETs (mean 26.99), even though differences did not reach statistical significance (p-value 0.0584). *Conclusions*: Although feasible, mutation-based ctDNA analysis was of limited clinical utility for patients with advanced WdNETs. The rates of PAs and mMAFs were higher in non-WdNETs. While patients with WdNETs could still be offered genomic profiling (if available and reimbursed), it is important to manage patients' expectations regarding the likelihood of the results impacting their treatment.

Keywords: neuroendocrine; molecular profiling; targeted therapies; mutation; fusion; ctDNA

1. Introduction

Neuroendocrine neoplasms (NENs) are broadly classified according to their morphological differentiation and proliferative rate in well-differentiated neuroendocrine tumours (WdNETs) (grade (G)1–2 (Ki-67 < 20%) or G3 (Ki-67 $\geq$ 20%, usually $\leq$50%)) and in poorly differentiated neuroendocrine carcinomas (PdNECs) (always G3, Ki-67 $\geq$ 20%) [1]. However, this histopathological classification only partially captures the biological heterogeneity within this family of tumours, and a more granular biological subtyping is needed to deliver more personalised treatment to patients with NENs.

The molecular profiling of tumours is becoming of increasing relevance in the management of patients with advanced cancer due to its potential to identify targetable molecular alterations and predictive biomarkers that can inform new treatments. In relation to the use of next-generation sequencing (NGS) technologies in neuroendocrine neoplasms (NENs), the current recommendation from the European Society for Medical Oncology (ESMO) is to assess the tumour mutational burden (TMB), an estimate of the rate of somatic mutations within a tumour genome, in WdNETs [2], as this may predict the tumour's response to immunotherapy. This recommendation is based on the results of a prospective exploratory analysis of the multi-cohort phase II KEYNOTE-158 trial, which assessed the activity of the programmed death-1 inhibitor Pembrolizumab in previously treated patients with 10 different cancer types, including NETs. This analysis reported a response rate of 29% in patients with a high TMB ($\geq$10 mutations/megabase (Mb)) using targeted NGS in diagnostic tumour tissues, as opposed to 6% in patients with a lower TMB [3].

Overall, the published literature supports the use of the multi-omic profiling of NENs as a tool to better understand their underlying biology and to identify the NEN molecular subtypes with potential clinical implications [4]. One of the largest studies in this regard was published by Scarpa and colleagues, who explored the whole-genome landscape of 102 sporadic pancreatic NETs (PanNETs) [5]. This study showed that 17% of PanNETs harbour germline mutations affecting DNA repair genes (e.g., *MUTYH*, *CHEK2* and *BRCA2*), or the genes *MEN1* and *VHL*. Somatic mutations or fusions are most commonly found in genes involved in four pathways: chromatin remodelling, DNA damage repair, mTOR signalling activation and telomere maintenance. Integrative transcriptomic analysis identified an additional PanNET subgroup associated with hypoxia and HIF signalling.

Van Riet and colleagues explored the genomic landscape of 85 advanced NENs (69 WdNETs and 16 PdNECs) of different primary origin: 68 from different gastro-entero-pancreatic (GEP) sites, 7 from the lung and 12 of unknown origin [6]. They showed a relatively high average TMB of 5.45 somatic mutations/Mb, with *TP53*, *KRAS*, *RB1*, *CSMD3*, *APC*, *CSMD1*, *LRATD2*, *TRRAP* and *MYC* as major drivers in PdNECs, compared to an overall low TMB in WdNETs (average of 1.09 somatic mutations/Mb), with the different repertoires of gene drivers affected by somatic aberrations in pancreatic (*MEN1*, *ATRX*, *DAXX*, *DMD* and *CREBBP*) and midgut (*CDKN1B*) NETs.

Hong et al. assessed the mutational and copy number variation (CNV) profiles of 211 PanNETs, confirming that insulinomas had different genomic features than other non-functional (NF)-PanNETs [7], and reclassified these tumours into novel molecular subtypes. Some of the subgroups identified were associated with a higher relapse risk.

The newly defined G3-WdNETs [8] have also been genomically characterised. Williamson and colleagues showed that G3-WdNETs of pancreatic origin exhibited a *TSC1*-disrupting fusion and a *CHD7–BEND2* fusion, and lacked any somatic variants in *ATRX*, *DAXX* and *MEN1* [9].

There are two main challenges to incorporating the molecular profiling of NENs into standard clinical practice. Firstly, the clinical utility of molecular profiling beyond the determination of TMB remains unclear, especially from a therapeutic perspective [2]. In relation to the targetable alterations identified, 42 of 85 samples (49%) from the patients with advanced NEN, in a series explored by Van Riet and colleagues, harboured a potential therapeutic target, with a predominance of NEC within these patients (15/42; 36%), followed by PanNETs (11/42; 26%) [6]. These targetable alterations were associated with the available "on-label" treatment options in 21 cases; in the other 21, they were associated with "off-label" therapies. Secondly, adequate profiling requires a minimum of 20% of tumour content; this might be difficult to achieve as the NEN tumour tissue remaining after a standard histopathological diagnostic work-up is usually of poor quantity or quality, and the efficient recovery of DNA/RNA from archival tumour tissues is challenging. In addition, it is extremely difficult to make a decision about the right technology to apply (whole-genome, whole-exome or RNA-sequencing) in an extremely volatile context regarding the cost and constant evolution of technology. Cell-free DNA may offer an easily accessible, alternative source of fresh tumour material for genomic characterisation; the profiling of its DNA fraction, namely ctDNA, has proven informative and clinically useful in different cancer types, and may also find application in patients with NENs [10,11]. In addition, ctDNA readouts, if detectable, can be measured over time to monitor changes in tumour burden and genomic profile.

This study aimed to assess the feasibility of ctDNA molecular profiling using a targeted NGS platform in patients with WdNETs, and its potential to guide clinical management.

2. Methods

Patients previously diagnosed with advanced NENs underwent molecular profiling (ctDNA) using the FoundationLiquid® testing platform (72 cancer-related genes) between April and November 2019, in the framework of a collaboration between The Christie NHS Foundation Trust (Manchester, UK) and Foundation Medicine (Roche®, Basel, Switzerland). This platform allows for the identification of pathogenic and likely pathogenic somatic and germline variants, herein defined as "pathological alterations," including base substitutions, insertions, deletions, copy number alterations and chromosomal rearrangements. It also reports on high microsatellite instability (MSI-h). Patients provided written informed consent for molecular profiling to be performed; in addition, the retrospective analysis of these data was approved by the institutional Audit Committee (approval number 19/2634).

Patients with a histologically confirmed WdNET diagnosis, as per the 2019 World Health Organisation Classification parameters (WHO editorial Board, 2019), were included in this analysis; patients diagnosed with non-WdNETs, such as paraganglioma, goblet cell adenocarcinoma or PdNECs, were used for comparative purposes only. Clinical baseline characteristics, demographic and treatment data were collected. Molecular profiling information was extracted, including the success of sample analysis, the presence or absence of pathological alterations and the mutant allele frequency (MAF) for pathological alterations.

The aim of the study was to assess the feasibility and the clinical impact of ctDNA molecular profiling in WdNETs. The primary end-point was to assess the percentage of WdNET ctDNA samples that failed testing (defined as those scenarios where insufficient DNA was isolated for analysis). Secondary end-points included defining the proportion of the sample in which pathological findings were identified, and the percentage of patients for whom management changed based on molecular profiling results.

Descriptive statistical analysis using STATA v.12 was performed. The Chi-Square test, Fisher's exact test and t-test were used, when appropriate. A two-sided p-value < 0.05 was considered statistically significant.

3. Results

Samples from 45 patients were included: 15 WdNETs and 30 non-WdNETs.

3.1. Patient Characteristics

Within the total of the 15 individual patients with WdNETs (accounting for 18 ctDNA samples) (Table 1), 8 were female (53.33%), with a median age of 63.2 years (range 23.5–86.8).

Most were small-bowel-primary patients (8 patients; 53.33%) (pancreas (5; 33.33%), gastric (1; 6.67%) and unknown primary (1; 6.67%)) and grade 2 patients (9; 60.00%) (grade 1 (5; 33.33%), grade 3 (1; 6.67%)), with a median Ki-67 of 5% (range 1–30). All patients with WdNET had a metastatic disease and seven were on treatment (three somatostatin analogues; four chemotherapy) at the time of the ctDNA sample acquisition.

Table 1. Baseline characteristics for patients who underwent ctDNA-based molecular profiling (WdNETs).

Baseline Characteristics (WdNETs)		Patients with Advanced WdNETs ($n = 15$)	
		n	%
Age (time of sample taken)	Median (range)	63.2	23.5–86.8
Gender	Female	8	53.3
	Male	7	46.7
Site of primary	Small bowel	8	53.3
	Pancreas	5	33.3
	Gastric	1	6.7
	Unknown primary	1	6.7
Grade	Grade 1	5	33.3
	Grade 2	9	60.0
	Grade 3	1	6.7
Ki-67	Median (range)	5	1–30
Concomitant treatment at time of ctDNA sampling	Yes	7	46.7

3.2. Feasibility and Main Findings of ctDNA-Based Molecular Profiling

A total of 5 WdNETs samples (27.78%) failed analysis (vs. 17.65% in non-WdNETs; *p*-value 0.395) (Figure 1).

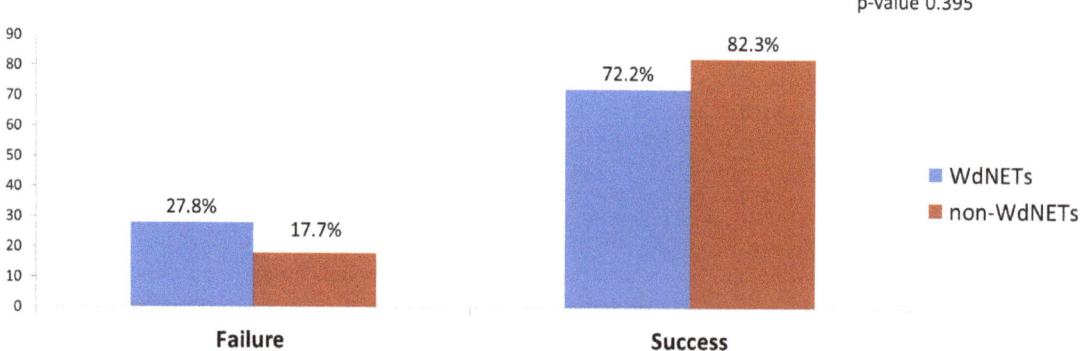

Figure 1. Failure and success rate of molecular profiling analysis by population being analysed.

Of the 13 WdNET samples with a successful ctDNA analysis, pathological alterations were identified in 6 (46.15%) (vs. 82.14% in non-WdNETs; *p*-value 0.018) (Figure 2). In addition, there was a lower maximum MAF in WdNETs (mean 0.33) vs. non-WdNETs (mean 26.99), even though differences did not reach statistical significance (*p*-value 0.0584) (Figure 3). The rate of findings of unclear significance was similar between WdNETs (69.23%) and non-WdNETs (78.57%) (*p*-value 0.517).

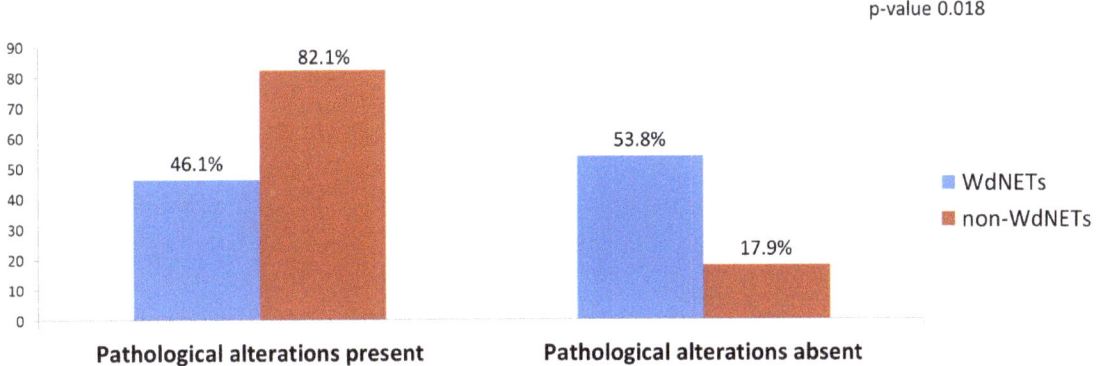

Figure 2. Presence and absence of pathological alterations in ctDNA by population being analysed.

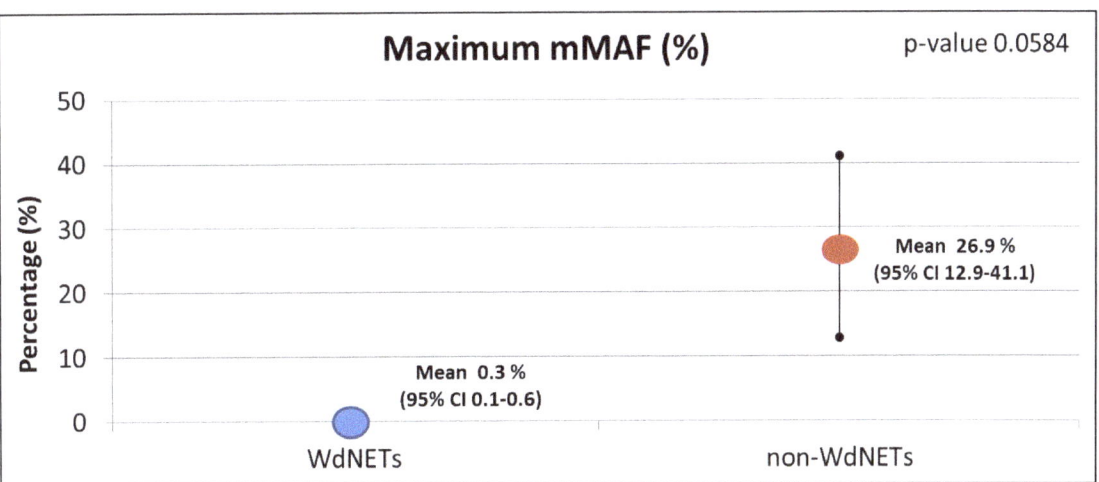

Figure 3. Maximum mutant allele frequency (mMAF) by population analysed.

Within the WdNET cohort, there was a higher presence of pathological mutations in G2 tumours (grade 1: 0%, grade 2: 66.67%; p-value 0.07) and in patients who were not receiving ongoing, concomitant anti-cancer systemic therapy at the time of the ctDNA sampling (no treatment: 66.67%, on treatment: 28.57%; p-value 0.286; Figure 4).

3.3. Identified Pathological Alterations and Impact on Management

A total of six pathological alterations were identified within the WdNET samples, including the *CDKN2A* mutation (one sample), *CHEK2* mutation (one sample), *TP53* mutation (two samples), *FGFR2* amplification (one sample), *IDH2* mutation (one sample), *CTNNB1* mutation (one sample), *NF1* mutation (one sample) and *PALB2* mutation (one sample). Concomitant alterations were identified in two samples (one had two alterations (the *CHEK2* and *TP53* mutations) and another had three (the *CTNNB1*, *NF1* and *PALB2* mutations)). The other four samples had one unique pathological alteration each.

None (0% of samples) of the identified pathological findings were considered potentially targetable. Thus, ctDNA-based molecular profiling did not change therapeutic management for any of the patients with a WdNET (0% of patients).

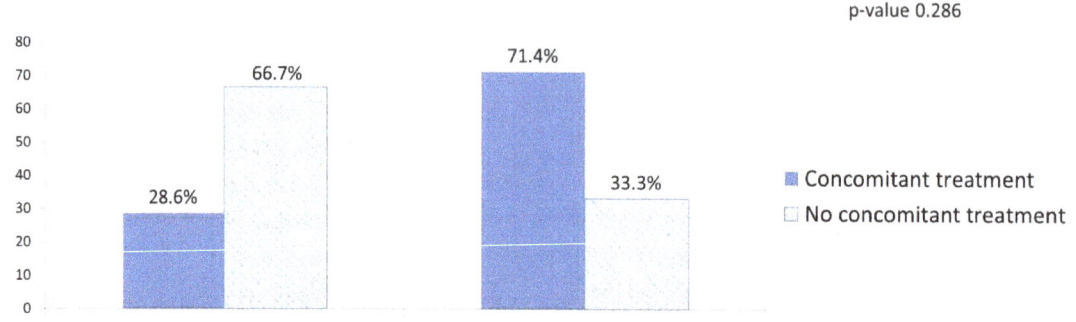

Figure 4. Presence and absence of pathological alterations in ctDNA by concomitant systemic treatment (WdNETs cohort).

4. Discussion

Although feasible, the role of molecular profiling using ctDNA seems to be limited in clinical decision making for patients with advanced WdNETs. The rate of identification of pathological alterations and the reported mMAF were significantly lower than in non-WdNETs. This is despite WdNETs having a similar sample failure rate to that described for non-Wd NETs, suggesting that the results are not associated with an increased rate of analysis failure in WdNETs (or a small amount of tumour-derived DNA in the bloodstream), but rather with a lower prevalence of significant alterations in this group of patients. Therefore, molecular profiling may be more relevant in non-WdNETs than in WdNETs. This is in line with the findings of genomic profiling studies of NEN tumour tissue showing that somatic mutations are less frequent in WdNETs than in PdNECs [6,12].

Although molecular profiling of WdNETs has been widely utilised to better understand the biology of these malignancies, true precision medicine therapeutic approaches in this patient group are currently non-existent [13]. Other series exploring targetable alterations in WdNETs have reported a higher rate of targetable alterations [6,10], which may be due to the differing definitions of "targetable" used, which ideally should follow evidence-based definitions [14]. It would also be of interest to understand how many of those patients were actually matched to a specific treatment based on the molecular alteration identified. While there are widely available data on this for other malignancies, data in WdNETs are scarce. The MOSCATO-01 clinical trial prospectively evaluated the clinical benefit of utilising high-throughput genomic analyses to identify actionable molecular alterations and match patients with a specific targeted therapy [15]. Of the total of 1035 patients included, 199 patients were matched with a specific treatment; within the group that received matched treatment, 11% of patients achieved an objective response, and a progression-free survival (PFS)2/PFS1 ratio of >1.3 was identified in 33% of patients. Ten patients with "thyroid and other endocrine glands" were included in this study. Of these, only two received a "matched" treatment. This corroborates the challenges of identifying targetable alterations in NENs.

Despite in-depth research on the identification of relevant molecular pathways in NETs [16], the development of precision medicine approaches represents one of the most relevant challenges in the current management of patients with NENs [17]. Beyond developments in the arena of nuclear medicine, which is rapidly developing new theragnostic approaches [18], predictive biomarkers for systemic therapy selection in WdNETs are lacking [19–21].

Interestingly, the findings of this study corroborate previous evidence suggesting that the dysregulation of cell-cycle/DNA damage repair (e.g., *TP53, CDKN2A, CHEK2, PALB2*) is a recurrent, critical biological vulnerability of WdNETs [5], highlighting the rationale for its therapeutic exploitation. Ongoing trials are evaluating the potential role of targeting such alterations. In addition, trials evaluating peptide-receptor radionuclide therapies in combination with DNA damage repair inhibitors, for patients with WdNETs expressing somatostatin receptors (e.g., ClinicalTrials.gov NCT04086485, NCT05053854), do also exist.

In addition to the potential therapeutic impact of molecular alterations, the identification of specific, presumed somatic mutations in ctDNA should trigger germ-line testing in selected cases, where there is the potential for a known underlying hereditary syndrome in patients with WdNETs, such as multiple endocrine neoplasia (MEN) syndromes, Von Hippel–Lindau disease (VHL), Neurofibromatosis 1 (NF1) syndrome and Tuberous sclerosis (TS) [22].

The limitations of this study include the small sample size, the heterogeneity of the tumour type and treatment administered and the potential selection bias at the time of selecting patients for molecular profiling, as non-consecutive patients were considered for this. In addition, the series included a mix of advanced-stage and prior-line therapy patients, and there was no access to concomitant tissue profiling, which would have been of interest. However, a strength of this study was that all patients were tested with identical technologies and within the same time frame. In addition, the presence of a cohort of patients with non-WdNETs allowed us to put the findings into context, providing our results with more robustness and allowing for clinical interpretation.

Finally, the NGS platform used here included 70 'pan-cancer'-related genes, yet excluded a number of genes commonly altered in WdNETs, such as *MUTYH*, *ATRX*, *DAXX* and *MEN1*; a WdNET-specific gene panel, developed on the basis of more recent NGS data from large NEN datasets, may allow for the increased sensitivity of ctDNA detection in these patients.

5. Conclusions

The use of molecular profiling utilising ctDNA in WdNETs is feasible, but the results are currently unlikely to identify targetable alterations that may impact patient management. While patients with WdNETs should still be offered molecular profiling (if available and reimbursed), it is important to manage patient expectations in relation to the likelihood of the results impacting their management. It is possible that, due to the nature of these malignancies, which have generally low numbers of somatic mutations, the evolution of the field from exclusive ctDNA profiling to a combination of mutational analyses and epigenetic changes (including methylation analyses) will have an impact on the expansion of molecular profiling's use as a tool for neuroendocrine tumours, expanding from prognosis to the uncovering of new targets.

Author Contributions: Study design: A.L.; Data collection: A.L., J.B. and M.F.; Data analysis: A.L.; Preparation of first manuscript draft: A.L.; Recruitment of patients: A.L., J.B., M.F., Z.K., W.M., M.G.M., R.A.H. and J.W.V.; Review and approval of final manuscript: A.L., J.B., M.F., Z.K., W.M., M.G.M., R.A.H. and J.W.V. All authors have read and agreed to the published version of the manuscript.

Funding: This research received no external funding; access to FoundationOne Liquid was provided by Roche®.

Institutional Review Board Statement: The retrospective analysis of these data was approved by the institutional Audit Committee (approval number 19/2634) on 4 December 2019.

Informed Consent Statement: Patients provided written informed consent for molecular profiling to be performed.

Data Availability Statement: Data can be made available upon request.

Acknowledgments: Angela Lamarca has been partially-funded by The Christie Charity. Access to FoundationOne Liquid was provided by Roche®. The salary of Zain Kapacee was funded by The Christie Charity. The salary of Melissa Frizziero was funded by a European Neuroendocrine Tumour Society Centre of Excellence Young Investigator grant.

Conflicts of Interest: The funders had no role in the design of the study; in the collection, analyses, or interpretation of data; in the writing of the manuscript, or in the decision to publish the results.

Access to FoundationOne Liquid® was provided by Roche®. Angela Lamarca: travel and educational support from Ipsen, Pfizer, Bayer, AAA, Sirtex, Novartis, Mylan and Delcath; speaker honoraria from Merck, Pfizer, Ipsen, Incyte, AAA, QED, Servier, Astra Zeneca and EISAI; advisory and consultancy honoraria from EISAI, Nutricia Ipsen, QED, Roche, Servier, Boston Scientific and Albireo Pharma; member of the Knowledge Network and NETConnect Initiatives funded by Ipsen. Melissa Frizziero has no conflicts of interest to declare. Jorge Barriuso: J.B. reports grants, personal fees and non-financial support from Ipsen; personal fees and non-financial support from Pfizer, Novartis; non-financial support from AAA, Nanostring, Roche; grants and personal fees from Servier; and personal fees from Nutricia outside the submitted work. Zainul Kapacee has received educational support from EISAI. Mairéad G McNamara: received research grant support from Servier, Ipsen and NuCana. She has received travel and accommodation support from Bayer and Ipsen and speaker honoraria from Advanced Accelerator Applications (UK & Ireland) Ltd., Pfizer, Ipsen, NuCana and Mylan. She has served on advisory boards for Celgene, Ipsen, Sirtex and Baxalta. Richard Hubner has served on the advisory board for Roche, BMS, Eisai, Celgene, Beigene, Ipsen and BTG. He has received speaker fees from Eisai, Ipsen, Mylan and PrimeOncology, and has received travel and educational support from Bayer, BMS, IPSEN and Roche, all outside of the scope of this work. Juan W Valle: consulting or advisory role for Agios, AstraZeneca, Delcath Systems, Keocyt, Genoscience Pharma, Incyte, Ipsen, Merck, Mundipharma EDO, Novartis, PCI Biotech, Pfizer, Pieris Pharmaceuticals, QED and Wren Laboratories; member of the Speakers' Bureau for Imaging Equipment Limited Ipsen Novartis Nucana; and received travel grants from Celgene and Nucana.

References

1. Nagtegaal, I.; Odze, R.D.; Klimstra, D.; Paradis, V.; Rugge, M.; Schirmacher, P.; Washington, M.K.; Carneiro, F.; Cree, I.A.; the WHO Classification of Tumours Editorial Board. The 2019 WHO classification of tumours of the digestive system. *Histopathology* **2020**, *76*, 182–188. [CrossRef] [PubMed]
2. Mosele, F.; Remon, J.; Mateo, J.; Westphalen, C.; Barlesi, F.; Lolkema, M.; Normanno, N.; Scarpa, A.; Robson, M.; Meric-Bernstam, F.; et al. Recommendations for the use of next-generation sequencing (NGS) for patients with metastatic cancers: A report from the ESMO Precision Medicine Working Group. *Ann. Oncol.* **2020**, *31*, 1491–1505. [CrossRef]
3. Marabelle, A.; Fakih, M.; Lopez, J.; Shah, M.; Shapira-Frommer, R.; Nakagawa, K.; Chung, H.C.; Kindler, H.L.; Lopez-Martin, J.A.; Miller, W.H.; et al. Association of tumour mutational burden with outcomes in patients with advanced solid tumours treated with pembrolizumab: Prospective biomarker analysis of the multicohort, open-label, phase 2 KEYNOTE-158 study. *Lancet Oncol.* **2020**, *21*, 1353–1365. [CrossRef]
4. Jiang, R.; Hong, X.; Zhao, Y.; Wu, W. Application of multiomics sequencing and advances in the molecular mechanisms of pancreatic neuroendocrine neoplasms. *Cancer Lett.* **2021**, *499*, 39–48. [CrossRef]
5. Scarpa, A.; Chang, D.K.; Nones, K.; Corbo, V.; Patch, A.-M.; Bailey, P.; Lawlor, R.T.; Johns, A.L.; Miller, D.K.; Mafficini, A.; et al. Whole-genome landscape of pancreatic neuroendocrine tumours. *Nature* **2017**, *543*, 65–71. [CrossRef]
6. Van Riet., J.; Van De Werken, H.J.G.; Cuppen, E.; Eskens, F.A.L.M.; Tesselaar, M.; Van Veenendaal, L.M.; Klümpen, H.J.; Dercksen, M.W.; Valk, G.D.; Lolkema, M.P. The genomic landscape of 85 advanced neuroendocrine neoplasms reveals subtype-heterogeneity and potential therapeutic targets. *Nat. Commun.* **2021**, *12*, 4612. [CrossRef]
7. Hong, X.; Qiao, S.; Li, F.; Wang, W.; Jiang, R.; Wu, H.; Chen, H.; Liu, L.; Peng, J.; Wang, J.; et al. Whole-genome sequencing reveals distinct genetic bases for insulinomas and non-functional pancreatic neuroendocrine tumours: Leading to a new classification system. *Gut* **2020**, *69*, 877–887. [CrossRef]
8. De Mestier, L.; Lamarca, A.; Hernando, J.; Zandee, W.; Alonso-Gordoa, T.; Perrier, M.; Walenkamp, A.M.; Chakrabarty, B.; Landolfi, S.; Van Velthuysen, M.L.F.; et al. Treatment outcomes of advanced digestive well-differentiated grade 3 NETs. *Endocr. Relat. Cancer* **2021**, *28*, 549–561. [CrossRef]
9. Williamson, L.M.; Steel, M.; Grewal, J.K.; Thibodeau, M.L.; Zhao, E.Y.; Loree, J.M.; Yang, K.C.; Gorski, S.M.; Mungall, A.J.; Mungall, K.L.; et al. Genomic characterization of a well-differentiated grade 3 pancreatic neuroendocrine tumor. *Mol. Case Stud.* **2019**, *5*, a003814. [CrossRef]
10. Burak, G.I.; Ozge, S.; Cem, M.; Gulgun, B.; Zeynep, D.Y.; Atil, B. The emerging clinical relevance of genomic profiling in neuroendocrine tumours. *BMC Cancer* **2021**, *21*, 234. [CrossRef]
11. Shah, D.; Lamarca, A.; Valle, J.; McNamara, M. The Potential Role of Liquid Biopsies in Advancing the Understanding of Neuroendocrine Neoplasms. *J. Clin. Med.* **2021**, *10*, 403. [CrossRef]
12. Venizelos, A.; Elvebakken, H.; Perren, A.; Nikolaienko, O.; Deng, W.; Lothe, I.M.B.; Couvelard, A.; Hjortland, G.O.; Sundlöv, A.; Svensson, J.; et al. The molecular characteristics of high-grade gastroenteropancreatic neuroendocrine neoplasms. *Endocr. Relat. Cancer* **2021**, *29*, 1–14. [CrossRef]
13. Rindi, G.; Wiedenmann, B. Neuroendocrine neoplasia of the gastrointestinal tract revisited: Towards precision medicine. *Nat. Rev. Endocrinol.* **2020**, *16*, 590–607. [CrossRef]

14. Mateo, J.; Chakravarty, D.; Dienstmann, R.; Jezdic, S.; Gonzalez-Perez, A.; Lopez-Bigas, N.; Ng, C.K.Y.; Bedard, P.; Tortora, G.; Douillard, J.-Y.; et al. A framework to rank genomic alterations as targets for cancer precision medicine: The ESMO Scale for Clinical Actionability of molecular Targets (ESCAT). *Ann. Oncol.* **2018**, *29*, 1895–1902. [CrossRef]
15. Massard, C.; Michiels, S.; Ferté, C.; Le Deley, M.-C.; Lacroix, L.; Hollebecque, A.; Verlingue, L.; Ileana, E.; Rosellini, S.; Ammari, S.; et al. High-Throughput Genomics and Clinical Outcome in Hard-to-Treat Advanced Cancers: Results of the MOSCATO 01 Trial. *Cancer Discov.* **2017**, *7*, 586–595. [CrossRef]
16. Patel, P.; Galoian, K. Molecular challenges of neuroendocrine tumors. *Oncol. Lett.* **2018**, *15*, 2715–2725. [CrossRef]
17. Barriuso, J.; Lamarca, A. Clinical and Translational Research Challenges in Neuroendocrine Tumours. *Curr. Med. Chem.* **2020**, *27*, 4823–4839. [CrossRef]
18. Langbein, T.; Weber, W.A.; Eiber, M. Future of Theranostics: An Outlook on Precision Oncology in Nuclear Medicine. *J. Nucl. Med.* **2019**, *60*, 13S–19S. [CrossRef]
19. Megdanova-Chipeva, V.G.; Lamarca, A.; Backen, A.; McNamara, M.G.; Barriuso, J.; Sergieva, S.; Gocheva, L.; Mansoor, W.; Manoharan, P.; Valle, J.W. Systemic Treatment Selection for Patients with Advanced Pancreatic Neuroendocrine Tumours (PanNETs). *Cancers* **2020**, *12*, 1988. [CrossRef]
20. Barriuso, J.; Custodio, A.; Afonso, R.; Alonso, V.; Astudillo, A.; Capdevila, J.; García-Carbonero, R.; Grande, E.; Jimenez-Fonseca, P.; Marazuela, M.; et al. Prognostic and predictive biomarkers for somatostatin analogs, peptide receptor radionuclide therapy and serotonin pathway targets in neuroendocrine tumours. *Cancer Treat. Rev.* **2018**, *70*, 209–222. [CrossRef]
21. De Dosso, S.; Treglia, G.; Pascale, M.; Tamburello, A.; Santhanam, P.; Kroiss, A.S.; Pereira Mestre, R.; Saletti, P.; Giovanella, L. Detection rate of unknown primary tu-mour by using somatostatin receptor PET/CT in patients with metastatic neuroendocrine tumours: A meta-analysis. *Endocrine* **2019**, *64*, 456–468. [CrossRef]
22. Bocchini, M.; Nicolini, F.; Severi, S.; Bongiovanni, A.; Ibrahim, T.; Simonetti, G.; Grassi, I.; Mazza, M. Biomarkers for Pancreatic Neuroendocrine Neoplasms (PanNENs) Management—An Updated Review. *Front. Oncol.* **2020**, *10*, 831. [CrossRef]

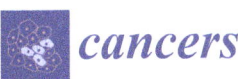

Article

Predictive and Prognostic Role of Pre-Therapy and Interim 68Ga-DOTATOC PET/CT Parameters in Metastatic Advanced Neuroendocrine Tumor Patients Treated with PRRT

Rexhep Durmo [1,2,*], Angelina Filice [1], Federica Fioroni [3], Veronica Cervati [4], Domenico Finocchiaro [3], Chiara Coruzzi [1], Giulia Besutti [5], Silvia Fanello [6], Andrea Frasoldati [7] and Annibale Versari [1]

[1] Nuclear Medicine Unit, Azienda USL-IRCCS of Reggio Emilia, 42123 Reggio Emilia, Italy; Angelina.Filice@ausl.re.it (A.F.); Chiara.Coruzzi@ausl.re.it (C.C.); Annibale.Versari@ausl.re.it (A.V.)
[2] PhD Program in Clinical and Experimental Medicine (CEM), University of Modena and Reggio Emilia, 41125 Modena, Italy
[3] Medical Physics Unit, Azienda USL-IRCCS of Reggio Emilia, 42123 Reggio Emilia, Italy; Federica.Fioroni@ausl.re.it (F.F.); Domenico.Finocchiaro@ausl.re.it (D.F.)
[4] Nuclear Medicine Unit, Azienda Ospedaliero-Universitaria di Parma, 43126 Parma, Italy; vcervati@ao.pr.it
[5] Radiology Unit, Azienda USL-IRCCS of Reggio Emilia, 42123 Reggio Emilia, Italy; Giulia.Besutti@ausl.re.it
[6] Medical Oncology Unit, Azienda USL-IRCCS of Reggio Emilia, 42123 Reggio Emilia, Italy; Silvia.Fanello@ausl.re.it
[7] Department of Endocrinology and Metabolism, Azienda USL-IRCCS of Reggio Emilia, 42123 Reggio Emilia, Italy; Andrea.Frasoldati@ausl.re.it
* Correspondence: Rexhep.Durmo@ausl.re.it; Tel.: +39-0522296284

Simple Summary: Although a significant improvement has been achieved in the management of metastatic neuroendocrine tumor (NET), disease progression is observed in 20–30% of patients treated with peptide receptor radionuclide therapy (PRRT). Therefore, the early identification of patients who are at high risk of treatment failure is important to avoid futile therapy toxicities. The aim of this study was to identify biomarkers derived from baseline and interim 68Ga-DOTATOC PET/CT in patients undergoing PRRT. In 46 metastatic NET patients with available baseline and interim PET, only baseline total tumor volume (bTV) was able to discriminate responders to PRRT (partial response or stable disease) vs. non-responders. Patients with high bTV had also the worst overall survival. bTV, an imaging biomarker, integrated in the initial workup of NET patients could improve risk stratification and contribute to a tailored therapy approach.

Abstract: Peptide receptor radionuclide therapy (PRRT) is an effective therapeutic option in patients with metastatic neuroendocrine tumor (NET). However, PRRT fails in about 15–30% of cases. Identification of biomarkers predicting the response to PRRT is essential for treatment tailoring. We aimed to evaluate the predictive and prognostic role of semiquantitative and volumetric parameters obtained from the 68Ga-DOTATOC PET/CT before therapy (bPET) and after two cycles of PRRT (iPET). A total of 46 patients were included in this retrospective analysis. The primary tumor was 78% gastroenteropancreatic (GEP), 13% broncho-pulmonary and 9% of unknown origin. 35 patients (76.1%) with stable disease or partial response after PRRT were classified as responders and 11 (23.9%) as non-responders. Logistic regression analysis identified that baseline total volume (bTV) was associated with therapy outcome (OR 1.17; 95%CI 1.02–1.32; p = 0.02). No significant association with PRRT response was observed for other variables. High bTV was confirmed as the only variable independently associated with OS (HR 12.76, 95%CI 1.53–107, p = 0.01). In conclusion, high bTV is a negative predictor for PRRT response and is associated with worse OS rates. Early iPET during PRRT apparently does not provide information useful to change the management of NET patients.

Keywords: neuroendocrine tumor; GEP-NET; PET/CT; PRRT; DOTATOC

1. Introduction

Neuroendocrine tumors (NETs) are relatively rare neoplasms that originate from endocrine cells, mostly of the gastroenteropancreatic tract (GEP) and the pulmonary system. Due to their indolent natural course, NETs are identified as locally advanced or with distant metastasis in 40–50% of patients [1].

Peptide receptor radionuclide therapy (PRRT) is an effective systemic therapeutic option for patients with advanced, metastatic, or unresectable NETs with high somatostatin receptor (SSTR) expression. PRRT consists in the intravenous systemic administration of somatostatin analogs (SSAs) labeled with a βminus (β-) emitting radioisotope (90Y and 177Lu), that binds SSTRs overexpressed in tumors with high affinity and specificity. The compound is internalized by endocytosis and retained in lysosomes of cells allowing the delivery of cytotoxic radiation directly on target cells, therefore producing the breakdown of intracellular DNA chains and cell death [2]. Although a significant improvement has been reported in progression free survival (PFS) and overall survival (OS), disease progression is still observed in 20–30% of patients treated with PRRT [3]. Moreover, PRRT can be associated with hematologic, renal, and hepatic toxicities [4]. Therefore, the early identification of patients who are at high risk of treatment failure represents an unmet need.

Positron emission tomography/computed tomography with 68Ga-DOTA-labelled somatostatin analogues (68Ga-DOTA-peptide PET/CT) is the elective imaging technique for diagnosis and management of NETs [5]. In clinical practice PET/CT plays a pivotal role also for properly selecting patients as candidates for PRRT. 68Ga-DOTA-peptide PET imaging is used for both evaluation of somatostatin receptor expression and correct staging of disease [6].

In addition, PET derived parameters, such as the semiquantitative standardized uptake values (SUVs), have been widely studied as prognostic and predictive factors in NET patients treated with PRRT [7]. In several other malignancies, FDG-PET-derived metabolic tumor volume (MTV) and total lesion glycolysis (TLG), which is the product of SUVmean × MTV, have shown a major role in prognosis and treatment monitoring compared to SUVs parameters [8]. MTV and TLG provide a direct estimation of the whole-body tumor burden and have been validated as quantitative imaging biomarkers in several tumors [9]. Furthermore, early changes in tumor burdens are a promising index of response to treatment and could be the basis of a more individualized treatment approach [10,11].

Hence, the aim of this study is to evaluate the predictive and prognostic value of semiquantitative and volumetric parameters calculated from 68Ga-DOTATOC PET/CT performed before PRRT. Moreover, we assessed the potential role of the change (Δ) between baseline and interim PET parameters after two cycles of PRRT for early prediction of response.

2. Materials and Methods

2.1. Study Design

We conducted a retrospective subgroup analysis of patients enrolled in a prospective, monocentric, non-randomized phase II clinical trial (EudraCT:2013-002605-65). All patients signed a written informed consent form. For this study we included biopsy-proven, unresectable, metastatic GEP or bronchopulmonary or unknown primary site NET patients, who were treated with PRRT in our institution (Azienda USL-IRCCS of Reggio Emilia, Italy). All patients underwent screening with 68Ga-DOTATOC PET/CT to confirm the adequate expression of SSTR type 2 on tumor sites and an interim PET/CT scan 7 weeks after the second cycle of PRRT. The association between PET parameters and outcomes (PRRT response and OS) was evaluated.

2.2. Ga-DOTATOC PET/CT

A baseline 68Ga-DOTATOC PET/CT (bPET) 1–3 weeks before PRRT and after two cycles of PRRT (interimPET) was performed with a hybrid scanner (Discovery STE; GE Healthcare). Image acquisition started 60 ± 10 min after administration of 2 MBq/kg of

68Ga-DOTATOC. All DOTATOC-avid lesions were semiautomatically segmented by an experienced board-certified nuclear medicine physician (V.C.) using a commercial software (PET VCAR, GE Healthcare). Subsequently, all regions of physiological or non-disease related uptake were manually removed. From the remaining volume-of interests (VOIs), containing all 68Ga-DOTATOC avid tumor lesions, maximum standardized uptake value (SUVmax), mean standardized uptake value (SUVmean), the somatostatin receptor-derived tumor volume (TV) and total lesion SSR expression (Total Lesion Activity-TLA, defined as SUVmean × TV) were measured. Based on the experience of metabolic tumor volume in FDG PET/CT studies a threshold above 41% of SUVmax was used to calculate TV. The whole-body tumor volume (bTV) was calculated by summing TV measurements of all lesions in each patient. The whole-body TLA (bTLA) was calculated by summing TLA of all lesions. Also, the ratio of the lesion SUVmax to the SUVmax in the spleen (SUVratio T/S) was calculated. Differences (Δ) in SUVmax, SUVmean, bTV, bTLA and SUVratio T/S were evaluated by calculating the percentage in variation of each parameter using the following formula: Delta = (interimPET − bPET)/bPET × 100.

2.3. PRRT

PRRT was performed according to the joint International Atomic Energy Agency (IAEA; Vienna, Austria), European Association of Nuclear Medicine (EANM; Vienna, Austria), and Society of Nuclear Medicine and Molecular Imaging (SNMMI; Reston, VA, USA) practical guidance ([12]). Briefly, the inclusion criteria for treatment with PRRT were histologically confirmed, unresectable, metastatic GEP or bronchopulmonary or unknown primary site NET patients; high expression of somatostatin receptor on baseline 68Ga-DOTATOC PET/CT (defined as greater than or equal to that of normal liver); a glomerular filtration rate greater than 50 mL/min/1.73 m^2; a white blood cell count greater than 2.5×10^9/L; a platelet count greater than 90×10^9/L; bilirubin levels less than 2.5 mg/dL and ECOG performance status ≤ 2. A fractionated treatment protocol, with an activity of 1850–2590 MBq 90Y-DOTATOC or 3700–5550 MBq 177Lu-DOTATOC per treatment cycle every eight weeks, aimed at four to six courses with an interval of eight weeks, was followed. The activity prescription was determined on the basis of the Biological Effective Dose (BED) delivered to kidneys and on the basis of the absorbed dose to bone marrow, considered as the main organs at risk. Dosimetry was scheduled during the first course of therapy after a therapeutic administration of ^{177}Lu-DOTATOC. The cumulative dose limit to kidneys was set to 46 Gy of BED for patients with no risk factors, and at 28 Gy for patients with risk factors, while the absorbed dose limit to bone marrow was set to 2 Gy for both. Documented disease progression at any time led to the cessation of PRRT and the classification of the patient as having progressive disease.

2.4. Assessment of Treatment Response

Response assessment was performed three months after completion of PRRT courses. Combination of anatomical imaging (CT/MRI), functional (PET) and clinical data in a multidisciplinary tumor board setting was used to define response. Response Evaluation criteria in Solid Tumors (RECIST version 1.1) criteria was used in determining anatomical response to PRRT. PET response was assessed using the European Organization for Research and Treatment of Cancer (EORTC) criteria. For the study analysis, responders were defined as patients with a complete/partial response or stable disease, and non-responders had progressive disease.

2.5. Statistical Analysis

Quantitative variables were expressed as median with range or mean with SD. Categorical variables are presented with absolute and relative frequencies. Mann-Whitney U test was used for comparing continuous variables between responders and non-responders. Chi-square test was used to analyze differences in discrete variables between responders and non-responders. Binary logistic regression was performed to identify factors predictive of treatment. Receiver operating characteristics (ROC) analysis was performed to identify optimal cut-off values for PET/CT quantitative parameters. The area under the curves (AUC), sensitivity, specificity and accuracy were reported. Survival curves were estimated according to the Kaplan-Meier method. A log-rank test was used to compare survival curves. Cox proportional-hazards model was used for univariate and multivariate survival analysis and results were reported as hazard ratio (HR), 95% confidence interval (95%CI) and p-Value based on statistical Wald-test. OS was defined as the time (months) from the first PRRT cycle to death from any cause. Surviving patients were censored at the last date of follow-up. All statistical tests were two-sided and $p < 0.05$ was considered a statistically significant result. Statistical analysis was performed using IBM SPS Statistics 25 (IBM, New York, NY, USA) and MedCalc Statistical Software 14.8.1 (Ostend, Belgium) for Windows.

3. Results

3.1. Patients

A total of 46 patients with available bPET and iPET were included in this retrospective analysis. The median age was 60 (range 25–85) and 21 patients (46%) were female. Primary tumor was for 78% GEP, 13% broncho-pulmonary and 9% of unknown origin. All patients had stage IV disease. Liver and lymph nodes were the most frequent sites of metastasis. Patients' main characteristics are reported in Table 1.

Table 1. Main characteristics of the study population.

Patients	($n = 46$)
Age, median (range) in years	60 (25–85)
Gender, n (%)	
Male	25 (54%)
Female	21 (46%)
Primary tumour, n (%)	
GEP	36 (78%)
Stomach	3 (8%)
Pancreas	8 (22%)
Intestine	25 (70%)
Broncho-Pulmonary	6 (13%)
Unkown	4 (9%)
GEP NETs WHO grade, n (%)	
G1 ((Ki-67 0–2%)	21 (46%)
G2 (Ki-67 3–20%)	19 (41%)
G3 (Ki-67 >20%)	2 (4%)
NA	4 (9%)
Metastasis, n	
Liver	21
Lymph nodes	23
Bone	15
Lung	7
Other	9
Cycles of PRRT, n (%)	
2	2 (4%)
3	1 (2%)
4	5 (11%)
5	11 (24%)
6	27 (59%)
Type of PRRT	
Only 177Lu	5 (11%)
177Lu + 90Y	41 (89%)

Abbreviations: GEP: gastroenteropancreatic; PRRT: peptide receptor radionuclide therapy; NET: neuroendocrine tumor.

3.2. PRRT and PET/CT

Forty-three patients (94%) received four to six cycles of PRRT. Five patients (11%) were treated with 177Lu-DOTATOC radiopeptide, while the 41 remaining subjects underwent a combination of 90Y-DOTATOC and 177Lu-DOTATOC therapy.

The observed response rates were 21% (*n* = 10) partial response, 55.1% (*n* = 25) stable disease, and 23.9% (*n* = 11) progressive disease for the entire cohort. Considering GEP NET cohort response rates were 27% (*n* = 10) partial response, 51% (*n* = 18) stable disease, and 22% (*n* = 8) progressive disease. Complete response was not observed. For the analysis of this study, 35 patients (76.1%) with either stable disease or partial response after PRRT were classified as responders and 11 (23.9%) patients with progressive disease as non-responders.

The median values of SUVmax, SUVmean, SUVt/s, bTV and bTLA were 34 (IQR, 23.1–55.8), 9.9 (IQR, 7.6–16.4), 1.1 (IQR, 0.7–2.3), 143.8 mL (IQR, 32.9–354), and 1834 (IQR, 342–6309), respectively. The median percentage in variation between baseline and inter-imPET after two cycles of PRTT reported as ΔSUVmax, ΔSUVmean, ΔSUVratioT/S, ΔbTV, ΔbTLA were 1.1% (IQR, −21.2–22.1), 4.2% (IQR, −17.8–39.4), −1.1% (IQR, −41.5–24.5), 32.4% (IQR, −10.2–70.6), 25% (−12.5–80.9), respectively. Figure 1 shows a baseline and interim PET.

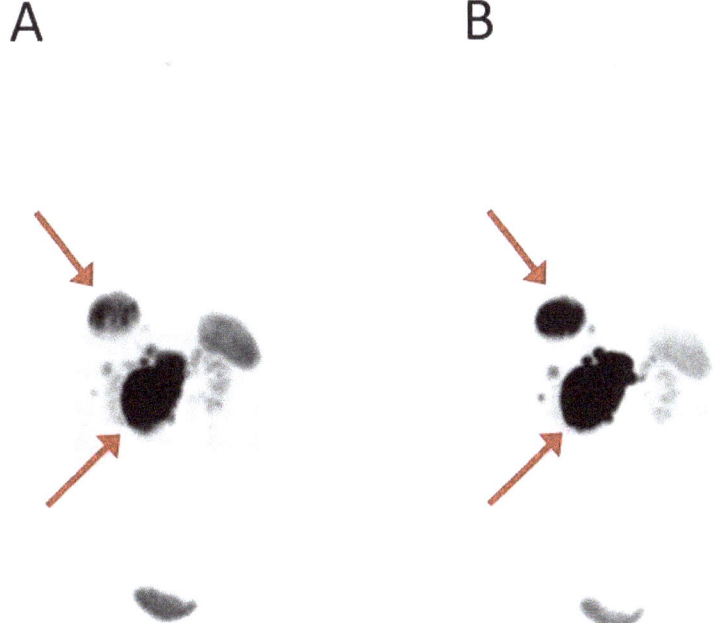

Figure 1. Baseline (**A**) and interim (**B**) PET scan of a 54-year-old patient with G1 pancreatic NET. Red arrows indicate the primary pancreatic tumor and the most representative liver metastasis. Interim 68Ga-DOTATOC PET after the second PRRT cycle shows disease progression. The patient was treated with a total of six PRRT courses (four cycles of 177Lu-DOTATOC + 2 cycles of 90Y-DOTATOC) for a total of 28,534 MBq activity and classified as partial response at the assessment following treatment.

The bTV and bTLA values of patients that did not respond to PRRT were significantly higher than those of patients with response to PRRT therapy (496.2 IQR 218.3–2029.4 vs. 77.6 IQR 31–186.6, $p < 0.001$ and 6078.3 IQR 2813–18,959 vs. 1341 IQR 272.3–3865, $p = 0.001$, respectively: Figure 2).

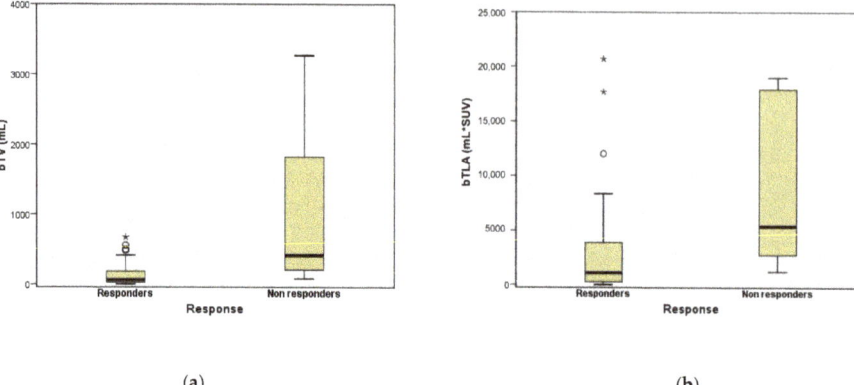

(a) (b)

Figure 2. Box Plot comparing bTV (**a**) and bTLA (**b**) between PRRT responder and non-responder patients. "★" and "○" symbols represent outlier cases.

No association between semiquantitative PET parameters and response were observed. Percentage variations (Δ) of PET semiquantitative and volumetric parameters were not significantly different between PRRT responders and non-responders. PET parameters and comparison between responders vs. non-responders are summarized in Table 2.

Table 2. Characteristic of calculated PET parameters. Data of all patients ($n = 46$) and a comparison between responders ($n = 35$) vs. non-responders ($n = 11$) groups are reported. Values are expressed in mean (SD) and median (IQR). Mann-Whitney U test was used to compare variables. The p-Values shown in boldface correspond to $p < 0.05$.

PET Parameters	All ($n = 46$)	Responders ($n = 35$)	Non-Responders ($n = 11$)	p Value
SUVmax				
Mean (SD)	40 (24.9)	41.5 (27.1)	35.5 (35.5)	0.58
Median (IQR)	34 (23.1–55.8)	34.5 (23.7–56.2)	33.5 (21.8–53.9)	
SUVmean				
Mean (SD)	11.6 (5.9)	10.3 (4.1)	11.9 (6.3)	0.57
Median (IQR)	9.9 (7.6–16.4)	9.9 (7.2–17.3)	10 (7.8–13.5)	
SUVratio T/S				
Mean (SD)	1.8 (0.9)	1.4 (0.7)	1.9 (2.2)	0.93
Median (IQR)	1.1 (0.7–2.3)	1.2 (0.6–2.3)	1 (0.8–2.2)	
bTV				
Mean (SD)	371 (665.5)	143.7 (177.6)	1073.5 (1061,4)	**<0.001**
Median (IQR)	143.8 (32.9–354)	77.6 (31–186.8)	496.2 (218.3–2029.4)	
bTLA				
Mean (SD)	5339.5 (8171.4)	3108.13 (4971.1)	12,236.4 (11,959)	**0.001**
Median (IQR)	1834 (342–6309)	1341 (272.3–3865)	6078.3 (2813–18,959)	
ΔSUVmax				
Mean (SD)	23.9 (117.7)	25.2 (129,6)	18.1 (62)	0.89
Median (IQR)	1.1 (−21.2–22.1)	−2.5 (−21.2–22.2)	3.5 (−26.6–22.1)	
ΔSUVmean				
Mean (SD)	25.5 (79.2)	45.6 (128)	19 (55,9)	0.84
Median (IQR)	4.2 (−17.8–39.4)	6.2 (−16.5–25.4)	−10.2 (−27.4–47.6)	
ΔSUVratioT/S				
Mean (SD)	1.3 (2)	1.9 (0.8)	1.4 (0.9)	0.42
Median (IQR)	−1.1 (−41.5–24.5)	−11.5 (−40.5–20.9)	1.9 (−46.8–32.3)	

Table 2. Cont.

PET Parameters	All (n = 46)	Responders (n = 35)	Non-Responders (n = 11)	p Value
ΔTV				
Mean (SD)	61 (170)	27.1 (55,6)	71.5 (756,7)	0.51
Median (IQR)	32.4 (−10.2–70.6)	32.4 (−5.5–69.2)	32.4 (−23.9–79.9)	
ΔTLA				
Mean (SD)	143 (668,4)	45.7 (79,1)	171.9 (756.7)	0.92
Median (IQR)	25 (−12.5–80.9)	24.3 (−0.4–80)	36 (−22.5–111)	

Abbreviations: SUV: standardized uptake value; T/S: tumor/spleen; TV: total volume; TLA: total lesion activity.

Logistic regression analysis of bPET derived parameters and ΔPET values identified that only bTV was associated with therapy outcome (OR 1.17; 95%CI 1.02–1.32; p = 0.02). No significant association with PRRT response was observed for other variables (Table 3).

Table 3. Logistic Regression Analysis.

PET Parameters	Univariate Analysis	
	OR (95%CI)	p Value
SUVmax	1.06 (0.99–1.13)	0.09
SUVmean	0.8 (0.55–1.15)	0.23
SUVratio T/S	0.84 (0.52–1.35)	0.48
bTV	1.17 (1.02–1.32)	**0.02**
bTLA	0.99 (0.93–1.01)	0.08
ΔSUVmax	0.97 (0.93–1.01)	0.25
ΔSUVmean	1.007 (0.98–1.01)	0.259
ΔSUVratioT/S	0.99 (0.98–1.01)	0.839
ΔTV	0.99 (0.98–1.01)	0.922
ΔTLA	0.99 (0.98–1.01)	0.70

Abbreviations: SUV: standardized uptake value; T/S: tumor/spleen; TV: total volume; TLA: total lesion activity. The p-Values shown in boldface correspond to p < 0.05.

3.3. Overall Survival Analysis

During the follow-up period (mean 31 months; ranged from eight to 86 months), seven (15.2%) patients died. Mean survival time was 69.4 (SD, 5.3) months, the median was non reached for the entire cohort.

ROC analysis showed a best cut-off point for bTV of >244.5 mL (sensitivity 85.7%; specificity 79.5%) and AUC of 0.77 (95% CI 0.62–0.88, p = 0.036) for identification of patients with worse OS. For bTLA best cut-off point was 2659 (sensitivity 85.7%; specificity 64.1%) and AUC of 0.71 (95% CI 0.56–0.84, p = 0.092). The complete ROC curves analysis of PET parameters is shown in Table S1.

In univariate analysis, higher bTV and bTLA were associated with lower survival probability (HR 13 95%CI 2.6–64.1, p = 0.001; HR 9.08 95%CI 1.09–75.76, p = 0.04) (Figure 3).

Moreover, a difference in SUVmax above 5.5% between iPET and bPET (ΔSUVmax) was associated with a favourable outcome (HR 0.15 95% CI0.03–0.67; p = 0.04). In Cox multivariate analysis, only a high bTV was confirmed as an independent prognostic factor (HR 12.76 95%CI 1.53–107, p = 0.01) (Table 4).

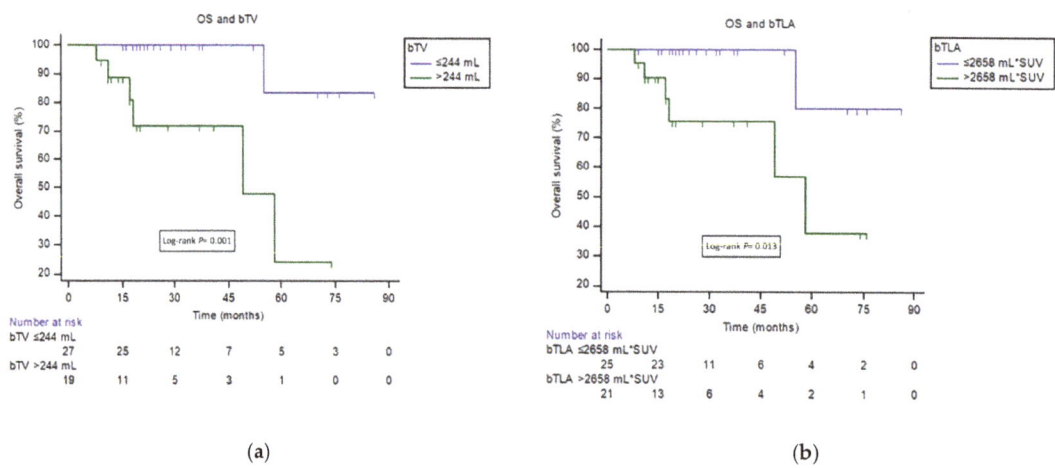

Figure 3. (**a**) Kaplan-Meier curves for overall survival (OS) among patients with high- and low-bTV defined on the basis of the ROC curve (244 mL). (**b**) Kaplan-Meier curves for OS among patients with high- and low-bTLA defined on the basis of the ROC curve (2658 mL*SUV).

Table 4. Univariate and multivariate Cox regression analysis for OS.

PET Parameter	Univariate Analysis		Multivariate Analysis	
	HR (95%CI)	p Value	HR (95%CI)	p Value
SUVmax (<22.02)	0.99 (0.12–8.20)	0.99	-	-
SUVmean (≤5.45)	0.31 (0.06–1.51)	0.26	-	-
SUVratioT/S (≤1.31)	0.84 (0.08–8.23)	0.87	-	-
bTV (>244.48)	13 (2.6–64.1)	**0.001**	12.76 (1.53–107)	**0.01**
bTLA (>2658.62)	9.08 (1.09–75.76)	**0.04**	7.15 (0.96–68.1)	0.98
ΔSUVmax (>5.5598)	0.15 (0.03–0.67)	**0.04**	0.17 (0.02–1.46)	0.1
ΔSUVmean (>24.4984)	0.65 (0.05–7.87)	0.68	-	-
ΔSUVratioT/S (>−0.75)	0.14 (0.017–1.28)	0.08	-	-
ΔTV (≤−15.876)	0.23 (0.02–1.86)	0.354	-	-
ΔTLA (>80.2)	0.45 (0.082–2.48)	0.2737	-	-

Abbreviations: SUV: standardized uptake value; T/S: tumor/spleen; TV: total volume; TLA: total lesion activity. The p-Values shown in boldface correspond to $p < 0.05$.

4. Discussion

After about 20 years of retrospective and phase I/II trials, PRRT was finally approved by regulatory authorities. Since its approval for the treatment of inoperable or metastatic GEP-NETs with progressive disease by the European Medicine Agency in 2017, PRRT has been widely used [13,14]. The phase III NETTER-1 trial has established that PRRT prolongs

PFS compared to high dose octreotide LAR and improved quality of life. [3,15] In our study, 76.1% of NET patients had stable disease or partial response and 23.9% patients showed progressive disease after PRRT. These findings are in line with the response rates reported in a recent large meta-analysis where the disease control rate (complete or partial response and stable disease) was 83% in metastatic NET patients treated with PRRT [16]. Despite the increasing role of PRRT in metastatic NETs, what is clear both from our results and literature is that we need parameters to improve the selection of patient candidates to PRRT.

In this study, we evaluated the predictive and prognostic significance of semiquantitative and volumetric baseline PET imaging parameters in patients with advanced, metastatic NET undergoing PRRT. We also investigated the role of interim PET after two cycles of PRRT as an early predictor.

Several retrospective studies have assessed the role of semiquantitative parameters, mostly SUVmax, as prognostic markers for NETs. However, conflicting results have been published regarding the role of SUV on baseline 68Ga-DOTA-SSA PET in PRRT response prediction. Several authors demonstrated that a high SUVmax in baseline PET is associated with a favorable outcome and a wide range of different cut-off values are reported to separate responders to PRRT vs. non responders [17–20].

In our cohort we did not find any association between SUVs obtained in the baseline PET and PRRT response. This finding is in line with published results by Gabriel et al. and Soydal et al., who similarly found that SUVs showed no additional value for PRRT response prediction [21,22]. This controversial result may be because SUVs are measured in a single region of interest and thus they are not representative of the total tumor burden. Indeed, the lesion heterogeneity in NET patients, and the well-known limits of semiquantitative parameters, might further limit SUVs utility [23].

We found that patients who did not respond to PRRT had significantly higher bTV compared to responders. Moreover, bTV was the only PET parameter that confirmed a predictive role for PRRT response on logistic regression analysis (OR 1.17). Furthermore, bTV was an independent prognostic factor associated with worse OS rates in Cox regression analysis.

To our knowledge, only two other studies have previously evaluated the role of baseline volumetric PET parameters in patients treated with PRRT. Ohlendorf et al. found that PFS was shorter in patients with high bTV and high bTLA in 32 NET patients treated with PRRT [22]. Pauwels et al. reported that a bTV higher than 578 mL was associated with worse OS [23]. In our study population, the bTV cut-off that better identified patients with shorter OS was 244 mL. This difference in cut-offs could be explained by different segmentation methods. Indeed, Pauwels used a SUV threshold customized per patient through visual inspection to segment the tumor. In contrast, we used a semiautomatic method applying a threshold above 41% of the SUVmax for calculation of TV and TLA, based on the experience with FDG PET studies [24]. Further studies are warranted to define and harmonize 68Ga-Dota-peptide PET/CT tumor burden segmentation.

Our findings are in line with several previous studies that assessed the prognostic significance of PET volumetric parameters in settings other than PRRT [25–30]. Thus, bTV seems to be a powerful prognostic parameter in NET patients. However, bTV should be validated in further prospective studies including more homogeneous populations in terms of primary site, disease course and treatment setting.

In contrast, we did not find any relationship between changes in PET semiquantitative and volumetric parameters between baseline and interim PET after two cycles of PRRT. However, changes in SUVmax (ΔSUVmax) showed a significance in OS univariate analysis ($p = 0.04$) that was not confirmed in multivariate analysis. These results, in accordance with previous studies, show no utility of iPET in guiding the management of metastatic NET patients treated with PRRT [11,27].

There are several limitations of the present study that should be acknowledged. First are the retrospective nature and the small sample size. Second, we included patients with different NET sites. Furthermore, we did not evaluate FDG PET findings in our analysis. It is known that some patients with grade 2–3 NET can show higher affinity for FDG rather than 68Ga-DOTATOC PET [28]. This can result in an underestimation of the actual tumor burden by 68Ga-DOTATOC PET. A combination of these two tracers can be considered to address this issue. In addition, it should be noted that the generalizability of our findings with 68Ga-DOTATOC to the other often used 68Ga-DOTATATE PET ligand need to be confirmed. Indeed, while 68Ga-DOTATATE shows only affinity to SSTR2, 68Ga-DOTATOC also exhibits some affinity to SSTR5. However, despite differences in receptor affinities, a head-to-head comparison showed no clinically significant difference between the two tracers [29]. Finally, it is worth mentioning that other PET tracers like 64Cu-DOTATATE, providing better resolution and potentially a better lesion detection rate than 68Ga-DOTATOC, may improve tumor burden quantification [30]. However, the 64Cu-labeled tracers are not in use in the clinical routine and require further work.

5. Conclusions

In metastatic NET patients addressed to PRRT, higher total body tumor volume measured from baseline 68Ga-DOTATOC PET/CT scans is a negative predictor for therapy response and is associated with worse OS rates. Interim 68Ga-DOTATOC PET/CT after two cycles of PRRT did not allow the identification of patients with poorer prognosis that would justify a change in treatment strategy.

Supplementary Materials: The following are available online at https://www.mdpi.com/article/10.3390/cancers14030592/s1, Table S1: ROC curve analysis for OS.

Author Contributions: Conceptualization and supervision A.V. and A.F. (Angelina Filice); data acquisitions, V.C. and C.C.; data analysis, F.F. and D.F.; writing—original draft preparation, R.D.; revision of the article for important intellectual content, A.F. (Andrea Frasoldati), S.F. and G.B. All authors have read and agreed to the published version of the manuscript.

Funding: This research received no external funding.

Institutional Review Board Statement: The study was conducted according to the guidelines of the Declaration of Helsinki and approved by the Ethics Committee of AUSL-IRCCS of Reggio Emilia (protocol code 24871).

Informed Consent Statement: Informed consent was obtained from all subjects involved in the study.

Data Availability Statement: The data presented in this study are available on request from the corresponding author. The data are not publicly available due to privacy-related issues.

Conflicts of Interest: A.V.: Novartis and Advanced Accelerator Applications for advisory role. The other authors declare no conflict of interest.

References

1. Dasari, A.; Shen, C.; Halperin, D.; Zhao, B.; Zhou, S.; Xu, Y.; Shih, T.; Yao, J.C. Trends in the incidence, prevalence, and survival outcomes in patients with neuroendocrine tumors in the United States. *JAMA Oncol.* **2017**, *3*, 1335–1342. [CrossRef]
2. Eychenne, R.; Bouvry, C.; Bourgeois, M.; Loyer, P.; Benoist, E.; Lepareur, N. Overview of Radiolabeled Somatostatin Analogs for Cancer Imaging and Therapy. *Molecules* **2020**, *25*, 4012. [CrossRef] [PubMed]
3. Strosberg, J.; El-Haddad, G.; Wolin, E.; Hendifar, A.; Yao, J.; Chasen, B.; Mittra, E.; Kunz, P.L.; Kulke, M.H.; Jacene, H.; et al. Phase 3 Trial of 177 Lu-Dotatate for Midgut Neuroendocrine Tumors. *N. Engl. J. Med.* **2017**, *376*, 125–135. [CrossRef] [PubMed]
4. Bodei, L.; Kidd, M.; Paganelli, G.; Grana, C.M.; Drozdov, I.; Cremonesi, M.; Lepensky, C.; Kwekkeboom, D.J.; Baum, R.P.; Krenning, E.P.; et al. Long-term tolerability of PRRT in 807 patients with neuroendocrine tumours: The value and limitations of clinical factors. *Eur. J. Nucl. Med. Mol. Imaging* **2015**, *42*, 5–19. [CrossRef] [PubMed]
5. Shah, M.H.; Goldner, W.S.; Halfdanarson, T.R.; Bergsland, E.; Berlin, J.D.; Halperin, D.; Chan, J.; Kulke, M.H.; Benson, A.B.; Blaszkowsky, L.S.; et al. Neuroendocrine and adrenal tumors, version 2.2018 featured updates to the nccn guidelines. *JNCCN J. Natl. Compr. Cancer Netw.* **2018**, *16*, 693–702. [CrossRef] [PubMed]
6. Filice, A.; Fraternali, A.; Frasoldati, A.; Asti, M.; Grassi, E.; Massi, L.; Sollini, M.; Froio, A.; Erba, P.A.; Versari, A. Radiolabeled Somatostatin Analogues Therapy in Advanced Neuroendocrine Tumors: A Single Centre Experience. *J. Oncol.* **2012**, *2012*, 320198. [CrossRef] [PubMed]

7. Albertelli, M.; Dotto, A.; Di Dato, C.; Malandrino, P.; Modica, R.; Versari, A.; Colao, A.; Ferone, D.; Faggiano, A. PRRT: Identikit of the perfect patient. *Rev. Endocr. Metab. Disord.* **2021**, *22*, 563–579. [CrossRef] [PubMed]
8. Cottereau, A.S.; Versari, A.; Loft, A.; Casasnovas, O.; Bellei, M.; Ricci, R.; Bardet, S.; Castagnoli, A.; Brice, P.; Raemaekers, J.; et al. Prognostic value of baseline metabolic tumor volume in early-stage Hodgkin lymphoma in the standard arm of the H10 trial. *Blood* **2018**, *131*, 1456–1463. [CrossRef] [PubMed]
9. Hofheinz, F.; Li, Y.; Steffen, I.G.; Lin, Q.; Lili, C.; Hua, W.; van den Hoff, J.; Zschaeck, S. Confirmation of the prognostic value of pretherapeutic tumor SUR and MTV in patients with esophageal squamous cell carcinoma. *Eur. J. Nucl. Med. Mol. Imaging* **2019**, *46*, 1485–1494. [CrossRef] [PubMed]
10. Ohlendorf, F.; Werner, R.A.; Henkenberens, C.; Ross, T.L.; Christiansen, H.; Bengel, F.M.; Derlin, T. Predictive and prognostic impact of blood-based inflammatory biomarkers in patients with gastroenteropancreatic neuroendocrine tumors commencing peptide receptor radionuclide therapy. *Diagnostics* **2021**, *11*, 504. [CrossRef] [PubMed]
11. Ortega, C.; Wong, R.K.S.; Schaefferkoetter, J.; Veit-Haibach, P.; Myrehaug, S.; Juergens, R.; Laidley, D.; Anconina, R.; Liu, A.; Metser, U. Quantitative 68 Ga-DOTATATE PET/CT Parameters for the Prediction of Therapy Response in Patients with Progressive Metastatic Neuroendocrine Tumors Treated with 177 Lu-DOTATATE. *J. Nucl. Med.* **2021**, *62*, 1406–1414. [CrossRef] [PubMed]
12. Zaknun, J.J.; Bodei, L.; Mueller-Brand, J.; Pavel, M.E.; Baum, R.P.; Hörsch, D.; O'Dorisio, M.S.; O'Dorisiol, T.M.; Howe, J.R.; Cremonesi, M.; et al. The joint IAEA, EANM, and SNMMI practical guidance on peptide receptor radionuclide therapy (PRRNT) in neuroendocrine tumours. *Eur. J. Nucl. Med. Mol. Imaging* **2013**, *40*, 800–816. [CrossRef] [PubMed]
13. CHMP Lutathera, INN-Lutetium (177Lu) Oxodotreotide. Available online: https://www.ema.europa.eu/en/documents/product-information/lutathera-epar-product-information_en.pdf (accessed on 23 January 2022).
14. Cives, M.; Strosberg, J. Radionuclide Therapy for Neuroendocrine Tumors. *Curr. Oncol. Rep.* **2017**, *19*, 1–9. [CrossRef] [PubMed]
15. Strosberg, J.; Wolin, E.; Chasen, B.; Kulke, M.; Bushnell, D.; Caplin, M.; Baum, R.P.; Kunz, P.; Hobday, T.; Hendifar, A.; et al. Health-related quality of life in patients with progressive midgut neuroendocrine tumors treated with 177 lu-dotatate in the phase III netter-1 trial. *J. Clin. Oncol.* **2018**, *36*, 2578–2584. [CrossRef] [PubMed]
16. Wang, L.; Lin, L.; Wang, M.; Li, Y. The therapeutic efficacy of 177Lu-DOTATATE/DOTATOC in advanced neuroendocrine tumors. *Medicine* **2020**, *99*, e19304. [CrossRef] [PubMed]
17. Öksüz, M.Ö.; Winter, L.; Pfannenberg, C.; Reischl, G.; Müssig, K.; Bares, R.; Dittmann, H. Peptide receptor radionuclide therapy of neuroendocrine tumors with 90Y-DOTATOC: Is treatment response predictable by pre-therapeutic uptake of 68Ga-DOTATOC? *Diagn. Interv. Imaging* **2014**, *95*, 289–300. [CrossRef] [PubMed]
18. Kratochwil, C.; Stefanova, M.; Mavriopoulou, E.; Holland-Letz, T.; Dimitrakopoulou-Strauss, A.; Afshar-Oromieh, A.; Mier, W.; Haberkorn, U.; Giesel, F.L. SUV of [68Ga]DOTATOC-PET/CT Predicts Response Probability of PRRT in Neuroendocrine Tumors. *Mol. Imaging Biol.* **2014**, *17*, 313–318. [CrossRef] [PubMed]
19. Gabriel, M.; Oberauer, A.; Dobrozemsky, G.; Decristoforo, C.; Putzer, D.; Kendler, D.; Uprimny, C.; Kovacs, P.; Bale, R.; Virgolini, I.J. 68Ga-DOTA-Tyr3-octreotide PET for assessing response to somatostatin-receptor-mediated radionuclide therapy. *J. Nucl. Med.* **2009**, *50*, 1427–1434. [CrossRef] [PubMed]
20. Soydal, Ç.; Peker, A.; Özkan, E.; Küçük, Ö.N.; Kir, M.K. The role of baseline Ga-68 DOTATATE positron emission tomography/computed tomography in the prediction of response to fixed-dose peptide receptor radionuclide therapy with lu-177 DOTATATE. *Turk. J. Med. Sci.* **2016**, *46*, 409–413. [CrossRef]
21. Werner, R.A.; Ilhan, H.; Lehner, S.; Papp, L.; Zsótér, N.; Schatka, I.; Muegge, D.O.; Javadi, M.S.; Higuchi, T.; Buck, A.K.; et al. Pre-therapy Somatostatin Receptor-Based Heterogeneity Predicts Overall Survival in Pancreatic Neuroendocrine Tumor Patients Undergoing Peptide Receptor Radionuclide Therapy. *Mol. Imaging Biol.* **2019**, *21*, 582–590. [CrossRef] [PubMed]
22. Ohlendorf, F.; Henkenberens, C.; Brunkhorst, T.; Ross, T.L.; Christiansen, H.; Bengel, F.M.; Derlin, T. Volumetric 68Ga-DOTATATE PET/CT for assessment of whole-body tumor burden as a quantitative imaging biomarker in patients with metastatic gastroenteropancreatic neuroendocrine tumors. *Q. J. Nucl. Med. Mol. Imaging* **2020**. [CrossRef] [PubMed]
23. Pauwels, E.; Van Binnebeek, S.; Vandecaveye, V.; Baete, K.; Vanbilloen, H.; Koole, M.; Mottaghy, F.M.; Haustermans, K.; Clement, P.M.; Nackaerts, K.; et al. Inflammation-based index and 68ga-dotatoc pet-derived uptake and volumetric parameters predict outcome in neuroendocrine tumor patients treated with 90y-dotatoc. *J. Nucl. Med.* **2020**, *61*, 1014–1020. [CrossRef] [PubMed]
24. Meignan, M.; Sasanelli, M.; Casasnovas, R.O.; Luminari, S.; Fioroni, F.; Coriani, C.; Masset, H.; Itti, E.; Gobbi, P.G.; Merli, F.; et al. Metabolic tumour volumes measured at staging in lymphoma: Methodological evaluation on phantom experiments and patients. *Eur. J. Nucl. Med. Mol. Imaging* **2014**, *41*, 1113–1122. [CrossRef] [PubMed]
25. Tirosh, A.; Papadakis, G.Z.; Millo, C.; Hammoud, D.; Sadowski, S.M.; Herscovitch, P.; Pacak, K.; Marx, S.J.; Yang, L.; Nockel, P.; et al. Prognostic Utility of Total 68Ga-DOTATATE-Avid Tumor Volume in Patients with Neuroendocrine Tumors. *Gastroenterology* **2018**, *154*, 998–1008.e1. [CrossRef] [PubMed]
26. Abdulrezzak, U.; Kurt, Y.K.; Kula, M.; Tutus, A. Combined imaging with 68Ga-DOTA-TATE and 18F-FDG PET/CT on the basis of volumetric parameters in neuroendocrine tumors. *Nucl. Med. Commun.* **2016**, *37*, 874–881. [CrossRef] [PubMed]
27. Haug, A.R.; Auernhammer, C.J.; Wängler, B.; Schmidt, G.P.; Uebleis, C.; Göke, B.; Cumming, P.; Bartenstein, P.; Tiling, R.; Hacker, M. 68Ga-DOTATATE PET/CT for the early prediction of response to somatostatin receptor-mediated radionuclide therapy in patients with well-differentiated neuroendocrine tumors. *J. Nucl. Med.* **2010**, *51*, 1349–1356. [CrossRef] [PubMed]

28. Binderup, T.; Knigge, U.; Johnbeck, C.B.; Loft, A.; Berthelsen, A.K.; Oturai, P.; Mortensen, J.; Federspiel, B.; Langer, S.W.; Kjaer, A. 18F-FDG PET is Superior to WHO Grading as a Prognostic Tool in Neuroendocrine Neoplasms and Useful in Guiding PRRT: A Prospective 10-Year Follow-up Study. *J. Nucl. Med.* **2021**, *62*, 808–815. [CrossRef] [PubMed]
29. Poeppel, T.D.; Binse, I.; Petersenn, S.; Lahner, H.; Schott, M.; Antoch, G.; Brandau, W.; Bockisch, A.; Boy, C. 68Ga-DOTATOC versus 68Ga-DOTATATE PET/CT in functional imaging of neuroendocrine tumors. *J. Nucl. Med.* **2011**, *52*, 1864–1870. [CrossRef] [PubMed]
30. Johnbeck, C.B.; Knigge, U.; Loft, A.; Berthelsen, A.K.; Mortensen, J.; Oturai, P.; Langer, S.W.; Elema, D.R.; Kjaer, A. Head-to-Head Comparison of 64Cu-DOTATATE and 68Ga-DOTATOC PET/CT: A Prospective Study of 59 Patients with Neuroendocrine Tumors. *J. Nucl. Med.* **2017**, *58*, 451–457. [CrossRef] [PubMed]

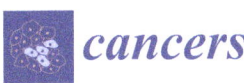

Article

Active Surveillance in *RET* Gene Carriers Belonging to Families with Multiple Endocrine Neoplasia

Alessandro Prete [1], Antonio Matrone [1], Carla Gambale [1], Valeria Bottici [1], Virginia Cappagli [1], Cristina Romei [1], Liborio Torregrossa [2], Laura Valerio [1], Elisa Minaldi [1], Maria Cristina Campopiano [1], Loredana Lorusso [1], Laura Agate [1], Eleonora Molinaro [1], David Viola [1], Teresa Ramone [1], Chiara Mulè [1], Raffaele Ciampi [1], Fulvio Basolo [2] and Rossella Elisei [1,*]

[1] Endocrine Unit, Department of Clinical and Experimental Medicine, University Hospital of Pisa, Via Paradisa 2, 56124 Pisa, Italy; alessandro.prete22@gmail.com (A.P.); antonio.matrone@med.unipi.it (A.M.); gambalecarla@libero.it (C.G.); v.bottici@ao-ao-pisa.toscana.it (V.B.); virginia.cappagli@med.unipi.it (V.C.); cristina.romei@unipi.it (C.R.); lau.val@hotmail.it (L.V.); elisa.minaldi@med.unipi.it (E.M.); cristina.campopiano@med.unipi.it (M.C.C.); lorussoloredana@hotmail.it (L.L.); laura.agate@virgilio.it (L.A.); e.molinaro@ao-pisa.toscana.it (E.M.); violadavid@hotmail.it (D.V.); teresa.ramone@hotmail.it (T.R.); c.mule@studenti.unipi.it (C.M.); raffaele.ciampi@unipi.it (R.C.)
[2] Pathology Unit, Department of Surgical, Medical, Molecular Pathology and Critical Area, University of Pisa, 56124 Pisa, Italy; l.torregrossa@ao-pisa.toscana.it (L.T.); fulvio.basolo@med.unipi.it (F.B.)
* Correspondence: rossella.elisei@med.unipi.it; Tel.: +39-050-544-723; Fax: +39-050-578-772

Citation: Prete, A.; Matrone, A.; Gambale, C.; Bottici, V.; Cappagli, V.; Romei, C.; Torregrossa, L.; Valerio, L.; Minaldi, E.; Campopiano, M.C.; et al. Active Surveillance in *RET* Gene Carriers Belonging to Families with Multiple Endocrine Neoplasia. *Cancers* **2021**, *13*, 5554. https://doi.org/10.3390/cancers13215554

Academic Editors: Alfredo Berruti, Vito Amoroso and Nicola Fazio

Received: 30 September 2021
Accepted: 4 November 2021
Published: 5 November 2021

Publisher's Note: MDPI stays neutral with regard to jurisdictional claims in published maps and institutional affiliations.

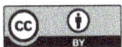

Copyright: © 2021 by the authors. Licensee MDPI, Basel, Switzerland. This article is an open access article distributed under the terms and conditions of the Creative Commons Attribution (CC BY) license (https://creativecommons.org/licenses/by/4.0/).

Simple Summary: MEN2 has a very high penetrance for the development of medullary thyroid cancer. However, intra- and inter-familial variabilities have been described. Accordingly, in this precision medicine era, a personalized approach should be adopted in subjects harboring *RET* mutations. In these subjects, we showed that thyroid surgery could be safely timed according to basal and stimulated calcitonin, especially in children who can reach adulthood, avoiding the risks of thyroid surgery and decreasing the period of a long-life hypothyroidism treatment.

Abstract: Multiple Endocrine Neoplasia 2 (MEN2) is a hereditary cancer syndrome for developing medullary thyroid cancer (MTC) due to germline mutations of *RET* gene. Subjects harboring a germline *RET* mutation without any clinical signs of MTC are defined as gene carriers (GCs), for whom guidelines propose a prophylactic thyroid surgery. We evaluate if active surveillance of GCs, pursuing early thyroid surgery, can be safely proposed and if it allows safely delaying thyroid surgery in children until adolescence/adulthood. We prospectively followed 189 GCs with moderate or high risk germline *RET* mutation. Surgery was planned in case of: elevated basal calcitonin (bCT) and/or stimulated CT (sCT); surgery preference of subjects (or parents, if subject less than 18 years old); other reasons for thyroid surgery. Accordingly, at *RET* screening, we sub-grouped GCs in subjects who promptly were submitted to thyroid surgery (Group A, $n = 67$) and who were not (Group B, $n = 122$). Group B was further sub-grouped in subjects who were submitted to surgery during their active surveillance (Group B1, $n = 22$) and who are still in follow-up (Group B2, $n = 100$). Group A subjects presented significantly more advanced age, bCT and sCT compared to Group B. Mutation *RET*^{V804M} was the most common variant in both groups but it was significantly less frequent in Group A than B. Analyzing age, bCT, sCT and genetic landscape, Group B1 subjects differed from Group B2 only for sCT at last evaluation. Group A subjects presented more frequently MTC foci than Group B1. Moreover, Group A MTCs presented more aggressive features (size, T and N) than Group B1. Accordingly, at the end of follow-up, all Group B1 subjects presented clinical remission, while 6 and 12 Group A MTC patients had structural and biochemical persistent disease, respectively. Thank to active surveillance, only 13/63 subjects younger than 18 years at *RET* screening have been operated on during childhood and/or adolescence. In Group B1, three patients, while actively surveilled, had the possibility to reach the age of 18 (or older) and two patients the age of 15, before being submitted to thyroid surgery. In Group B2, 12 patients become older than 18 years and 17 older than 15 years. In conclusion, we demonstrated that an active surveillance pursuing an early thyroid surgery could be safely recommended in GCs. This patient-centered approach permits postponing thyroid surgery in children until their adolescence/adulthood. At the same time, we confirmed that genetic screening allows finding hidden MTC cases that otherwise would be diagnosed much later.

Keywords: medullary thyroid cancer; calcitonin; MEN2; gene carriers

1. Introduction

Multiple Endocrine Neoplasia 2 (MEN2) is an hereditary cancer syndrome characterized by the development of medullary thyroid cancer (MTC), variably associated with other endocrine neoplasia, such as pheochromocytoma and primary hyperparathyroidism [1–3]. MEN2 is an autosomal dominant disease with a very high penetrance due to missense gain-of-function mutation of the *RET* gene (Rearranged during Transfection) [4,5]. Germline *RET* mutation is present in about 99% of familial and about 6.0% of apparently sporadic cases of MTC [6]. Accordingly, germline *RET* screening must be offered to all patients with MTC and, if positive, all first-degree relatives should be screened [7,8]. Subjects harboring a germline *RET* mutation without any clinical signs of MTC are defined as Gene Carriers (GCs) [8].

In the case of a GC, guidelines propose a prophylactic thyroid surgery as "the removal of the thyroid before MTC develops or while it is clinically unapparent and confined to the gland" [8]. Its timing is essentially based on subject *RET* mutation and age; in cases of *RET* mutation at highest risk (*M918T*) surgical therapy must be performed within the first year, in cases at high risk (*C634F/G/R/S/W/Y* and *A883F*) the timing of thyroidectomy can be based on serum calcitonin (CT). However, in any case before 5 years and in cases at moderate risk (other mutations), basal and stimulated CT (bCT and sCT) should guide thyroid surgery timing [8]. This latter suggestion is not always followed in the real clinical world and several centers still follow the indication to operate immediately after the *RET* screening, warning against the use of serum CT in this clinical scenario [9].

By many years, in the case of GCs harboring high and moderate risk mutations, in our center we are performing an active surveillance by timing the thyroid surgery on bCT and sCT levels, regardless of *RET* mutation and age, pursuing an early, instead of a prophylactic, thyroid surgery [10]. The main reasons are related to both the higher risk of surgical complications in children, particularly permanent hypoparathyroidism that implies long-life therapy [11], and to the need of early medication with levothyroxine during childhood and adolescence in subjects who actually have normal thyroid function.

In this study, we evaluated if an active surveillance with an early thyroid surgery can be safely proposed in *RET* GCs and for how many years the surgery could be safely delayed in children. Moreover, we looked also at the relevance of genetic screening in finding hidden MTC cases that, otherwise, would be diagnosed much later.

2. Materials and Methods

2.1. Subjects

After 1993, we performed *RET* genetic screening in all patients with diagnosis of MTC, either familial or apparently sporadic and, if positive, to all their first-grade relatives [6].

All adult patients signed informed consent to perform *RET* genetic screening. Parents or guardians signed the informed consent in the case of subjects less than 18 years of age. As per the policy of the University Hospital, all patients provided written informed consent to both the genetic screening and the use of their clinical and biochemical data for scientific purposes.

2.2. Clinical Evaluation

We evaluated GCs by using clinical, biochemical (i.e., bCT and sCT (pentagastrin (Pg) stimulation test up to 2013, and then calcium (Ca) stimulation test, as elsewhere described [12]), urinary metanephrine and normetanephrine, serum PTH, calcium and

25-hydroxyvitamin D (25[OH]D) and imaging examinations (i.e., neck and abdominal ultrasound and whenever necessary abdominal MRI).

2.3. Surgery Criteria

According to the most recent advances carried out by Elisei et al. [10], in our center the surgical treatment for GCs, independently from the type of germline mutation, is planned according to the following criteria:

(1) elevated bCT (i.e., higher than upper limit of normal range) and/or positive stimulation test;
(2) subjects (or parents when subjects were under the age of 18) who specifically asked for immediate surgery;
(3) other reasons for thyroidal surgery (e.g., Graves disease or symptomatic goiter).

Otherwise, patients without any of the above-mentioned criteria were followed every 6–12 months with clinical, biochemical, and morphological assays (namely neck ultrasound) as previously described.

2.4. Post-Surgery Follow-Up

Four/six months after surgery, all patients were submitted to biochemical analysis (bCT and, if necessary, Pg or Ca stimulation test for CT) and neck ultrasound. Whenever indicated, other imaging (e.g., CT scan, MRI etc.) were performed.

2.5. RET Genetic Analysis

RET genetic screening has been performed on DNA extracted from the blood of MTC patients and of their relatives according to a procedure previously reported [6]. MTC patients have been screened for the presence of RET mutations in exons 5, 8, 10, 11, 13, 14, 15, and 16 while relatives of RET positive index cases have been analyzed only for the presence of the mutation identified in their family. Actually, genomic DNA is amplified using KAPA2G Fast HotStart PCR Kit (Sigma-Aldrich, Saint Louis, MI, USA) in a final volume of 20 µL with 0.5 pmoli/µL of each primer and using a SimplyAmp thermal cycler (Thermofisher, Waltham, MA, USA). Amplification cycle is performed with an initial step of 95 °C for 2 min, followed by 35 cycles of 95 °C for 15 s, 60 °C for 15 s and 72 °C for 15 s. A final extension at 72 °C for 7 min was performed at the end of the amplification protocol. Sequence analysis was performed, and has been reported on previously. Primers'sequence can be provided upon request. Sequence reactions are performed according to the Sanger method using an ABI Prism 3130XL genetic analyzer (Thermofisher, Waltham, MA, USA).

2.6. Laboratory Evaluation

In the last 25 years CT measurement has been performed using two immunometric assays (ELSA-hCT, Cis-BioInternational, Gif sur Yvette, France, functional sensitivity 10.0 pg/mL, from 1993 to 2013 and chemoluminescent immunometric Immulite, Siemens Healthcare Diagnostic Products Ltd., Lianberis, Gwynedd LL55 4EL, UK, with analytic sensitivity 2.0 pg/mL reference values of up to 18.2 pg/mL for women and 11.5 pg/mL for men, from 2014 to the present).

2.7. Histopathology

All the specimens were submitted to routine pathological procedure and were reviewed by two pathologists (LT, FB). Briefly, the surgical specimens were fixed in 10% buffered formaldehyde and embedded in paraffin, and then 4-mm-thick sections were cut and stained with hematoxylin & eosin (H&E). For immunohistochemistry, paraffin sections (3–5 mm) were dewaxed in xylene, dehydrated through graded alcohols, and processed using the diaminobenzidine detection system. All of the immunohistochemical analyses for calcitonin were performed automatically using the Ventana Benchmark® immunostaining system (Ventana Medical Systems, Tucson, AZ, USA) and a rabbit monoclonal primary antibody direct against calcitonin polypeptide (Ventana Medical Systems, clone SP17; dilution 0.56 μg/mL).

Usually, on routine H&E stained-slides the "neoplastic" or "primary" CCH is easily identified by the presence of clusters of intrafollicular C-cells, composed of cells with mild or moderate cellular atypia, resembling those identified in an MTC [13]. According to the last edition of WHO Classification of Tumours of Endocrine Organs [14] the diagnosis of "primary" CCH is encountered when >6–8 C cells per cluster in several foci with >50 C cells per low power field are identified. Immunostaining for CT was performed in all cases to confirm the recognition of C-cells. Histologically, the main difference between the "primary" CCH and the microfocus of MTC is represented by extension of C cells through the basement membrane into the surrounding thyroid interstitium or when a desmoplastic stromal reaction surrounding the infiltrating neoplastic cells is evident [15].

2.8. Statistical Analysis

Statistical analysis was performed using Kruskal–Wallis, Mann–Whitney, t tests, ROC curves, univariate and multivariate regression analysis, according to the variables to be analyzed, using IBM SPSS Statistics (Armonk, NY, USA) for Macintosh, Version 25.0. A p value less than 0.05 was considered statistically significant.

3. Results

3.1. Study Groups: Epidemiological, Biochemical and Genetics Data

RET genetic screening allowed us to discover 189 GCs in 84 families. At first clinical evaluation, after the screening, we distinguished two groups of GCs: those who already met surgery criteria (n = 67, Group A) and those who did not (n = 122, Group B). Epidemiological, biochemical and US data of Group A and B, are reported in Table 1. Group A subjects were significantly older than Group B (median 44 vs. 18 years) (p < 0.0001). As expected, at *RET* genetics screening, Group A subjects presented significantly higher bCT (median 24 ng/L vs. below functional sensitivity) as well as sCT (median 276.5 vs. 10.6 ng/L) compared to Group B (p < 0.0001). US scan identified thyroid nodule in 71.2% (37/52) of Group A subjects and in 22.1% (23/104) of Group B (p < 0.0001) (Table 1).

Table 1. Epidemiological, biochemical and US data of Group A and B. bCT: basal calcitonin, sCT: calcitonin upon pentagastrin or calcium stimulation test, US: ultrasound, BFS: below functional sensitivity.

Determinants		Group A (n = 67)	Group B (n = 122)	p Value
Follow-up (years) median (IQR, intervals)		7 (1.5–12.5, 0.3–26)	3.6 (0.8–6.5, 0.08–21.8)	0.0001
Male: Female (number of patients)		31:36	57:65	0.952
Age at *RET* screening (years) median (IQR, intervals)		44.0 (30–56, 5–80)	18.0 (8–41.3, 1–86)	<0.0001
bCT at *RET* screening (ng/L) median (IQR, intervals)		24.0 (0–245, 0–33571)	BFS (BFS-3.9, BFS-19.4)	<0.0001
sCT at *RET* screening (ng/L) median (IQR, intervals)		276.5 (38–1175, 0–17810)	10.6 (BFS-21.4, BFS-193)	<0.0001
US assessment at *RET* screening	Presence of at least one nodule	71.2%	22.1%	<0.0001
	Negative	28.8%	77.9%	

We analyzed the genetic landscape of Group A and B. In agreement with our previous report [6], we confirmed that mutations occurring at 804 codon were the most common mutations in both groups, although they were significantly less frequent in Group A than B (26% vs. 42%, p = 0.034) (Figure 1A). Otherwise, we observed that mutations occurring at 634 codon were substantially, although not significantly, more frequent in Group A than B (12% vs. 5%, p = 0.083) (Figure 1A). Accordingly, at first evaluation, 57% of patients with RET^{C634X} mutation presented the criteria for surgery while only 37% with other mutations presented these criteria, although this difference was not statistically significant, probably due to relatively low number of subjects with RET^{C634X} mutation ($n = 14$) ($p = 0.22$) (Figure 1B).

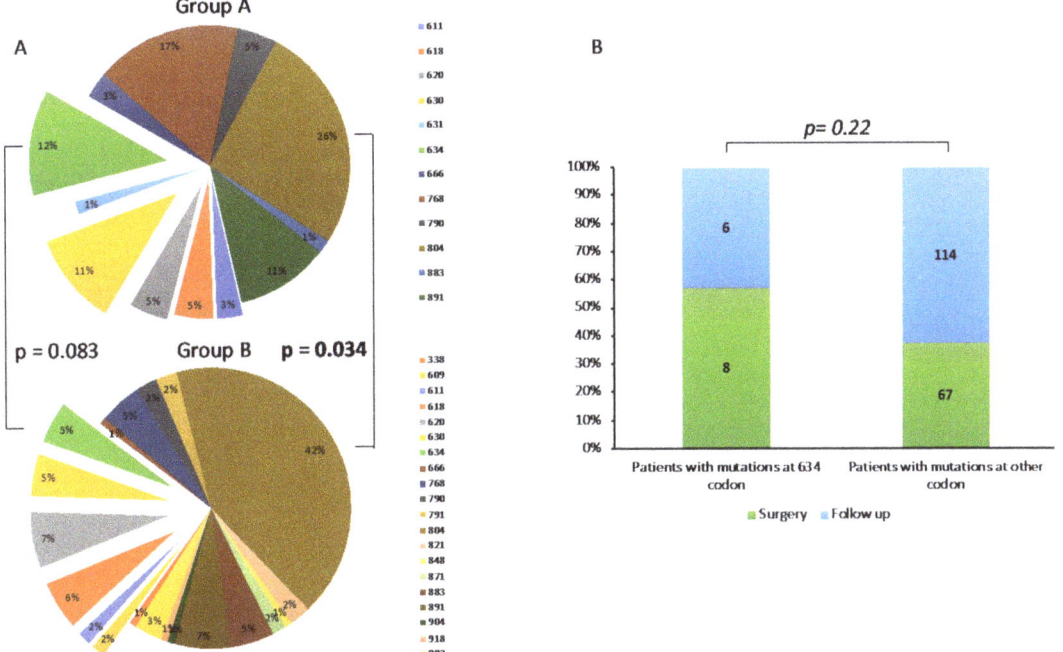

Figure 1. (**A**) Genetic landscape of Group A (upper graph) and B (lower graph). (**B**) Rate of patients submitted to surgery or follow-up, according to RET mutations (634 codon vs. other codons).

3.2. Follow-Up in Group B

After the *RET* genetics screening assessment, Group B subjects were followed every 6–12 months. During their follow-up, 22/122 (19%) subjects were submitted to surgery (Group B1) after a median time of 1.6 years (IQR 1.1–3.6, range 1.1–10.3 years) and 100/122 (81%) patients are still in follow-up (Group B2) after a median time of 2.9 years (IQR 0.9–6.3, range 0.1–21.8 years). We analyzed epidemiological, biochemical, and US-features of GCs of Groups B1 and B2 both at *RET* screening and last evaluation (either before surgery in Group B1 or at the end of follow-up in Group B2). At *RET* screening evaluation, Groups B1 and B2 subjects did not differ for age, bCT, and sCT (Figure 2). Otherwise, at the last evaluation, Group B1 subjects presented significantly higher levels of sCT compared to Group B2 (median 38 vs. 20 ng/L, respectively, $p = 0.035$), whereas bCT and age were not different (Figure 2). At US scan, thyroid nodules were substantially more frequent in Group B1 than Group B2 at *RET* screening evaluation (42%, 8/19 vs. 17.6%, 15/85; $p = 0.059$) and significantly at last evaluation (50%, 10/20 vs. 25%, 23/92; $p = 0.022$) (Figure 2D). Figure 2E summarized genetics landscapes of both groups. Mutations occurring at 804 codon were substantially, although not significantly, more frequent in Group B1 (61%, 14/23) than B2 (38%, 37/98) ($p = 0.067$). Mutations at 634 codon did not differ between the two groups.

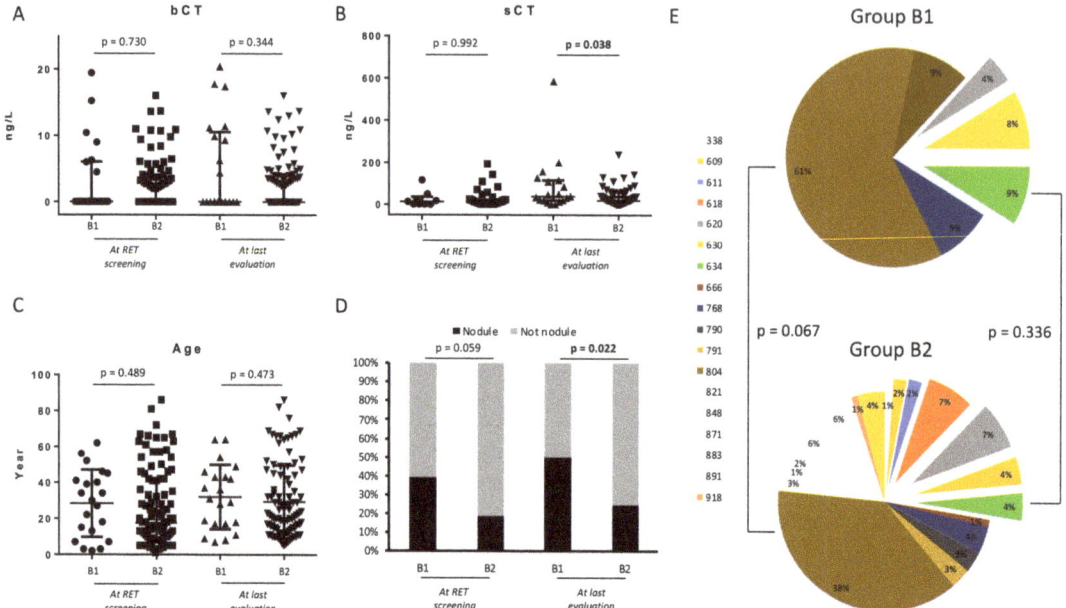

Figure 2. (**A**,**B**) basal CT (bCT) and stimulated CT (sCT) in Group B1 and B2 at *RET* screening and at last evaluation. (**C**) Age of subjects of Group B1 and Group B2 at *RET* screening and at last evaluation. (**D**) Rate of nodule at neck ultrasound in subjects of Group B1 and Group B2 at RET screening and at last evaluation. (**E**) Genetic landscape of subjects of Group B1 and Group B2.

3.3. MTC in Group A and B1: Anatomopathological Features, Prognosis and Surgical Complications

At histology, all cases showed MTC foci and/or CCH. We compared anatomopathological features between Groups A and B1 and we found that MTC foci ± CCH was significantly more present in Group A (58/67, 86.7%) than B1 (9/22, 40.9%), in which the CCH alone was prevalent (Figure 3) ($p < 0.0001$).

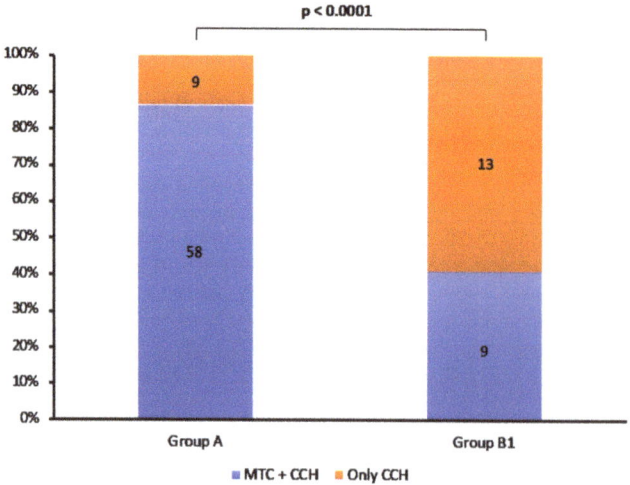

Figure 3. Rate of MTC + CCH and only CCH in Group A and B1 patients.

Among those patients who had MTC foci, Group A patients had MTC foci significantly larger than Group B1 (median 0.65 vs. 0.40 cm, p value = 0.036). At variance, MTC multifocality and bilaterality were not different in Groups A and B1 (Table 2). We, therefore, analyzed TNM classification system in patients of Group A and B1 with MTC (67 patients). Although most of the MTC patients belonging to Group A had T score of 1 (51/58, 88%), a significant portion (7/58, 12%) had T score > 1, whereas all MTC patients of Group B1 had a T score of 1. Lymph node metastasis occurred in 21 patients of Group A, while they did not occur in Group B1 patients (p = 0.045). In the case of lymph-node metastasis, they occurred in 15/21 patients (71.4%) in central and in 6/21 in latero-cervical (28.6%) compartments (Table 2). At the time of surgery, only one case of Group A presented metastasis spread to lungs, liver, and bones. All MTC patients of Group B1 experienced clinical remission during the follow-up after surgery (median 4 years, IQR 2–7 years, intervals 3–153 months), while 6/67 (9%) and 12/67 (18%) MTC patients of Group A had structural and biochemical persistent disease, respectively, during their follow-up (median 6.5 years, IQR 2.25–13 years, 3–311 months) (Table 2). All patients of both groups with CCH were cured at the data lock of this study (median follow up 4.6 years, IQR 2.5–11, 1–178) as assessed by undetectable levels of both bCT and sCT.

Table 2. Histopathological features of MTCs of Group A and B1 patients.

Histopathological Features	Group A n = 58/67 (86.7%)	Group B1 n = 9/22 (40.9%)	p Value
Diameter main MTC focus median (IQR, interval) (cm)	0.65 (0.25–1.05, 0.1–6.5)	0.40 (0.23–0.58, 0.10–0.60)	0.036
Multifocality	39 (65%)	6 (66%)	0.392
Bilaterality	17 (45%)	1 (15%)	0.676
T score more than 1	8 (14%)	0%	0.289
Lymph node metastasis at surgery	22 (38.6%)	0%	0.045
Distant metastasis at surgery	1 (1.85%)	0%	1.000

About surgical complications, they were observed in 15 (22.4%) patients of group A and in only one (6.3%) of group B1 (p = 0.059). Among group A patients, 14 of them presented only hypoparathyroidism and one patient both recurrent laryngeal nerve injury and hypoparathyroidism. Patient of group B1 developed only hypoparathyroidism.

3.4. Follow-Up of GCs under the Age of 18

Looking at GCs younger than 18 years at the time of RET genetic screening, we had a total of 63 subjects. Applying the aforementioned surgery criteria, 5/63 patients were submitted to surgery after first evaluation (belonging to Group A), 8/63 during their follow-up (belonging to Group B1), while 50/63 individuals are still on follow-up (belonging to Group B2). At RET genetics screening, there was not any difference between age of subjects belonging to Group A (median age 10 years old, IQR 6–14, intervals 5–15 years), to Group B1 (median age 7 years old, IQR 3–12.5, intervals 2–15 years) or to Group B2 (median age 8 years old, IQR 5–13, intervals 1–17 years). Otherwise, as expected, mutations occurring at 634 or cysteine codon were significantly more common in group A, although present also in Group B1 and B2 (p = 0.001 for 634 codon and p = 0.021 for cysteines); likewise, RET^{C634X} mutations were substantially more common in Group B1 than Group B2 (p = 0.075), whereas mutations occurring at cysteine or 804 codons did not differ in Group B1 and Group B2 (p = 0.935 and p = 0.847, respectively) (Figure 4).

Surgery was performed after a median time of 5 months (IQR 4–7, intervals 4–7 months) in subjects of Group A and of about 3 years (IQR 1.6–9.3, intervals 1.6–10.3 years) in subjects of Group B1. So far, only 11/63 (17.5%) patients have been operated during childhood and/or adolescence. At the study data lock, a total of 15/58 (25.9%) GCs who did not immediately meet the criteria for surgery reached the age of 18 and two of them have been operated at 18 and 22 versus 15 and 11 years at screening. Among Group B1 patients, at time of surgery, two of them (one patient with RET^{C634Y} and one with RET^{V804M}) became older than 18 years, one reached 18 years (with RET^{V804M}) and two older than 15 (two patients with RET^{E768D}) (Figure 5). Only one patient (age at surgery of 17 years) developed a surgical complication (hypoparathyroidism). Among patients who are still in follow-up (n = 50), (median time of 5 years, IQR 3–9, intervals 1–15 years) at study data lock, 12 patients became older than 18 years and 17 older than 15 years (Figure 5).

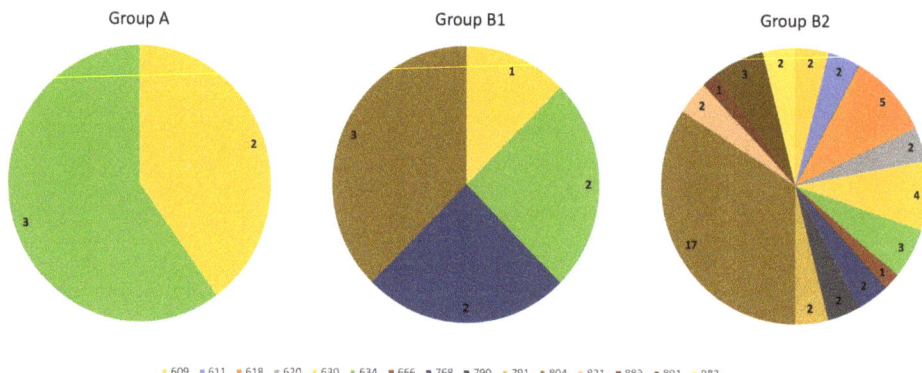

Figure 4. Genetic landscape of subjects younger than 18 years belonging to Group A, B1 or B2.

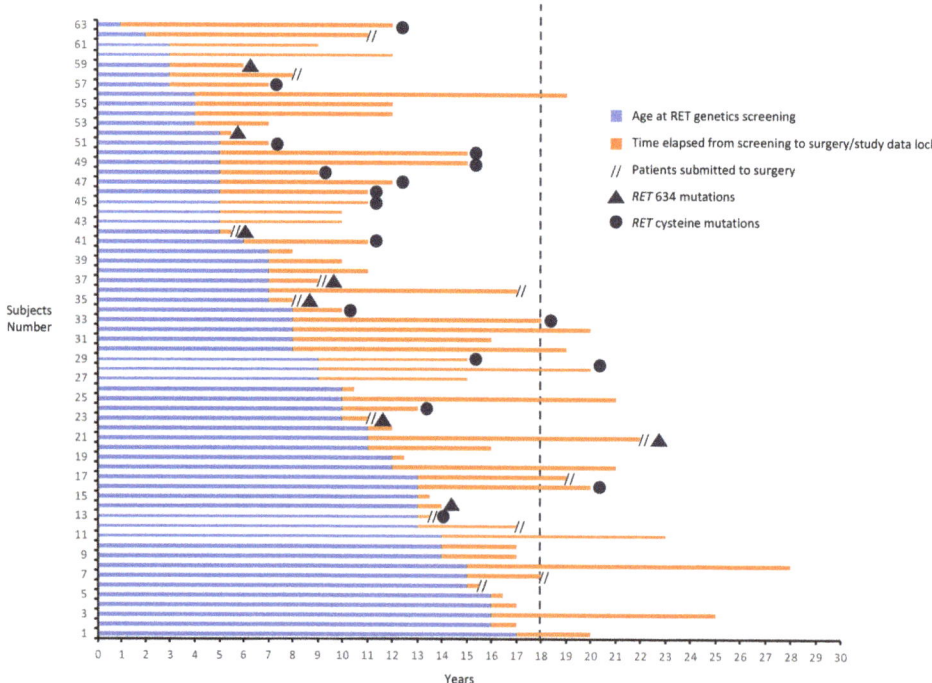

Figure 5. Genetic landscape, and duration of follow-up, of GCs younger than 18 at the time of *RET* genetic screening of Group A, B1 and B2.

4. Discussion

Oncology was radically revolutionized by screening of hereditary cancer diseases, diminishing the rate of patients with advanced disease at diagnosis and their mortality [16]. According to genetic and clinical characteristics of each hereditary disease, several approaches may be proposed: prophylactic surgery of involved organ, regular biochemical and/or morphological screening to promptly identify an arising neoplasia, and chemoprevention to hinder cancer development [16]. In MEN2, the suggested approach swings between the prophylactic surgery (in case of highest and very high risk *RET* mutations) and the regular follow-up (in case of moderate risk *RET* mutations), while chemoprevention has not gained space so far [8,17]. If the surgical approach must be proposed before 1 year of age in patients harboring RET^{M918T}, in case of other *RET* mutations a personalized approach should be persuaded [8,18].

In this prospective study looking at 189 GCs with high and moderate risk *RET* mutations, we showed that thyroid surgery might be safely planned following bCT and sCT. In particular, GCs who were submitted to surgery after a regular follow-up (Group B1) did not experience neither lymph-node nor distant metastasis, and neither biochemical nor structural persistence was observed, at least at study data lock (median follow-up 4 years). Although the median follow-up is rather short, we should consider that all these patients showed a negative CT stimulation test at 3–6 months after surgery, which implies a negligible risk of possible recurrence [19].

The disease status of GCs who already had the criteria for surgery at the time of *RET* genetic screening (Group A) was indeed more advanced with 21/67 (31.3%) patients having lymph-node and 1/67 (1.5%) distant metastasis. Despite the prompt thyroidectomy and lymphadenectomy, 9.0% and 18% of them had structural and biochemical persistent disease, respectively, after a median follow-up of 6.5 years. However, if we consider that the percentage of MTC patients with lymph-node metastasis and/or distant metastasis in big series of MTC is around 45.1–53% and 10–11.4%, respectively [19–21], our findings demonstrate that, even in already affected GCs, the *RET* genetic screening can anticipate the diagnosis when the MTC is still clinically silent. This evidence confirmed that *RET* genetic screening should be offered and solicited to all first-degree relatives of patients with MEN2, as recommended by MTC guidelines [7,8].

We also found a relevant difference of both disease stage and outcome between group A and B1, demonstrating that timing surgery according to the increase of bCT and sCT allows performing an early, but not prophylactic, thyroid surgery that is still safe, since all patients in group B1 were cured at the time of data lock but also justified since microfoci of MTC were already present in more than 40% of cases [10].

Recently, Machens et al. showed that the risk of lymph-nodes metastasis in patients harboring *RET* germline mutations increased by age and by *RET* risk category (e.g., low-moderate vs. moderate-high and high risk) [22]. In our series, patients of Group A, were effectively older than those of Group B while no significant differences were found in the type of RET mutations except for the fact that V804M was more frequent in Group B. This finding confirms the role of the advanced age in the development of the disease but reduces the impact of the type of *RET* mutation. New evidence showed that RETV804M mutation harbors a moderate risk of MTC development [23], although in our cohort this risk seems to not be negligible. Although age and *RET* mutation seem to be two milestones of MEN2 phenotypic variability, it is far long to be completely enlightened and inter- and intra-familial variability has been shown by many authors [24–28]. Accordingly, patients in Groups B1 and B2 did differ neither in age nor in *RET* genetics while they differ in the biological behavior of the tumor whose growth was faster in Group B1. These data argued that MEN2 genotypic-phenotypic relation is less stiff than imagined in the past and might be influenced by other factors: genetics (e.g., unbalanced expression of mutant and wild *RET* gene), epigenetics (e.g., DNA methylation, histone modification, or chromatin remodeling) and non-genetics (e.g., environmental factor) [29]. In this nebulous scenario, *RET* mutation and age should certainly guide clinical decisions, but these data argued that each clinical management must be individualized, and thyroid surgery should be timed according to bCT and sCT, avoiding prophylactic surgery that is necessarily followed by the medicalization of the patients and, sometimes, by surgical complications, especially in children.

Using this approach, 15 out 58 patients, who were younger than 18 years of age at the time of screening, reached adulthood without thyroid surgery, postponing the beginning of a long-life therapy with levothyroxine (LT4). LT4 is the only current recommended therapy for patients undergone to total thyroidectomy, both in adults and children [7,30]. However, although a biochemical euthyroidism is generally reached, LT4 seems to do not guarantee an euthyroidism state in all tissues [31,32]. In addition, biochemical features in athyreotic patients seem to be different from those in euthyroid ones, as demonstrated by Gullo and colleagues, who showed that athyreotic patients treated with LT4 had higher fT4 and lower fT3 levels than euthyroid control and about one third of them had lower than reference fT4/fT3 ratio [33]. It is unknown if this not physiological thyroid state might play a role in children growth.

Transient or permanent disruption of calcium metabolism may occur after thyroid surgery in more than 25% and 5% of patients, respectively [34]. De Jong and colleagues collected clinical and biochemical data of 106 children (younger than 18 years) submitted to thyroid surgery and described a hypocalcemia at discharge in 49.3% and at 6 months 21.7% of them [35]. The higher risk of hypoparathyroidism in children compared to adult was confirmed by other authors [36,37], in particular in those younger than 3 years old [37]. In our cohort of GCs younger than 18 years who were submitted to surgery (13), only one patient (1/13, 7.7%) is experiencing a permanent hypoparathyroidism. Otherwise, this risk seems to be minimized in high-volume facilities [38,39], especially in patients who do not need central neck dissection [40]. Accordingly, in order to minimize this risk, GCs should be referred to surgical centers experienced in pediatric surgery for thyroid cancer. In this scenario, safely postponing thyroid surgery across the childhood could be a winning choice.

A recent review observed that subjects who experienced cancer diagnosis during their childhood seemed to be at higher risk of impaired psychological development [41], as well as manifestations of anxiety, depression, inattention, and antisocial behavior [42]. Adult survivors of childhood cancer were described to be at higher risk of depression and anxiety symptoms, even many years after the end of therapies [43]. At the same time, adults with a history of cancer during childhood presented poorer social outcomes, such as the capacity of living independently or psychosexual milestones in both females and males [43–45]. According to this evidence, the psychological impact of thyroid surgery should be carefully evaluated in children, especially after this demonstration that by taking children in active surveillance once a year and postponing the thyroidectomy to an early phase of the disease development their outcome is still favorable like that obtained with prophylactic thyroidectomy.

Finally, this approach requires an adherence of GCs (and their parents, in case of children) to regular assessments, which could represent a limitation of this active surveillance approach in our mobile society. However, like in other chronic conditions, patient education and participation are vitally important [46,47]. Subjects with RET mutations (and their parents) must be highly informed about the advantages and the disadvantages of this approach. In this highly personalized approach, each GC must not be a passive character but an active and collaborative player and social and psychological needs of each subject should be considered.

5. Conclusions

Our data showed that an active surveillance pursuing an early thyroid surgery, based upon bCT and sCT, could be safely recommended in high and moderate risk *RET* GCs, both adults and children, thus reducing the lifespan of medicalization and the risk of surgical complications. This is particularly desirable in children and is independent from the type of *RET* mutation even if those with a high risk mutation likely will reach the need to be operated earlier than those with moderate risk mutations. Moreover, we confirmed that genetic screening allows finding hidden MTC cases that otherwise would be diagnosed much later.

Author Contributions: Conceptualization, A.P. and R.E.; methodology, R.E.; investigation, A.M., C.G., V.B., V.C., E.M. (Elisa Minaldi), L.A., D.V., C.R., T.R., C.M., and R.C.; resources, L.T. and F.B.; data curation, A.P., L.V., E.M. (Eleonora Molinaro), M.C.C., L.L., and R.E.; writing—original draft preparation, A.P. and R.E.; writing—review and editing, A.P. and R.E.; supervision, R.E.; funding acquisition, R.E. All authors have read and agreed to the published version of the manuscript.

Funding: This research was funded by Associazione Italiana per la Ricerca sul Cancro (AIRC, Investigator grant 2018, project code 21790).

Institutional Review Board Statement: This study has been conducted according to the guidelines of the Declaration of Helsinki. Since it is a retrospective collection and analysis of clinical and biochemical data, it does not require the approval by Ethics Committee.

Informed Consent Statement: Informed consent was obtained from all subjects involved in the study. Parents or guardians signed the informed consent in case of subjects less than 18 years of age.

Data Availability Statement: The data presented in this study are available on request from the corresponding author. The data are not publicly available due to ethical issues.

Acknowledgments: The authors would thank all the families who had faith in us and in this clinical behavior. Their incessant support was essential for this article.

Conflicts of Interest: The authors declare no conflict of interest.

References

1. Raue, F.; Frank-Raue, K. Update on Multiple Endocrine Neoplasia Type 2: Focus on Medullary Thyroid Carcinoma. *J. Endocr. Soc.* **2018**, *2*, 933–943. [CrossRef]
2. Amodru, V.; Taieb, D.; Guerin, C.; Romanet, P.; Paladino, N.; Brue, T.; Cuny, T.; Barlier, A.; Sebag, F.; Castinetti, F. MEN2-Related Pheochromocytoma: Current State of Knowledge, Specific Characteristics in MEN2B, and Perspectives. *Endocrine* **2020**, *69*, 496–503. [CrossRef]
3. Romei, C.; Pardi, E.; Cetani, F.; Elisei, R. Genetic and Clinical Features of Multiple Endocrine Neoplasia Types 1 and 2. *J. Oncol.* **2012**, *2012*, 1–15. [CrossRef]
4. Wells, S.A. Advances in the management of MEN2: From Improved Surgical and Medical Treatment to Novel Kinase Inhibitors. *Endocr. Relat. Cancer* **2018**, *25*, T1–T13. [CrossRef]
5. Romei, C.; Ciampi, R.; Elisei, R. A Comprehensive Overview of the Role of the RET Proto-Oncogene in Thyroid Carcinoma. *Nat. Rev. Endocrinol.* **2016**, *12*, 192–202. [CrossRef] [PubMed]
6. Elisei, R.; Tacito, A.; Ramone, T.; Ciampi, R.; Bottici, V.; Cappagli, V.; Viola, D.; Matrone, A.; Lorusso, L.; Valerio, L.; et al. Twenty-Five Years Experience on RET Genetic Screening on Hereditary MTC: An Update on The Prevalence of Germline RET Mutations. *Genes* **2019**, *10*, 698. [CrossRef]
7. Elisei, R.; Alevizaki, M.; Conte-Devolx, B.; Frank-Raue, K.; Leite, V.; Williams, G.R. 2012 European Thyroid Association Guidelines for Genetic Testing and Its Clinical Consequences in Medullary Thyroid Cancer. *Eur. Thyroid J.* **2012**, *1*, 216–231. [CrossRef] [PubMed]
8. Wells, S.A.; Asa, S.; Dralle, H.; Elisei, R.; Evans, D.B.; Gagel, R.F.; Lee, N.Y.; Machens, A.; Moley, J.F.; Pacini, F.; et al. Revised American Thyroid Association Guidelines for the Management of Medullary Thyroid Carcinoma. *Thyroid. Off. J. Am. Thyroid. Assoc.* **2015**, *25*, 567–610. [CrossRef]
9. Kuhlen, M.; Frühwald, M.C.; Dunsheimer, D.P.A.; Vorwerk, P.; Redlich, A. Revisiting the Genotype-Phenotype Correlation in Children with Medullary Thyroid Carcinoma: A Report from the GPOH-MET Registry. *Pediatr. Blood Cancer* **2020**, *67*, e28171. [CrossRef]
10. Elisei, R.; Romei, C.; Renzini, G.; Bottici, V.; Cosci, B.; Molinaro, E.; Agate, L.; Cappagli, V.; Miccoli, P.; Berti, P.; et al. The Timing of Total Thyroidectomy inRETGene Mutation Carriers Could Be Personalized and Safely Planned on the Basis of Serum Calcitonin: 18 Years Experience at One Single Center. *J. Clin. Endocrinol. Metab.* **2012**, *97*, 426–435. [CrossRef]
11. Sosa, J.A.; Tuggle, C.T.; Wang, T.S.; Thomas, D.C.; Boudourakis, L.; Rivkees, S.; Roman, S.A. Clinical and Economic Outcomes of Thyroid and Parathyroid Surgery in Children. *J. Clin. Endocrinol. Metab.* **2008**, *93*, 3058–3065. [CrossRef] [PubMed]
12. Mian, C.; Perrino, M.; Colombo, C.; Cavedon, E.; Pennelli, G.; Ferrero, S.; De Leo, S.; Sarais, C.; Cacciatore, C.; Manfredi, G.I.; et al. Refining Calcium Test for the Diagnosis of Medullary Thyroid Cancer: Cutoffs, Procedures, and Safety. *J. Clin. Endocrinol. Metab.* **2014**, *99*, 1656–1664. [CrossRef] [PubMed]

13. Perry, A.; Molberg, K.; Albores-Saavedra, J. Physiologic versus Neoplastic C-Cell Hyperplasia of the Thyroid: Separation of Distinct Histologic and Biologic Entities. *Cancer* **1996**, *77*, 750–756. [CrossRef]
14. Lloyd, R.V.; Osamura, R.; Kloppel, G.; Rosai, J. *WHO Classification of Tumours of the Endocrine Organs*, 2017th ed.; IARC Press: Lyon, France, 2017; Volume 10, pp. 210–239. ISBN 978-92-832-4493-6.
15. Kaserer, K.; Scheuba, C.; Neuhold, N.; Weinhäusel, A.; Haas, O.A.; Vierhapper, H.; Niederle, B. Sporadic versus Familial Medullary Thyroid Microcarcinoma. *Am. J. Surg. Pathol.* **2001**, *25*, 1245–1251. [CrossRef] [PubMed]
16. Couch, F.J.; Nathanson, K.L.; Offit, K. Two Decades After BRCA: Setting Paradigms in Personalized Cancer Care and Prevention. *Science* **2014**, *343*, 1466–1470. [CrossRef]
17. Mathiesen, J.S.; Effraimidis, G.; Rossing, M.; Rasmussen, K.; Hoejberg, L.; Bastholt, L.; Godballe, C.; Oturai, P.; Feldt-Rasmussen, U. Multiple Endocrine Neoplasia Type 2: A Review. *Semin. Cancer Biol.* **2021**. [CrossRef] [PubMed]
18. Li, S.-Y.; Ding, Y.-Q.; Si, Y.-L.; Ye, M.-J.; Xu, C.-M.; Qi, X.-P. 5P Strategies for Management of Multiple Endocrine Neoplasia Type 2: A Paradigm of Precision Medicine. *Front. Endocrinol.* **2020**, *11*, 698. [CrossRef]
19. Modigliani, E.; Cohen, R.; Campos, J.-M.; Conte-Devolx, B.; Maes, B.; Boneu, A.; Schlumberger, M.; Bigorgne, J.-C.; Dumontier, P.; Leclerc, L.; et al. Prognostic Factors for Survival and for Biochemical Cure in Medullary Thyroid Carcinoma: Results in 899 Patients. The GETC Study Group. Groupe d'étude Des Tumeurs à Calcitonine. *Clin. Endocrinol.* **1998**, *48*, 265–273. [CrossRef]
20. Matrone, A.; Gambale, C.; Prete, A.; Piaggi, P.; Cappagli, V.; Bottici, V.; Romei, C.; Ciampi, R.; Torregrossa, L.; De Napoli, L.; et al. Impact of Advanced Age on the Clinical Presentation and Outcome of Sporadic Medullary Thyroid Carcinoma. *Cancers* **2020**, *13*, 94. [CrossRef]
21. Mathiesen, J.S.; Kroustrup, J.P.; Vestergaard, P.; Stochholm, K.; Poulsen, P.L.; Rasmussen, Å.K.; Feldt-Rasmussen, U.; Schytte, S.; Londero, S.C.; Pedersen, H.B.; et al. Survival and Long-Term Biochemical Cure in Medullary Thyroid Carcinoma in Denmark 1997–2014: A Nationwide Study. *Thyroid* **2019**, *29*, 368–377. [CrossRef]
22. Machens, A.; Lorenz, K.; Weber, F.; Dralle, H. Genotype-Specific Progression of Hereditary Medullary Thyroid Cancer. *Hum. Mutat.* **2018**, *39*, 860–869. [CrossRef] [PubMed]
23. Loveday, C.; Josephs, K.; Chubb, D.; Gunning, A.; Izatt, L.; Tischkowitz, M.; Ellard, S.; Turnbull, C.P. Val804Met, the Most Frequent Pathogenic Mutation in RET, Confers a Very Low Lifetime Risk of Medullary Thyroid Cancer. *J. Clin. Endocrinol. Metab.* **2018**, *103*, 4275–4282. [CrossRef]
24. Mathiesen, J.S.; Nielsen, S.G.; Rasmussen, Å.K.; Kiss, K.; Wadt, K.; Hermann, A.P.; Nielsen, M.F.; Larsen, S.R.; Brusgaard, K.; Frederiksen, A.L.; et al. Variability in Medullary Thyroid Carcinoma in RET L790F Carriers: A Case Comparison Study of Index Patients. *Front. Endocrinol.* **2020**, *11*. [CrossRef] [PubMed]
25. Long, K.L.; Etzel, C.; Rich, T.; Hyde, S.; Perrier, N.D.; Graham, P.H.; Lee, J.E.; Hu, M.I.; Cote, G.J.; Gagel, R.; et al. All in the Family? Analyzing the Impact of Family History in Addition to Genotype on Medullary Thyroid Carcinoma Aggressiveness in MEN2A Patients. *Fam. Cancer* **2017**, *16*, 283–289. [CrossRef]
26. Signorini, P.S.; França, M.I.C.; Camacho, C.P.; Lindsey, S.C.; Valente, F.O.F.; Kasamatsu, T.S.; Machado, A.L.; Salim, C.P.; Delcelo, R.; Hoff, A.O.; et al. A Ten-Year Clinical Update of a LargeRETp.Gly533Cys Kindred with Medullary Thyroid Carcinoma Emphasizes the Need for an Individualized Assessment of Affected Relatives. *Clin. Endocrinol.* **2014**, *80*, 235–245. [CrossRef]
27. Lindskog, S.; Nilsson, O.; Jansson, S.; Nilsson, B.; Illerskog, A.; Ysander, L.; Ahlman, H.; Tisell, L. Phenotypic Expression of a Family with Multiple Endocrine Neoplasia Type 2A due to a RET Mutation at Codon 618. *Br. J. Surg* **2004**, *91*, 713–718. [CrossRef]
28. Lombardo, F.; Baudin, E.; Chiefari, E.; Arturi, F.; Bardet, S.; Caillou, B.; Conte, C.; Dallapiccola, B.; Giuffrida, D.; Bidart, J.-M.; et al. Familial Medullary Thyroid Carcinoma: Clinical Variability and Low Aggressiveness Associated withRETMutation at Codon 804. *J. Clin. Endocrinol. Metab.* **2002**, *87*, 1674–1680. [CrossRef]
29. Taeubner, J.; Wieczorek, D.; Yasin, L.; Brozou, T.; Borkhardt, A.; Kuhlen, M. Penetrance and Expressivity in Inherited Cancer Predisposing Syndromes. *Trends Cancer* **2018**, *4*, 718–728. [CrossRef]
30. Leung, A.K.C.; Leung, A.A.C. Evaluation and Management of the Child with Hypothyroidism. *World J. Pediatr.* **2019**, *15*, 124–134. [CrossRef]
31. Wiersinga, W.M. Paradigm Shifts in Thyroid Hormone Replacement Therapies for Hypothyroidism. *Nat. Rev. Endocrinol.* **2014**, *10*, 164–174. [CrossRef] [PubMed]
32. Ettleson, M.D.; Bianco, A.C. Individualized Therapy for Hypothyroidism: Is T4 Enough for Everyone? *J. Clin. Endocrinol. Metab.* **2020**, *105*, e3090–e3104. [CrossRef]
33. Gullo, D.; Latina, A.; Frasca, F.; Le Moli, R.; Pellegriti, G.; Vigneri, R. Levothyroxine Monotherapy Cannot Guarantee Euthyroidism in All Athyreotic Patients. *PLoS ONE* **2011**, *6*, e22552. [CrossRef]
34. Russell, M.D.; Kamani, D.; Randolph, G.W. Modern Surgery for Advanced Thyroid Cancer: A Tailored Approach. *Gland Surg.* **2020**, *9*, S105–S119. [CrossRef] [PubMed]
35. De Jong, M.; Nounou, H.; García, V.R.; Christakis, I.; Brain, C.; Abdel-Aziz, T.E.; Hewitt, R.J.; Kurzawinski, T.R. Children are at a High Risk of Hypocalcaemia and Hypoparathyroidism after Total Thyroidectomy. *J. Pediatr. Surg.* **2020**, *55*, 1260–1264. [CrossRef]
36. Kluijfhout, W.P.; van Beek, D.-J.; Stuart, A.A.V.; Lodewijk, L.; Valk, G.D.; van der Zee, D.C.; Vriens, M.R.; Rinkes, I.H.B. Postoperative Complications After Prophylactic Thyroidectomy for Very Young Patients With Multiple Endocrine Neoplasia Type 2.: Retrospective Cohort Analysis. *Medcine* **2015**, *94*, e1108. [CrossRef] [PubMed]
37. Machens, A.; Dralle, H. Advances in Risk-Oriented Surgery for Multiple Endocrine Neoplasia Type 2. *Endocr.-Relat. Cancer* **2018**, *25*, T41–T52. [CrossRef] [PubMed]

38. Youngwirth, L.M.; Adam, M.A.; Thomas, S.M.; Roman, S.A.; Sosa, J.A.; Scheri, R.P. Pediatric Thyroid Cancer Patients Referred to High-Volume Facilities have Improved Short-Term Outcomes. *Surgery* **2018**, *163*, 361–366. [CrossRef]
39. Tuggle, C.T.; Roman, S.A.; Wang, T.S.; Boudourakis, L.; Thomas, D.C.; Udelsman, R.; Sosa, J.A. Pediatric endocrine surgery: Who is operating on our children? *Surgery* **2008**, *144*, 869–877. [CrossRef] [PubMed]
40. Wu, S.-Y.; Chiang, Y.-J.; Fisher, S.B.; Sturgis, E.M.; Zafereo, M.E.; Nguyen, S.; Grubbs, E.G.; Graham, P.H.; Lee, J.E.; Waguespack, S.G.; et al. Risks of Hypoparathyroidism After Total Thyroidectomy in Children: A 21-Year Experience in a High-Volume Cancer Center. *World J. Surg.* **2020**, *44*, 442–451. [CrossRef]
41. Brinkman, T.M.; Recklitis, C.J.; Michel, G.; Grootenhuis, M.A.; Klosky, J.L. Psychological Symptoms, Social Outcomes, Socioeconomic Attainment, and Health Behaviors Among Survivors of Childhood Cancer: Current State of the Literature. *J. Clin. Oncol.* **2018**, *36*, 2190–2197. [CrossRef] [PubMed]
42. Brinkman, T.M.; Li, C.; Vannatta, K.; Marchak, J.G.; Lai, J.-S.; Prasad, P.K.; Kimberg, C.; Vuotto, S.; Di, C.; Srivastava, D.; et al. Behavioral, Social, and Emotional Symptom Comorbidities and Profiles in Adolescent Survivors of Childhood Cancer: A Report From the Childhood Cancer Survivor Study. *J. Clin. Oncol.* **2016**, *34*, 3417–3425. [CrossRef]
43. Zeltzer, L.K.; Recklitis, C.; Buchbinder, D.; Zebrack, B.; Casillas, J.; Tsao, J.C.I.; Lu, Q.; Krull, K. Psychological Status in Childhood Cancer Survivors: A Report from the Childhood Cancer Survivor Study. *J. Clin. Oncol.* **2009**, *27*, 2396–2404. [CrossRef] [PubMed]
44. Ford, J.S.; Kawashima, T.; Whitton, J.; Leisenring, W.; Laverdière, C.; Stovall, M.; Zeltzer, L.; Robison, L.L.; Sklar, C.A. Psychosexual Functioning among Adult Female Survivors of Childhood Cancer: A Report From the Childhood Cancer Survivor Study. *J. Clin. Oncol.* **2014**, *32*, 3126–3136. [CrossRef]
45. Ritenour, C.W.; Seidel, K.D.; Leisenring, W.; Mertens, A.C.; Wasilewski-Masker, K.; Shnorhavorian, M.; Sklar, C.A.; Whitton, J.A.; Stovall, M.; Constine, L.S.; et al. Erectile Dysfunction in Male Survivors of Childhood Cancer—A Report From the Childhood Cancer Survivor Study. *J. Sex. Med.* **2016**, *13*, 945–954. [CrossRef] [PubMed]
46. Allan, F.N. Education of the Diabetic Patient. *New Engl. J. Med.* **1963**, *268*, 93–95. [CrossRef] [PubMed]
47. Koch, L. Efficacy of behavioral interventions in patients with poorly controlled diabetes mellitus. *Nat. Rev. Endocrinol.* **2011**, *7*, 691. [CrossRef]

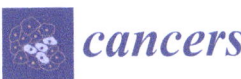

Article

Epithelial and Mesenchymal Markers in Adrenocortical Tissues: How Mesenchymal Are Adrenocortical Tissues?

Iuliu Sbiera [1], Stefan Kircher [2], Barbara Altieri [1], Martin Fassnacht [1,3,4], Matthias Kroiss [1,4,5,*] and Silviu Sbiera [1,*]

1 Department of Internal Medicine I, Division of Endocrinology and Diabetes, University Hospital Würzburg, 97080 Würzburg, Germany; e_sbiera_i@ukw.de (I.S.); Altieri_B@ukw.de (B.A.); Fassnacht_M@ukw.de (M.F.)
2 Institute for Pathology, University of Würzburg, 97080 Würzburg, Germany; stefan.kircher@uni-wuerzburg.de
3 Clinical Chemistry and Laboratory Medicine, University Hospital Würzburg, 97080 Würzburg, Germany
4 Comprehensive Cancer Center Mainfranken, University of Würzburg, 97080 Würzburg, Germany
5 Department of Internal Medicine IV, University Hospital Munich, Ludwig-Maximilians-Universität München, 80336 Munich, Germany
* Correspondence: Matthias.Kroiss@med.uni-muenchen.de (M.K.); Sbiera_S@ukw.de (S.S.)

Simple Summary: Recent studies have hinted to an involvement of epithelial to mesenchymal transition, a mechanism often associated with metastasis in epithelial cancers, in adrenocortical carcinoma. We assessed, in a large number of normal, benign and malignant adrenocortical tissues, the expression of canonical epithelial and mesenchymal markers and compared it with their expression in typical epithelial and mesenchymal tissues. Surprisingly, both normal and neoplastic adrenocortical tissues lacked expression of epithelial markers but strongly expressed mesenchymal markers, suggesting a higher similarity of adrenocortical tissues to mesenchymal compared to epithelial tissues, reminiscent of the adrenocortical origin from the intermediate mesoderm. Despite their ubiquitous expression in all adrenocortical tissues, mesenchymal markers had a variable expression in ACC, associating either directly or inversely with different clinical markers of tumor aggressiveness. Our data are an important step in better understanding the adrenocortical tissues in general and adrenocortical tumorigenesis in particular, and could be exploited therapeutically in the future.

Abstract: A clinically relevant proportion of adrenocortical carcinoma (ACC) cases shows a tendency to metastatic spread. The objective was to determine whether the epithelial to mesenchymal transition (EMT), a mechanism associated with metastasizing in several epithelial cancers, might play a crucial role in ACC. 138 ACC, 29 adrenocortical adenomas (ACA), three normal adrenal glands (NAG), and control tissue samples were assessed for the expression of epithelial (E-cadherin and EpCAM) and mesenchymal (N-cadherin, SLUG and SNAIL) markers by immunohistochemistry. Using real-time RT-PCR we quantified the alternative isoform splicing of FGFR 2 and 3, another known indicator of EMT. We also assessed the impact of these markers on clinical outcome. Results show that both normal and neoplastic adrenocortical tissues lacked expression of epithelial markers but strongly expressed mesenchymal markers N-cadherin and SLUG. FGFR isoform splicing confirmed higher similarity of adrenocortical tissues to mesenchymal compared to epithelial tissues. In ACC, higher SLUG expression was associated with clinical markers indicating aggressiveness, while N-cadherin expression inversely associated with these markers. In conclusion, we could not find any indication of EMT as all adrenocortical tissues lacked expression of epithelial markers and exhibited closer similarity to mesenchymal tissues. However, while N-cadherin might play a positive role in tissue structure upkeep, SLUG seems to be associated with a more aggressive phenotype.

Keywords: adrenocortical tissues; EMT; epithelial markers; mesenchymal markers; recurrence-free survival

Citation: Sbiera, I.; Kircher, S.; Altieri, B.; Fassnacht, M.; Kroiss, M.; Sbiera, S. Epithelial and Mesenchymal Markers in Adrenocortical Tissues: How Mesenchymal Are Adrenocortical Tissues?. *Cancers* 2021, 13, 1736. https://doi.org/10.3390/cancers13071736

Academic Editor: Christofer Juhlin

Received: 17 March 2021
Accepted: 4 April 2021
Published: 6 April 2021

Publisher's Note: MDPI stays neutral with regard to jurisdictional claims in published maps and institutional affiliations.

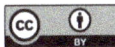

Copyright: © 2021 by the authors. Licensee MDPI, Basel, Switzerland. This article is an open access article distributed under the terms and conditions of the Creative Commons Attribution (CC BY) license (https://creativecommons.org/licenses/by/4.0/).

1. Introduction

Adrenocortical carcinoma (ACC) is a rare endocrine malignancy and its pathogenesis is poorly understood. Complete surgical resection is the treatment of choice in localized ACC and is virtually the only option to achieve a cure. As recurrence is frequent, adjuvant therapy is recommended in most patients [1–4]. Several genomic studies have been performed in adrenocortical tumors with the goal to better understand the mechanisms that lead to tumorigenesis, hormone excess and malignancy [5–8]. Using clustering of genome wide data, these studies consistently identified a subgroup of highly malignant tumors characterized by enhanced genomic variability and altered gene expression [9,10].

In irresectable and metastatic disease, cytotoxic chemotherapy is the standard treatment. The first and largest randomized phase III study in advanced ACC established etoposide, doxorubicin, cisplatin plus mitotane (EDP-M) as the cytotoxic chemotherapy of first choice in metastatic ACC [11]. With a median progression-free survival of only 5.0 months and an overall survival of only 14.8 months in the group receiving EDP-M, the prognosis is still poor. In the meantime, several other therapeutic approaches have been investigated [12–16], but a clinically meaningful breakthrough has not yet been achieved.

Epithelial-mesenchymal transition (EMT) is a process that was first recognized as a feature of embryogenesis and, together with its reverse process MET (mesenchymal-epithelial transition), plays a crucial role in the development of many tissues and organs [17,18]. Most importantly, the mechanism of EMT, which allows the epithelial tumor cells to acquire a motile mesenchymal phenotype [19], is diverted by several types of cancer to promote metastasis and resistance to treatment [20]. This process has been considered to be implicated in metastatic spread of such a large variety of human cancers like breast, prostate, lung etc. [21–23] (Figure 1).

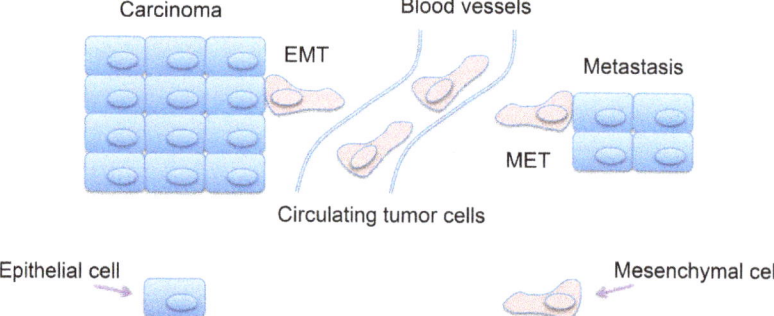

Figure 1. Classical EMT in cancer cells. Upper panel: EMT (Epithelial to Mesenchymal Transition) and MET (Mesenchymal to Epithelial Transition) processes in metastatic spread. Lower panel: Canonical markers of epithelial (left) and mesenchymal (right) cells.

Around 90% of all malignancies originate from epithelial tissue. The adrenocortical tissue is also classically categorized as an epithelial tissue. Studies on the adrenal cortex place its origins in the intermediate mesoderm (mesenchymal) [24], but it is considered to have undergone MET to an epithelial tissue [25]. Accordingly, adrenal tumors are also classified as carcinomas (tumors of an epithelial tissue) [26] as opposed to sarcomas (tumors of a mesenchymal tissue) [27]. Two studies have provided a first indication that adrenocortical tissues are expressing some mesenchymal markers [28,29]. However, the number of adrenocortical carcinoma tissues analyzed in these studies was low (24 cases in each study) and a correlation between EMT marker expression and clinicopathological markers indicative of tumor aggressiveness was not possible.

A number of distinct molecular processes participate in EMT like activation of transcription factors, expression of specific cell-surface proteins, reorganization and expression of cytoskeletal proteins etc. In many cases, the factors involved are also used as biomarkers to demonstrate that a specific cell is undergoing EMT [20]. For example, E-cadherin and epithelial cell adhesion molecule (EpCAM) are considered as classical epithelial markers while N-cadherin, SNAIL and SLUG are considered mesenchymal markers [30]. In addition, at mRNA level, the expression of the epithelial (IIIB) and mesenchymal (IIIC) isoforms of FGFR 2 and 3 can be also used to characterize EMT [31] (Figure 1).

Epithelial cell adhesion molecule (EpCAM) is a transmembrane glycoprotein mediating Ca^{2+}-independent homotypic cell–cell adhesion in epithelia [32] associating with the actin cytoskeleton via an intermediate molecule [33]. Epithelial tumors are often characterized by strong expression of EpCAM while its expression is downregulated during EMT but then upregulated once the metastasis reaches its future tumor site, where the MET process is supposed to take place [34].

E-cadherin and N-cadherin are classical cadherins and share similar structures. They form cadherin-catenin complex where the cytoplasmic domain consists of EC repeats that bind with catenins to moderate the cytoskeletal filament containing actin. The structural difference between E-cadherin and N-cadherin is that E-cadherin binds with the shorter isoform of p120 catenin while N-cadherin binds with the longer isoform and the switch from E-cadherin expression to N-cadherin, which mediates weaker cell-cell interactions is classically used as a mesenchymal marker to define EMT [35]. N-cadherin is also present in few epithelial tissues such as hepatocytes but only together with a much stronger E-cadherin expression [30].

Snail and Slug (SNAI1 and SNAI 2), are two transcription factors that suppress E-cadherin and lead to a decrease in cell-to-cell adhesion and are also commonly used to detect EMT [36,37]. Knockout models for both SNAIL and SLUG showed significant reduction in cancer invasiveness [38,39].

At mRNA level, the fibroblast growth factors receptors (FGFR) isoform switching is another model that can be used as a marker for EMT. Fibroblast growth factor receptors (FGFRs) are a family of receptor tyrosine kinases expressed on the cell membrane that play crucial roles in both developmental and adult cells. The fibroblast growth factor receptor family has 4 members, FGFR1, FGFR2, FGFR3, and FGFR4 [40]. The FGFRs consist of three extracellular immunoglobulin-type domains (D1-D3), a single-span trans-membrane domain and an intracellular split tyrosine kinase domain. FGFs interact with the D2 and D3 domains, with the D3 interactions primarily responsible for ligand-binding specificity [40]. The receptors 1 to 3 have the unique feature of having two isoforms due to alternative splicing of the D3 domain which changes the specificity [41]. For the FGFRs 2 and 3 it has been shown that the isoform IIIB is mainly present in epithelial cells while the isoform IIIC is mostly mesenchymal [31,42].

We hypothesized that EMT may be relevant for the subgroup of highly aggressive ACCs and investigated the expression of several EMT markers in a large cohort of adrenocortical carcinoma tissue samples (including also normal adrenals and benign adrenocortical tumors) and correlated them with clinical features and patient outcome.

2. Materials and Methods
2.1. Patient Material

Formalin fixed, paraffin embedded (FFPE) tissue samples of ACC (n = 138; a total of 122 samples were previously assembled in seven tissue microarrays/TMAs [43]), adrenocortical adenomas (ACA, n = 29), as well as normal adrenal glands resulting from kidney cancer surgery (NAG, n = 3) were analyzed. All patients gave informed consent and the study was approved by the ethical committee of the University of Würzburg (88/11). This cohort was clinically annotated and the data were collected through the registry of the

European Network for the Study of Adrenal Cancer (ENSAT). A short clinical description of the patients can be found in Table 1. For establishment of the detection of the different epithelial markers we used tissues from two normal thyroid, three thyroid carcinoma and three colon carcinoma. For establishment of the detection of the different mesenchymal markers we used tissues from one osteosarcoma, one liposarcoma, one leiomyosarcoma and one pleomorphic sarcoma.

Table 1. Patient clinical characteristics.

	Normal Adrenal Gland	ACA	ACC
n	3	29	138
Sex [male/female]	1/2	11/18	45/93
Age [yr (sd)]	49 (11)	51 (14)	50 (15)
Size of the tumor [cm (sd)]		3.3 (1.2)	10 (4.4)
Hormone secretion			
Cortisol—n (%)		11 (38%)	50 (37%)
Androgen—n (%)		0 (0%)	10 (7%)
Aldosterone—n (%)		7 (24%)	4 (3%)
Inactive—n (%)		11 (38%)	21 (15%)
Unknown—n (%)		0 (0%)	53 (38%)
Tumor localization—n (%)			
Primary—ENSAT stage I+II			44 (32%)
Primary—ENSAT stage III			37 (27%)
Primary—ENSAT stage IV			25 (18%)
Local recurrences			21 (15%)
Distant metastases			11 (8%)
Ki67 index [median (range)]			10 (1–70)
Weiss Score [median (range)]			5 (2–9)

For the evaluation of the FGFR 1-3 isoforms at mRNA levels, we used available frozen tissue from 18 ACA and NAG, 21 ACC, 6 sarcoma (2× osteosarcoma, 2× liposarcoma, 1× synovialsarcoma, 1× rhabdomyosarcoma), 5 epithelial tumors (3 colon carcinoma, 1 thyroid carcinoma, 1 ovarian carcinoma), as well as four different ACC cell lines (NCI-H295R [44], MUC-1 [45], CU-ACC1 and CU-ACC2 [46]).

2.2. Immunohistochemistry

The immunohistochemistry procedure is explained in more detail elsewhere [43]. In short, the FFPE TMA and full tissue slices of ~2 μm thickness were mounted on SuperFrost glass slides (Langenbrinck, Emmendingen, Germany), deparaffinized in xylene, and rehydrated in a series of water in alcohol dilutions. Antigen retrieval was achieved by boiling in 1 mM citrate buffer (pH 6.5) inside a pressure cooker for 13 min. Endogenous peroxidase was blocked with a 3% solution of hydrogen peroxide in methanol for 10 min, followed by the blocking of non-specific binding for another 10 min with the help of a 20% solution of human AB serum in PBS. The primary antibodies used were: E-Cadherin (Sigma-Aldrich, St. Louis, MO, USA, mouse monoclonal, clone CL1172, 1:2250 dilution), EpCAM (abcam, Cambridge, UK, rabbit polyclonal (ab71916), 1:20000 dilution), N-Cadherin (Santa Cruz Biotechnology, Dallas, TX, USA, mouse monoclonal, clone D-4, 1:125 dilution), SLUG (Novus Biologicals, Centennial, CO, USA, mouse monoclonal, clone OTI1A6, 1:300 dilution) and SNAIL (kindly provided as a gift from Dr. A. García de Herreros, University Pompeu Fabra, Barcelona, Spain; clone EC3, subclone EC11, 1:50 dilution [47]). Incubation time for the primary antibodies was 1 h at room temperature in PBS. Signal amplification was done with "HiDef Detection HRP Polymer System" (Cell Marque, Rocklin, CA, USA) and the signal was developed using the chromogen DAB substrate kit (Cell Marque) for 10 min. Counterstaining of nuclei was performed using Meyer's Hematoxylin for 2 min (Carl Roth, Karlsruhe, Germany), followed by washing in running tap water for 5 min. After dehydration, slides were mounted using Entellan (Merck, Darmstadt, Germany) and borosilicate glass coverslips (A. Hartenstein, Würzburg, Germany).

Stained tissue slides were imaged with the Leica Aperio Versa brightfield scanning microscope (Leica, Wetzlar, Germany) and evaluated using a semi-quantitative H-Score [48] that estimated the intensity of the staining [scored as negative (0), low (1), medium (2) and high (3)] and the percentage of positive cells (scored as 0, 0.1, 0.5, or 1 if 0%, 1–9%, 10–49%, or $\geq$50% of the cells were positive, respectively). All slides were evaluated by two independent investigators blinded to clinical data. Low expression was defined as H-score < 2 and high score as H-score $\geq$ 2.

2.3. Cell Culture

NCI-H295R cells were obtained from ATCC and cultured in DMEM/F12 supplemented with 1× Insulin-Transferrin-Selenium and Nu-Serum (2.5%). CU-ACC1 and CU-ACC2 cells were obtained from Katja Kiseljak-Vassiliades and cultured as described [46]. In brief, a 1:3 mixture of F12 Ham and DMEM high glucose (both Thermo Fisher Scientific, Waltham, MA, USA) was supplemented with 10% FCS, 0.4 µg/mL hydrocortisone (Sigma-Aldrich), 5 µg/mL insulin (Sigma-Aldrich), 8.4 ng/mL cholera toxin (Sigma-Aldrich), 24 µg/mL adenine (Sigma-Aldrich) and 10 ng/mL EGF (Thermo Fisher Scientific). MUC-1 were obtained from Constanze Hantel and cultured in DMEM Advance 1% penicilin/streptomycin and 10% FCS as described [45].

2.4. Real-Time PCR

RNA was first extracted from frozen tissues using the RNeasy Lipid Tissue Kit (Qiagen, Düsseldorf, Germany) and reverse transcribed using the High-Capacity cDNA Reverse Transcription Kit (Thermo Fisher Scientific). TaqMan Gene Expression Assay (Thermo Fisher Scientific) was used with the Hs01005396_m1 (FGFR3 IIIB) and Hs00997397_m1 (FGFR3 IIIC) probes and the following custom primers/probes for FGFR2 receptor isoforms [49]:

FGFR2 IIIb fw: 5'-GGCTCTGTTCAATGTGACCGA-3'; rev: 5'-GTTGGCCTGCCCTAT ATAATTGGA-3'; TaqMan probe: 5'-TTTCCCCAGCATCCGCC-3'

FGFR2 IIIc up: 5'-CACGGACAAAGAGATTGAGGTTCT-3'; low: 5'-CCGCCAAGCA CGTATATTCC-3'; TaqMan probe: 5'-CCAGCGTCCTCAAAAG-3'

The expression of β-actin (Hs9999903_m1) was used for normalization. Amplification and results evaluation were performed using a Bio-Rad CFX-96 Dx system (Bio-Rad Laboratories, Hercules, CA, USA).

2.5. Statistical Analyses

The relationship between two categorical variables was determined using the Chi square test. For non-parametrical multiple comparisons between groups the Kruskal-Wallis test with Dunn's post-hoc comparison was used. A p-value < 0.05 was considered statistically significant. p-values between 0.05 and 0.15 were considered indicative of a statistical trend. All statistical analyses were performed with Graph Pad Prism v 7 for Windows (GrapPad Software Inc., La Jolla, CA, USA). For ACC patients, the Kaplan-Meier method was used to estimate overall survival (OS, in all patients with primary tumors) and recurrence-free survival (RFS, in patients with complete resection of the primary tumor) using IBM SPSS v 26 for Windows (SPSS Inc., Chicago, IL, USA). After $\approx$10% of subjects remaining at risk the Kaplan-Meier survival was curtailed.

3. Results

3.1. Typical Epithelial Adhesion Markers Are Not Expressed in Adrenocortical Tissues

The expression of E-cadherin, was absent in all adrenal tissues analyzed (n = 170), both normal and tumoral (Figure 2B–E), while this marker showed a normal, membrane expression in 14 different epithelial tissues analyzed (Figure 2A,E). Similar results were also observed for EpCAM, which was also completely missing in all adrenocortical tissues analyzed (Figure 2G–J) while strong expression of this marker in classical epithelial tissues was observed that were used as positive controls (Figure 2F,J).

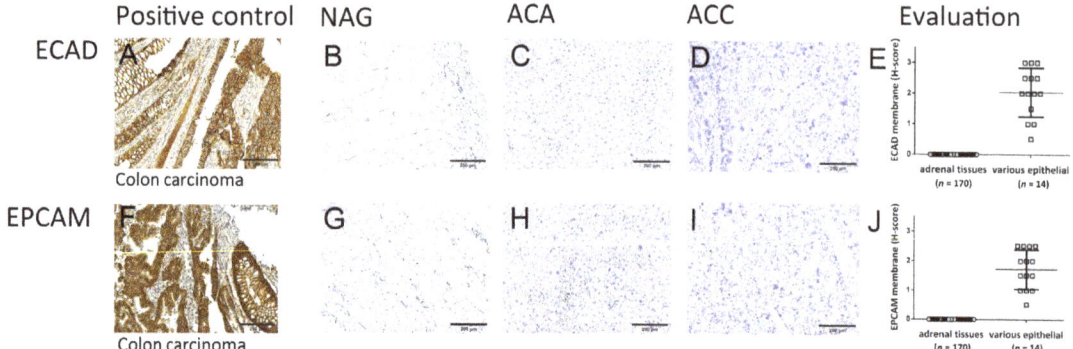

Figure 2. Expression of canonical immunohistochemical epithelial markers in adrenocortical tissues. Staining of epithelial markers E-cadherin (**A–E**) and Epithelial Cell Adhesion Molecule (EpCAM) (**F–J**) protein in classical epithelial tissues (**A,F**) vs. normal adrenal glands (NAG, $n = 3$; **B,G**) vs. adrenocortical adenomas (ACA, $n = 29$; **C,H**) vs. adrenocortical carcinomas (ACC, $n = 138$; **D,I**). Scale bar = 200 μm. Quantitative evaluation in (**E,J**), respectively.

3.2. Adrenocortical Tissues Are Characterized by Relatively High Expression of Mesenchymal Markers

Surprisingly, membrane N-cadherin expression was expressed in normal adrenocortical tissues at high levels (H-score 2.5 ± 0.5, Figure 3B,E). The expression was distributed rather equally between the three functional regions, with slightly lower expression in the zona fasciculata (Supplementary Figure S1A–C). Most adrenocortical adenomas and carcinomas demonstrated moderate to high expression (ACA mean H-score 1.8 ± 0.7; Figure 3C,E, ACC 1.6 ± 0.9; Figure 3D,E) similar to the mesenchymal sarcomas (1.9 ± 0.8; Figure 3A,E). There were no significant differences between the different adrenocortical tissues, only a trend (NAG vs. ACA: $p = 0.14$, NAG vs. ACC: $p = 0.09$ and ACA vs. ACC: $p = 0.20$), however, interestingly, the variability of expression of N-cadherin increased gradually from NAG to ACA and then to ACC (Figure 3E) as shown by increasing coefficients of variation (NAG 20.00%, ACA 39.25% and ACC 58.53%; mesenchymal 45.54%).

While Snail nuclear expression was found in most mesenchymal tissues tested (Figure 3F,J), detectable expression was not observed in any of the adrenocortical tissues (Figure 3G–I and evaluation in Figure 3J). In contrast, a strong expression of Slug was found in both mesenchymal tissues (mean H-score 2.3 ± 0.5; Figure 3K,O) and normal and benign adrenal tissues without statistically significant differences among groups (NAG mean H-score 2.3 ± 0.5, ACA 2.2 ± 0.7; Figure 3L,M,O) but variable expression in ACC (mean H-score 1.6 ± 1.1; Figure 3N,O).

Only the expression in ACC was significantly different compared to the other two adrenocortical sample sets (NAG vs. ACA: $p = 0.79$, NAG vs. ACC: $p = 0.02$ and ACA vs. ACC: $p = 0.01$*) but as with N-cadherin, the variability of expression of SLUG increased gradually from NAG to ACA and then to ACC (Figure 3O) as shown by increasing coefficients of variation (NAG 24.74%, ACA 34.29% and ACC 68.77%; mesenchymal 20.16%). Interestingly, in the normal adrenal gland tissue the most nuclei stained positive were localized in the subcapsular region, in the zona glomerulosa (Supplementary Figure S1D–F).

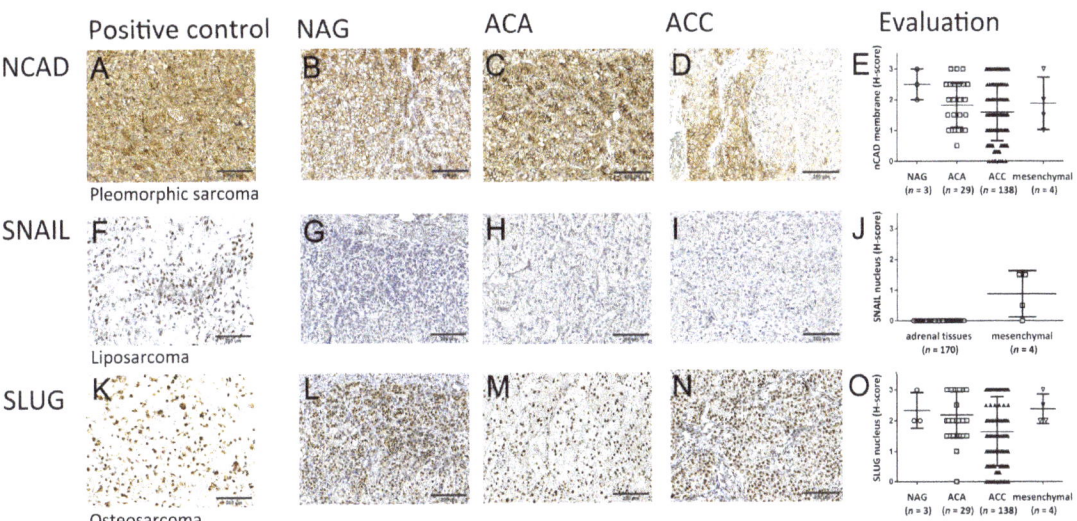

Figure 3. Expression of canonical immunohistochemical mesenchymal markers in adrenocortical tissues. Staining of mesenchymal markers N-cadherin (**A–E**), Zinc finger protein SNAI1 (SNAIL) (**F–J**) and Zinc finger protein SNAI2 (SLUG) (**K–O**) in classical mesenchymal cancers (**A,F,K**) vs. normal adrenal glands (NAG, $n = 3$; **B,G,L**) vs. adrenocortical adenomas (ACA, $n = 29$; **C,H,M**) and vs. adrenocortical carcinomas (ACC, $n = 138$; **D,I,N**). Scale bar = 200 µm. Quantitative evaluation in (**E,J,O**), respectively.

3.3. FGFR1-3 Isotype Expression Shows a Pattern Similar to Mesenchymal Tissues

To further elucidate the epithelial vs. mesenchymal phenotype of adrenocortical tumors, we used the ratio between the "mesenchymal" IIIC and the "epithelial" IIIB isotypes of FGFR 2-3 in a subgroup of fresh frozen adrenocortical tissue samples and cell lines. Isoform IIIC of FGFR 2 was expressed on average 4.6 times higher than IIIB in all adrenocortical tissues studied (Figure 4A) (ratio IIIC/IIIB: 5.1 ± 2.6 for the normal adrenal glands and adrenocortical adenomas vs. 4.2 ± 2 for the ACC samples vs. 4.8 ± 1.2 for ACC cell-lines) similar to the mesenchymal sarcomas (2.8 ± 0.8), but in contrast to the epithelial samples where the IIIB isoform was higher expressed than the IIIC isoform, as expected (ratio IIIB/IIIC: 3.9 ± 2.3). For FGFR 3 the IIIC/IIIB ratios were even higher (Figure 4B) (12.2 ± 5.5 for the normal adrenal glands and adrenocortical adenomas vs. 11.9 ± 7.7 for the ACC samples vs. 11.7 ± 3.2 for ACC cell-lines) similar again to the mesenchymal sarcomas (9.1 ± 7.1). The epithelial control tissues showed again, as expected, higher IIIB than IIIC expression (ratio IIIB/IIIC: 25.1 ± 18.4).

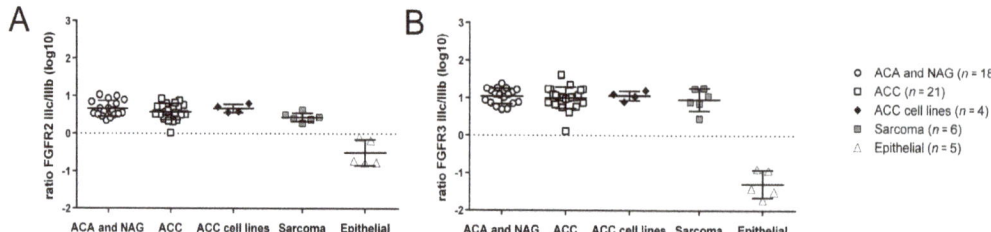

Figure 4. Differential expression of FGFR splice variants mRNA in adrenocortical tissues. Analysis of the ratios between the "mesenchymal" (IIIC) and "epithelial" (IIIB) splice variants for FGFR-2 (**A**) and 3 (**B**), in normal adrenal glands (NAG), adrenocortical adenomas (ACA) and carcinomas (ACC) as compared to mesenchymal sarcomas and canonical epithelial tissues; for better visualization of the isoform switch, results are represented in log10 base.

3.4. SLUG and N-Cadherine Are Associated in an Opposite Manner with Pathoclinical Tumor Aggressiveness Parameters

Since expression of NCAD and SLUG showed an increase in variability from normal, to benign, to malignant adrenocortical tissues, this suggested a modulation of these factors during the tumorigenesis and tumor progression. Therefore we looked for possible associations between different expression levels of NCAD and SLUG and indicators of tumoral metastatic potential. The presence of venous infiltration was associated with high (H-score $\geq$ 2) vs. low (H-score < 2) expression of SLUG (31 vs. 44%, χ^2 = 3.6, p = 0.05) (Figure 5A), but with lower expression of N-cadherin (28 vs. 46%, χ^2 = 6.9, p = 0.008) (Figure 5B). Similarly, lymph node infiltration was significantly more often present in tumors with high SLUG expression (23% vs. 12%, χ^2 = 4.2, p = 0.04) (Figure 5C) and with low N-cadherin expression (26% vs. 9%, χ^2 = 10.0, p = 0.001) (Figure 5D). Unsurprisingly, also the mixed pathomorphological diagnostic Weiss score, an indicator for tumor malignancy, was significantly higher for samples with low NCAD expression (6.0 $\pm$ 1.5 vs. 4.7 $\pm$ 1.6, p < 0.001) (Figure 5F), and for samples with high SLUG expression (6.0 $\pm$ 1.9 vs. 5.1 $\pm$ 1.5, p = 0.04) (Figure 5E). A Mann-Whitney test of the distribution of N-cadherin and SLUG expression in tumors with low and high expression of the proliferation marker Ki67, the best defined prognostic marker for the ACC [50], confirmed this association. In tumors with high Ki67 expression the SLUG expression was significantly higher (2.2 $\pm$ 0.9 vs. 1.5 $\pm$ 1.1, p = 0.03) (Figure 5G) while the expression of N-cadherin was significantly lower (1.1 $\pm$ 0.6 vs. 1.5 $\pm$ 0.9, p = 0.04) (Figure 5H).

3.5. SLUG and N-Cadherin Expression Have a Divergent Association with ACC Patients' Progression-Free Survival

We next investigated a potential association of SLUG and N-cadherin expression with patient outcome and found no difference on OS (low vs. high SLUG expression: Average survival time 64.20 $\pm$ 10.27 vs. 68.82 $\pm$ 9.14 months, HR = 1.15, 95%CI: 0.5–1.5, p = 0.79 and low vs. high N-cadherin expression: Mean survival time 65.11 $\pm$ 9.49 vs. 71.22 $\pm$ 10.66 months, HR = 0.81, 95%CI: 0.48–1.37, p = 0.44) (Figure 6A,B) and only a trend that high SLUG expression correlated with a less favorable RFS in ACC patients after complete resection (high vs. low SLUG expression: Mean survival time 25.96 $\pm$ 5.40 vs. 49.82 $\pm$ 10.12 months, HR = 2.15, 95% CI: 0.96–4.83, p = 0.056) (Figure 6C). For N-cadherin the situation was opposite, while again not statistically significant, there was a light trend that high N-cadherin expression correlated with a better progression-free survival (mean survival time 40.12 $\pm$ 8.35 vs. 21.32 $\pm$ 6.6 months, HR = 0.65, 95% CI: 0.34–1.11, p = 0.14) (Figure 6D).

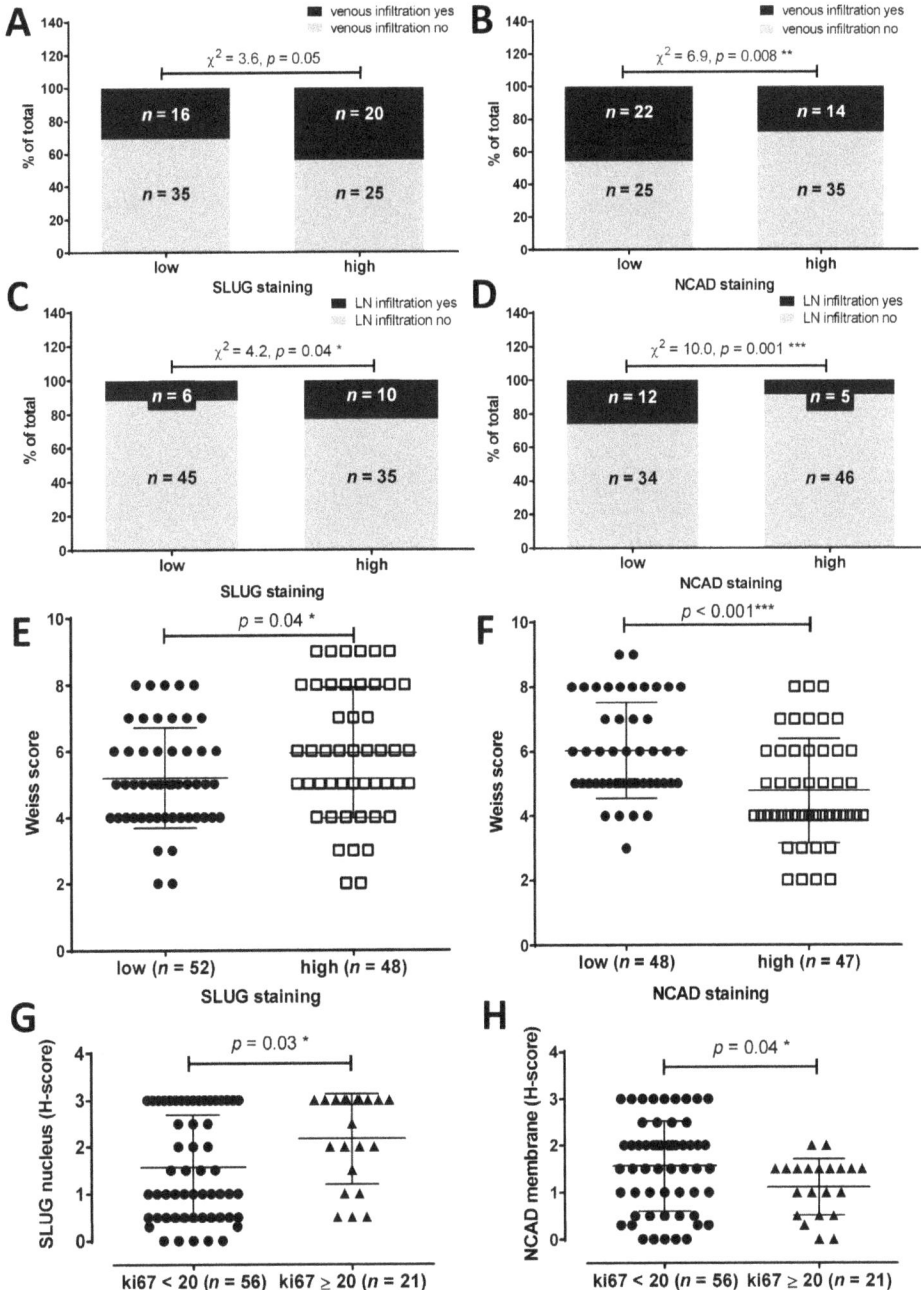

Figure 5. Comparison between relevant clinicopathological data and expression levels of mesenchymal markers SLUG and N-Cadherin. (**A**,**B**) venous tumor infiltration, (**C**,**D**) lymph node tumor infiltration, (**E**,**F**) Weiss score distribution and (**G**,**H**) proliferation marker Ki67. "*n*" numbers represent the absolute number of cases in each subgroup. χ^2 analyses have been performed between proportions (%) in each staining intensity group. * $p < 0.05$, ** $p < 0.01$, *** $p < 0.001$.

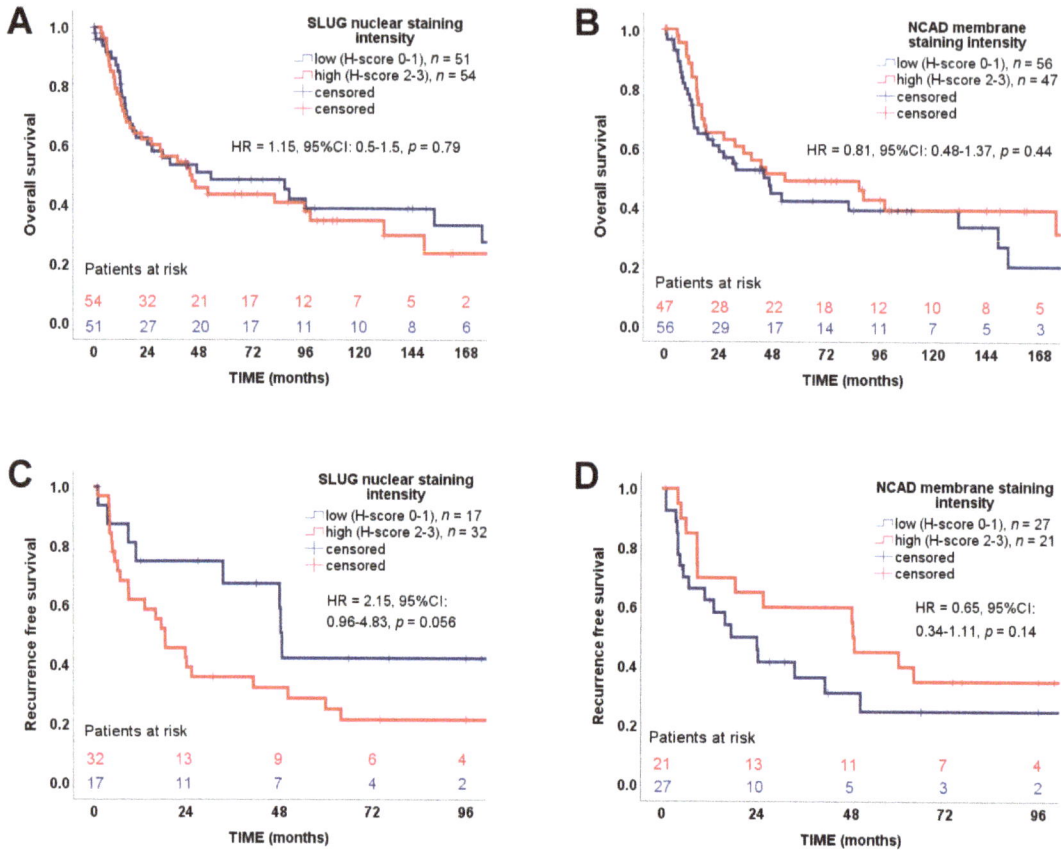

Figure 6. Correlation of patient survival with expression of mesenchymal markers SLUG and N-Cadherin. (**A**,**B**) overall survival (**C**,**D**) recurrence-free survival.

4. Discussion

In this study we investigated a series of both classical epithelial and mesenchymal markers in a large cohort of normal, benign and malignant adrenocortical tissues, and compared the expression of these markers with that in epithelial and mesenchymal control tissues. Against our hypothesis, our analysis revealed that in adrenocortical tumors EMT indicated by a more frequent occurrence of mesenchymal markers in neoplastic tissue, does not appear to play a role in tumor progression as suggested before in smaller studies [28,29]. Adrenocortical tissues do not express established epithelial markers like E-cadherin and EpCAM but express a series of "classical" mesenchymal markers like Slug and N-cadherin at similar levels as mesenchymal tissues.

By using the more recently discovered marker of alternative mRNA splicing of the FGFR2 and 3 [42,51–53] we confirmed that adrenocortical tissues are more similar to mesenchymal than to epithelial tissues. This may be due to the special case of adrenocortical tissue as it originates during embryogenesis from the intermediate mesoderm, but is considered to undergo MET to result in an epithelial tissue [25]. Obviously, this epithelial transformation is incomplete and the adrenal cortex keeps most of its mesenchymal characteristics at molecular level.

While expressed in all adrenocortical tissues, there may still be a role of mesenchymal differentiation status in tumor aggressiveness. While higher SLUG expression is associated with more aggressive behavior of the tumors as indicated by its association with markers for lymphatic and hematogenic metastasizing and high cell proliferation, N-cadherin appears to play the role of major cell- cell adhesion molecule in the adrenocortical tissue and thus is a counterplayer of SLUG. There are also other tissues where N-cadherin is the prevalent constituent of adherens junctions such as neural tissues [54]. It is hence likely that adherens junctions in adrenocortical tissue are predominantly mediated by N-cadherin instead of the E-cadherin, which is more commonly found in epithelial adherens junctions. However, only future studies at a deeper molecular level on the cell-to-cell interactions in the adrenal will be able to definitely answer this question.

Interestingly, SLUG nuclear expression in the normal adrenal gland was highest in the subcapsular area of the zona glomerulosa. This zone accommodates a subset of cells that have been reported to centripetally migrate towards the center of the gland and are responsible for the permanent renewal of the adrenocortical tissue [55]. The idea of a progenitor cell population that gives rise to all differentiated cell types within the adrenal cortex is old [56,57], but while its subcapsular localization has been clarified using animal models [58,59], there is not yet an universally accepted immunohistochemical marker that can be used to identify this population. It has been shown that Wnt, β-catenin and Shh all play an important role in this process [60–62], however, their expression in the adult adrenal cortex did not coincide with cell-proliferation markers [63] so they cannot be used to identify the progenitor cell population. The best candidate to date is the Notch atypical ligand Delta-like homologue 1 (DLK1) [64].

It would have been especially interesting to correlate in more detail the expression of SLUG and N-cadehrin in metastases with clinicopathological characteristics of the same, especially KI67. However, these data have been inconsistently retrieved in the past and the rarity of ACC renders the collection of such a larger series of clinically well-annotated cases prospectively quite challenging. Another limitation is the perceived limited choice of both epithelial and mesenchymal markers analyzed. While the list of possible specific markers is very long [20], we have concentrated on the best defined and used markers in each category. But we did not limit ourselves to immunohistological staining investigating also markers defined at mRNA level, thus covering quite a broad selection of pathways involved in cell adhesion, migration and response to external stimuli. The results of all these analyses corroborated with each other to give a synchronized picture on the role played by these markers in the adrenal tissues.

5. Conclusions

We could show that adrenocortical tissues, whether normal, benign or malignant, are characterized by lack of expression of classical epithelial tissues and are closer to mesenchymal tissues through high expression of classical mesenchymal markers like N-cadherin and SLUG. These factors also appear to play a role in cancer progression in ACC: While N-cadherin seems to have a positive role in the tissue structure sustainability and against metastatic spread, SLUG seems to promote this.

Supplementary Materials: The following are available online at https://www.mdpi.com/article/10.3390/cancers13071736/s1, Figure S1: Expression of canonical immunohistochemical mesenchymal markers in normal adrenal gland.

Author Contributions: Conceptualization, M.F., M.K. and S.S.; methodology, I.S.; software, I.S. and S.S.; validation, I.S., S.K. and B.A.; formal analysis, I.S. and S.S.; investigation, I.S.; resources, S.K. and B.A.; data curation, I.S. and B.A.; writing—original draft preparation, I.S., M.F., M.K. and S.S.; writing—review and editing, I.S., S.K., B.A., M.F., M.K. and S.S.; visualization, I.S. and S.S.; supervision, M.F., M.K., S.S.; project administration, S.S.; funding acquisition, M.F., M.K., S.S. All authors have read and agreed to the published version of the manuscript.

Funding: This study was supported by the Else Kröner-Fresenius Foundation (Else Kröner-Fresenius-Stiftung; project number: 2016_A96 to SS and MK and the German Research Foundation (Deutsche Forschungsgemeinschaft; project numbers 314061271—CRC/TRR 205 and 237292849 to MF and MK).

Institutional Review Board Statement: The study was conducted according to the guidelines of the Declaration of Helsinki, and approved by the Ethics Committee of the University of Würzburg (approval # 88/11).

Informed Consent Statement: Informed consent was obtained from all subjects involved in the study.

Data Availability Statement: All data presented in this study is contained within the article and supplementary material.

Acknowledgments: This publication was supported by the Open Access Publication Fund of the University of Würzburg.

Conflicts of Interest: The authors declare no conflict of interest. The funders had no role in the design of the study; in the collection, analyses, or interpretation of data; in the writing of the manuscript, or in the decision to publish the results.

References

1. Fassnacht, M.; Dekkers, O.M.; Else, T.; Baudin, E.; Berruti, A.; de Krijger, R.; Haak, H.R.; Mihai, R.; Assie, G.; Terzolo, M. European Society of Endocrinology Clinical Practice Guidelines on the management of adrenocortical carcinoma in adults, in collaboration with the European Network for the Study of Adrenal Tumors. *Eur. J. Endocrinol.* **2018**, *179*, G1–G46. [CrossRef]
2. Fassnacht, M.; Assie, G.; Baudin, E.; Eisenhofer, G.; de la Fouchardiere, C.; Haak, H.R.; de Krijger, R.; Porpiglia, F.; Terzolo, M.; Berruti, A.; et al. Adrenocortical carcinomas and malignant phaeochromocytomas: ESMO-EURACAN Clinical Practice Guidelines for diagnosis, treatment and follow-up. *Ann. Oncol.* **2020**, *31*, 1476–1490. [CrossRef]
3. Jasim, S.; Habra, M.A. Management of Adrenocortical Carcinoma. *Curr. Oncol. Rep.* **2019**, *21*, 20. [CrossRef]
4. Else, T.; Kim, A.C.; Sabolch, A.; Raymond, V.M.; Kandathil, A.; Caoili, E.M.; Jolly, S.; Miller, B.S.; Giordano, T.J.; Hammer, G.D. Adrenocortical carcinoma. *Endocr. Rev.* **2014**, *35*, 282–326. [CrossRef]
5. Assie, G.; Letouze, E.; Fassnacht, M.; Jouinot, A.; Luscap, W.; Barreau, O.; Omeiri, H.; Rodriguez, S.; Perlemoine, K.; Rene-Corail, F.; et al. Integrated genomic characterization of adrenocortical carcinoma. *Nat. Genet.* **2014**, *46*, 607–612. [CrossRef] [PubMed]
6. Giordano, T.J.; Kuick, R.; Else, T.; Gauger, P.G.; Vinco, M.; Bauersfeld, J.; Sanders, D.; Thomas, D.G.; Doherty, G.; Hammer, G. Molecular classification and prognostication of adrenocortical tumors by transcriptome profiling. *Clin. Cancer Res.* **2009**, *15*, 668–676. [CrossRef] [PubMed]
7. Zheng, S.Y.; Cherniack, A.D.; Dewal, N.; Moffitt, R.A.; Danilova, L.; Murray, B.A.; Lerario, A.M.; Else, T.; Knijnenburg, T.A.; Ciriello, G.; et al. Comprehensive Pan-Genomic Characterization of Adrenocortical Carcinoma (vol 29, pg 723, 2016). *Cancer Cell* **2016**, *30*, 363. [CrossRef] [PubMed]
8. Mohan, D.R.; Lerario, A.M.; Hammer, G.D. Therapeutic Targets for Adrenocortical Carcinoma in the Genomics Era. *J. Endocr. Soc.* **2018**, *2*, 1259–1274. [CrossRef] [PubMed]
9. Jouinot, A.; Bertherat, J. Management of endocrine disease: Adrenocortical carcinoma: Differentiating the good from the poor prognosis tumors. *Eur. J. Endocrinol.* **2018**, *178*, R215–R230. [CrossRef]
10. Crona, J.; Beuschlein, F. Adrenocortical carcinoma—Towards genomics guided clinical care. *Nat. Rev. Endocrinol.* **2019**, *15*, 548–560. [CrossRef]
11. Fassnacht, M.; Terzolo, M.; Allolio, B.; Baudin, E.; Haak, H.; Berruti, A.; Welin, S.; Schade-Brittinger, C.; Lacroix, A.; Jarzab, B.; et al. Combination Chemotherapy in Advanced Adrenocortical Carcinoma. *N. Engl. J. Med.* **2012**. [CrossRef] [PubMed]
12. Altieri, B.; Ronchi, C.L.; Kroiss, M.; Fassnacht, M. Next-generation therapies for adrenocortical carcinoma. *Best Pract. Res. Clin. Endocrinol. Metab.* **2020**, *34*, 101434. [CrossRef]
13. Cosentini, D.; Badalamenti, G.; Grisanti, S.; Basile, V.; Rapa, I.; Cerri, S.; Spallanzani, A.; Perotti, P.; Musso, E.; Lagana, M.; et al. Activity and safety of temozolomide in advanced adrenocortical carcinoma patients. *Eur. J. Endocrinol.* **2019**, *181*, 681–689. [CrossRef] [PubMed]
14. Megerle, F.; Kroiss, M.; Hahner, S.; Fassnacht, M. Advanced Adrenocortical Carcinoma-What to do when First-Line Therapy Fails? *Exp. Clin. Endocrinol. Diabetes* **2019**, *127*, 109–116. [CrossRef]
15. Henning, J.E.K.; Deutschbein, T.; Altieri, B.; Steinhauer, S.; Kircher, S.; Sbiera, S.; Wild, V.; Schlotelburg, W.; Kroiss, M.; Perotti, P.; et al. Gemcitabine-Based Chemotherapy in Adrenocortical Carcinoma: A Multicenter Study of Efficacy and Predictive Factors. *J. Clin. Endocrinol. Metab.* **2017**, *102*, 4323–4332. [CrossRef] [PubMed]
16. Fassnacht, M.; Berruti, A.; Baudin, E.; Demeure, M.J.; Gilbert, J.; Haak, H.; Kroiss, M.; Quinn, D.I.; Hesseltine, E.; Ronchi, C.L.; et al. Linsitinib (OSI-906) versus placebo for patients with locally advanced or metastatic adrenocortical carcinoma: A double-blind, randomised, phase 3 study. *Lancet. Oncol.* **2015**, *16*, 426–435. [CrossRef]
17. Thiery, J.P.; Acloque, H.; Huang, R.Y.; Nieto, M.A. Epithelial-mesenchymal transitions in development and disease. *Cell* **2009**, *139*, 871–890. [CrossRef]
18. Acloque, H.; Adams, M.S.; Fishwick, K.; Bronner-Fraser, M.; Nieto, M.A. Epithelial-mesenchymal transitions: The importance of changing cell state in development and disease. *J. Clin. Investig.* **2009**, *119*, 1438–1449. [CrossRef]
19. Puisieux, A.; Brabletz, T.; Caramel, J. Oncogenic roles of EMT-inducing transcription factors. *Nat. Cell Biol.* **2014**, *16*, 488–494. [CrossRef]

20. Kalluri, R.; Weinberg, R.A. The basics of epithelial-mesenchymal transition. *J. Clin. Investig.* **2009**, *119*, 1420–1428. [CrossRef]
21. Karlsson, M.C.; Gonzalez, S.F.; Welin, J.; Fuxe, J. Epithelial-mesenchymal transition in cancer metastasis through the lymphatic system. *Mol. Oncol.* **2017**, *11*, 781–791. [CrossRef] [PubMed]
22. Navas, T.; Kinders, R.J.; Lawrence, S.M.; Ferry-Galow, K.V.; Borgel, S.; Hollingshead, M.G.; Srivastava, A.K.; Alcoser, S.Y.; Makhlouf, H.R.; Chuaqui, R.; et al. Clinical Evolution of Epithelial-Mesenchymal Transition in Human Carcinomas. *Cancer Res.* **2020**, *80*, 304–318. [CrossRef] [PubMed]
23. Wang, Y.; Zhou, B.P. Epithelial-mesenchymal transition in breast cancer progression and metastasis. *Chin. J. Cancer* **2011**, *30*, 603–611. [CrossRef] [PubMed]
24. Keegan, C.E.; Hammer, G.D. Recent insights into organogenesis of the adrenal cortex. *Trends. Endocrinol. Metab.* **2002**, *13*, 200–208. [CrossRef]
25. Xing, Y.; Lerario, A.M.; Rainey, W.; Hammer, G.D. Development of adrenal cortex zonation. *Endocrinol. Metab. Clin. N. Am.* **2015**, *44*, 243–274. [CrossRef]
26. Rogalla, S.; Contag, C.H. Early Cancer Detection at the Epithelial Surface. *Cancer J.* **2015**, *21*, 179–187. [CrossRef]
27. Mohseny, A.B.; Hogendoorn, P.C. Concise review: Mesenchymal tumors: When stem cells go mad. *Stem Cells* **2011**, *29*, 397–403. [CrossRef]
28. Bulzico, D.; Faria, P.A.S.; Maia, C.B.; de Paula, M.P.; Torres, D.C.; Ferreira, G.M.; Pires, B.R.B.; Hassan, R.; Abdelhay, E.; Vaisman, M.; et al. Is there a role for epithelial-mesenchymal transition in adrenocortical tumors? *Endocrine* **2017**, *58*, 276–288. [CrossRef]
29. Rubin, B.; Regazzo, D.; Redaelli, M.; Mucignat, C.; Citton, M.; Iacobone, M.; Scaroni, C.; Betterle, C.; Mantero, F.; Fassina, A.; et al. Investigation of N-cadherin/beta-catenin expression in adrenocortical tumors. *Tumor Biol.* **2016**, *37*, 13545–13555. [CrossRef]
30. Zeisberg, M.; Neilson, E.G. Biomarkers for epithelial-mesenchymal transitions. *J. Clin. Investig.* **2009**, *119*, 1429–1437. [CrossRef]
31. Turner, N.; Grose, R. Fibroblast growth factor signalling: From development to cancer. *Nat. Rev. Cancer* **2010**, *10*, 116–129. [CrossRef] [PubMed]
32. Litvinov, S.V.; Velders, M.P.; Bakker, H.A.; Fleuren, G.J.; Warnaar, S.O. Ep-CAM: A human epithelial antigen is a homophilic cell-cell adhesion molecule. *J. Cell Biol.* **1994**, *125*, 437–446. [CrossRef] [PubMed]
33. Balzar, M.; Bakker, H.A.; Briaire-de-Bruijn, I.H.; Fleuren, G.J.; Warnaar, S.O.; Litvinov, S.V. Cytoplasmic tail regulates the intercellular adhesion function of the epithelial cell adhesion molecule. *Mol. Cell Biol.* **1998**, *18*, 4833–4843. [CrossRef]
34. van der Gun, B.T.; Melchers, L.J.; Ruiters, M.H.; de Leij, L.F.; McLaughlin, P.M.; Rots, M.G. EpCAM in carcinogenesis: The good, the bad or the ugly. *Carcinogenesis* **2010**, *31*, 1913–1921. [CrossRef]
35. Loh, C.Y.; Chai, J.Y.; Tang, T.F.; Wong, W.F.; Sethi, G.; Shanmugam, M.K.; Chong, P.P.; Looi, C.Y. The E-Cadherin and N-Cadherin Switch in Epithelial-to-Mesenchymal Transition: Signaling, Therapeutic Implications, and Challenges. *Cells* **2019**, *8*, 1118. [CrossRef] [PubMed]
36. Davidson, N.E.; Sukumar, S. Of Snail, mice, and women. *Cancer Cell* **2005**, *8*, 173–174. [CrossRef] [PubMed]
37. Nieto, M.A. The snail superfamily of zinc-finger transcription factors. *Nat. Rev. Mol. Cell Biol.* **2002**, *3*, 155–166. [CrossRef] [PubMed]
38. Olmeda, D.; Moreno-Bueno, G.; Flores, J.M.; Fabra, A.; Portillo, F.; Cano, A. SNAI1 is required for tumor growth and lymph node metastasis of human breast carcinoma MDA-MB-231 cells. *Cancer Res.* **2007**, *67*, 11721–11731. [CrossRef] [PubMed]
39. Emadi Baygi, M.; Soheili, Z.S.; Essmann, F.; Deezagi, A.; Engers, R.; Goering, W.; Schulz, W.A. Slug/SNAI2 regulates cell proliferation and invasiveness of metastatic prostate cancer cell lines. *Tumour Biol.* **2010**, *31*, 297–307. [CrossRef]
40. Dai, S.; Zhou, Z.; Chen, Z.; Xu, G.; Chen, Y. Fibroblast Growth Factor Receptors (FGFRs): Structures and Small Molecule Inhibitors. *Cells* **2019**, *8*, 614. [CrossRef]
41. Holzmann, K.; Grunt, T.; Heinzle, C.; Sampl, S.; Steinhoff, H.; Reichmann, N.; Kleiter, M.; Hauck, M.; Marian, B. Alternative Splicing of Fibroblast Growth Factor Receptor IgIII Loops in Cancer. *J. Nucleic. Acids* **2012**, *2012*, 950508. [CrossRef]
42. Ishiwata, T. Role of fibroblast growth factor receptor-2 splicing in normal and cancer cells. *Front. Biosci. (Landmark)* **2018**, *23*, 626–639. [CrossRef] [PubMed]
43. Sbiera, S.; Sbiera, I.; Ruggiero, C.; Doghman-Bouguerra, M.; Korpershoek, E.; de Krijger, R.R.; Ettaieb, H.; Haak, H.; Volante, M.; Papotti, M.; et al. Assessment of VAV2 Expression Refines Prognostic Prediction in Adrenocortical Carcinoma. *J. Clin. Endocrinol. Metab.* **2017**, *102*, 3491–3498. [CrossRef] [PubMed]
44. Gazdar, A.F.; Oie, H.K.; Shackleton, C.H.; Chen, T.R.; Triche, T.J.; Myers, C.E.; Chrousos, G.P.; Brennan, M.F.; Stein, C.A.; Larocca, R.V. Establishment and Characterization of a Human Adrenocortical Carcinoma Cell-Line That Expresses Multiple Pathways of Steroid-Biosynthesis. *Cancer Res.* **1990**, *50*, 5488–5496.
45. Hantel, C.; Shapiro, I.; Poli, G.; Chiapponi, C.; Bidlingmaier, M.; Reincke, M.; Luconi, M.; Jung, S.; Beuschlein, F. Targeting heterogeneity of adrenocortical carcinoma: Evaluation and extension of preclinical tumor models to improve clinical translation. *Oncotarget* **2016**, *7*, 79278–79290. [CrossRef]
46. Kiseljak-Vassiliades, K.; Zhang, Y.; Bagby, S.M.; Kar, A.; Pozdeyev, N.; Xu, M.; Gowan, K.; Sharma, V.; Raeburn, C.D.; Albuja-Cruz, M.; et al. Development of new preclinical models to advance adrenocortical carcinoma research. *Endocr.-Relat. Cancer* **2018**, *25*, 437–451. [CrossRef] [PubMed]
47. Franci, C.; Takkunen, M.; Dave, N.; Alameda, F.; Gomez, S.; Rodriguez, R.; Escriva, M.; Montserrat-Sentis, B.; Baro, T.; Garrido, M.; et al. Expression of Snail protein in tumor-stroma interface. *Oncogene* **2006**, *25*, 5134–5144. [CrossRef]

48. Altieri, B.; Sbiera, S.; Della Casa, S.; Weigand, I.; Wild, V.; Steinhauer, S.; Fadda, G.; Kocot, A.; Bekteshi, M.; Mambretti, E.M.; et al. Livin/BIRC7 expression as malignancy marker in adrenocortical tumors. *Oncotarget* **2017**, *8*, 9323–9338. [CrossRef] [PubMed]
49. D'Amici, S.; Ceccarelli, S.; Vescarelli, E.; Romano, F.; Frati, L.; Marchese, C.; Angeloni, A. TNF alpha Modulates Fibroblast Growth Factor Receptor 2 Gene Expression through the pRB/E2F1 Pathway: Identification of a Non-Canonical E2F Binding Motif. *PLoS ONE* **2013**, *8*, e61491. [CrossRef]
50. Beuschlein, F.; Weigel, J.; Saeger, W.; Kroiss, M.; Wild, V.; Daffara, F.; Libe, R.; Ardito, A.; Al Ghuzlan, A.; Quinkler, M.; et al. Major prognostic role of Ki67 in localized adrenocortical carcinoma after complete resection. *J. Clin. Endocrinol. Metab.* **2015**, *100*, 841–849. [CrossRef]
51. Shimizu, A.; Takashima, Y.; Kurokawa-Seo, M. FGFR3 isoforms have distinct functions in the regulation of growth and cell morphology. *Biochem. Bioph. Res. Commun.* **2002**, *290*, 113–120. [CrossRef]
52. Paur, J.; Nika, L.; Maier, C.; Moscu-Gregor, A.; Kostka, J.; Huber, D.; Mohr, T.; Heffeter, P.; Schrottmaier, W.C.; Kappel, S.; et al. Fibroblast Growth Factor Receptor 3 Isoforms: Novel Therapeutic Targets for Hepatocellular Carcinoma? *Hepatology* **2015**, *62*, 1767–1778. [CrossRef]
53. Zhao, Q.; Caballero, O.L.; Davis, I.D.; Jonasch, E.; Tamboli, P.; Yung, W.K.A.; Weinstein, J.N.; Shaw, K.; Strausberg, R.L.; Yao, J.; et al. Tumor-Specific Isoform Switch of the Fibroblast Growth Factor Receptor 2 Underlies the Mesenchymal and Malignant Phenotypes of Clear Cell Renal Cell Carcinomas. *Clin. Cancer Res.* **2013**, *19*, 2460–2472. [CrossRef]
54. Miyamoto, Y.; Sakane, F.; Hashimoto, K. N-cadherin-based adherens junction regulates the maintenance, proliferation, and differentiation of neural progenitor cells during development. *Cell Adhes. Migr.* **2015**, *9*, 183–192. [CrossRef]
55. Vinson, G.P. Functional Zonation of the Adult Mammalian Adrenal Cortex. *Front. Neurosci. (Switz.)* **2016**, *10*, 238. [CrossRef]
56. Arnold, J. Ein Beitrag zu der feineren Structur und dem Chemismus der Nebennieren. *Virchows. Arch.* **1866**, 64–117. [CrossRef]
57. Gottschau, M. Struktur und embryonale Entwicklung der Nebennieren bei Säugetieren. *Arch. Anat. Physiol.* **1883**, 412–458.
58. Chang, S.P.; Morrison, H.D.; Nilsson, F.; Kenyon, C.J.; West, J.D.; Morley, S.D. Cell Proliferation, Movement and Differentiation during Maintenance of the Adult Mouse Adrenal Cortex. *PLoS ONE* **2013**, *8*, e81865. [CrossRef] [PubMed]
59. Vidal, V.; Sacco, S.; Rocha, A.S.; da Silva, F.; Panzolini, C.; Dumontet, T.; Doan, T.M.P.; Shan, J.D.; Rak-Raszewska, A.; Bird, T.; et al. The adrenal capsule is a signaling center controlling cell renewal and zonation through Rspo3. *Gene Dev.* **2016**, *30*, 1389–1394. [CrossRef] [PubMed]
60. Walczak, E.M.; Kuick, R.; Finco, I.; Bohin, N.; Hrycaj, S.M.; Wellik, D.M.; Hammer, G.D. Wnt Signaling Inhibits Adrenal Steroidogenesis by Cell-Autonomous and Non-Cell-Autonomous Mechanisms. *Mol. Endocrinol.* **2014**, *28*, 1471–1486. [CrossRef] [PubMed]
61. King, P.; Paul, A.; Laufer, E. Shh signaling regulates adrenocortical development and identifies progenitors of steroidogenic lineages. *Proc. Natl. Acad. Sci. USA* **2009**, *106*, 21185–21190. [CrossRef] [PubMed]
62. Hammer, G.D.; Basham, K.J. Stem cell function and plasticity in the normal physiology of the adrenal cortex. *Mol. Cell Endocrinol.* **2021**, *519*, 111043. [CrossRef] [PubMed]
63. Lerario, A.M.; Finco, I.; LaPensee, C.; Hammer, G.D. Molecular Mechanisms of Stem/ Progenitor Cell Maintenance in the Adrenal Cortex. *Front. Endocrinol.* **2017**, *8*, 52. [CrossRef]
64. Hadjidemetriou, I.; Mariniello, K.; Ruiz-Babot, G.; Pittaway, J.; Mancini, A.; Mariannis, D.; Gomez-Sanchez, C.E.; Parvanta, L.; Drake, W.M.; Chung, T.T.; et al. DLK1/PREF1 marks a novel cell population in the human adrenal cortex. *J. Steroid. Biochem.* **2019**, *193*, 105422. [CrossRef] [PubMed]

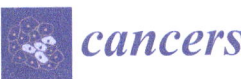

Review

Anaplastic Thyroid Carcinoma: An Update

Arnaud Jannin [1,2], Alexandre Escande [2,3], Abir Al Ghuzlan [4], Pierre Blanchard [5], Dana Hartl [6], Benjamin Chevalier [1,2], Frédéric Deschamps [7], Livia Lamartina [8], Ludovic Lacroix [9], Corinne Dupuy [10], Eric Baudin [8], Christine Do Cao [1] and Julien Hadoux [8,*]

1. Department of Endocrinology, Diabetology, Metabolism and Nutrition, Lille University Hospital, 59000 Lille, France; arnaud.jannin@chu-lille.fr (A.J.); benjamin.chevalier@chu-lille.fr (B.C.); christine.docao@chru-lille.fr (C.D.C.)
2. H. Warembourg School of Medicine, University of Lille, 59000 Lille, France; a-escande@o-lambret.fr
3. Academic Radiation Oncology Department, Oscar Lambret Center, 59000 Lille, France
4. Cancer Medical Pathology and Biology Department, Institute Gustave Roussy, 94805 Villejuif, France; abir.alghuzlan@gustaveroussy.fr
5. Department of Radiation Oncology, Institute Gustave Roussy, Université Paris Saclay, 94805 Villejuif, France; pierre.blanchard@gustaveroussy.fr
6. Département d'Anesthésie, Chirurgie et Interventionnel (DACI), Institute Gustave Roussy, Université Paris Saclay, 94805 Villejuif, France; dana.hartl@gustaveroussy.fr
7. Department of Head and Neck Oncology, Institute Gustave Roussy, Université Paris Saclay, 94805 Paris, France; frederic.deschamps@gustaveroussy.fr
8. Cancer Medicine Department, Institute Gustave Roussy, Université Paris Saclay, 94805 Villejuif, France; livia.lamartina@gustaveroussy.fr (L.L.); eric.baudin@gustaveroussy.fr (E.B.)
9. Department of Medical Oncology, Institute Gustave Roussy, Université Paris Saclay, 94805 Villejuif, France; ludovic.lacroix@gustaveroussy.fr
10. CNRS, UMR 9019, 94805 Villejuif, France; corinne.dupuy@gustaveroussy.fr
* Correspondence: julien.hadoux@gustaveroussy.fr; Tel.: +33-142116361

Simple Summary: Anaplastic thyroid carcinoma (ATC) has a dismal prognostic. Chemotherapy and radiotherapy are the mainstem options for patients with ATC. In selected cases with actionable genomic alterations or with favorable immune tumor microenvironment, new therapeutic options as targeted therapies and immunotherapy have led to better outcome and raised some hope for treatment of this deadly disease.

Abstract: Anaplastic thyroid carcinoma (ATC) is a rare and undifferentiated form of thyroid cancer. Its prognosis is poor: the median overall survival (OS) of patients varies from 4 to 10 months after diagnosis. However, a doubling of the OS time may be possible owing to a more systematic use of molecular tests for targeted therapies and integration of fast-track dedicated care pathways for these patients in tertiary centers. The diagnostic confirmation, if needed, requires an urgent biopsy reread by an expert pathologist with additional immunohistochemical and molecular analyses. Therapeutic management, defined in multidisciplinary meetings, respecting the patient's choice, must start within days following diagnosis. For localized disease diagnosed after primary surgical treatment, adjuvant chemo-radiotherapy is recommended. In the event of locally advanced or metastatic disease, the prognosis is very poor. Treatment should then involve chemotherapy or targeted therapy and decompressive cervical radiotherapy. Here we will review current knowledge on ATC and provide perspectives to improve the management of this deadly disease.

Keywords: anaplastic thyroid carcinoma; chemotherapy; immune checkpoint inhibitors; tumors associated macrophages; radiotherapy; molecular targeted therapy

1. Introduction

Anaplastic thyroid cancer (ATC) is a rare malignancy with a poor prognosis. It is characterized by a rapid onset with local and distant metastases, local progression and distant evolution [1]. Its treatment is an emergency, based on surgery (if feasible), radiation therapy and chemotherapy [2,3]. However, the prognosis remains very poor with a one-year overall survival (OS) rate between only 20 and 50% [4–7]. Recent results of the dabrafenib/trametinib combination for *BRAF*-mutated patients [8,9] and of immune checkpoint inhibitors (ICI), used alone or in combination with targeted therapies [10–13], have raised some hope toward an improvement of the prognosis of this deadly disease [14].

Here we will review current knowledge on the epidemiology, pathology/biology and standard treatment of ATC and discuss the recent progress and perspectives for their management.

2. Epidemiology and Clinical Presentation: A Rare Disease with a Rapid Onset and Poor Prognosis

ATC is a rare cancer as defined by the European Union rare cancer surveillance program (RARECARE) with an incidence far below six new cases per 100,000 person-years [15]. Indeed, recent epidemiological studies have confirmed an age-adjusted incidence in the US of 0.12 per 100,000 person-years (95% CI: 0.8–1.6) in 2014 in the Surveillance, Epidemiology, and End Results (SEER) database [16] and 0.1 to 0.3 per 100,000 person-years in Europe according to data from Denmark [4], Wales [17] and the Netherlands [18] registries. The SEER database and the Netherlands registries analyses have suggested an increase in the age-adjusted incidence with an average annual percent change of 3.0% per year (95% CI: 2.2–3.7%) and 1.3% per year (95% CI: 0.4–2.1%), respectively, over a 30–40-year period of time; this increase in incidence was not reported in the Danish and the Welsh databases [4,16–18]. The reasons for the discrepancies are unknown; however, incidence rates are consistent across the different studies in Europe and US. The increase in incidence is unlikely to be related to better screening/diagnosis because all ATC patients end up being diagnosed with cervical compressive symptoms.

ATC usually affects elderly patients, with the majority being over 60 years old with a female predominance (male/female sex ratio = 1.5:2). The advanced stage of the disease is the most common diagnosis presentation (localized (IVa) 10%, locally advanced (IVb) 35% and metastatic (IVc) 55%) displaying extremely aggressive behavior with rapid tumor progression, local invasion and/or distant metastases (lung, bone, liver and/or brain metastases) [1,2,19–21] (Figure 1).

Classically, patients report a rapid transformation of a long-standing goiter (30% of cases) within a few days to a few weeks. The others symptoms include neck pain as well as signs of neck tumoral invasion and compression: dyspnea, dysphonia and dysphagia.

On clinical examination, there is a large cervical mass, hardness on palpation, palpable lymphadenopathy and sometimes skin involvement. Invasion of the aerodigestive tract is frequent. Laryngeal dyspnea, dysphagia or superior vena cava syndrome which may require urgent treatment (placement of a tracheotomy and/or placement of a gastrostomy) as well as local pain can be associated. The repercussions of local tumor spread on the general condition immediately indicate the gravity of the situation.

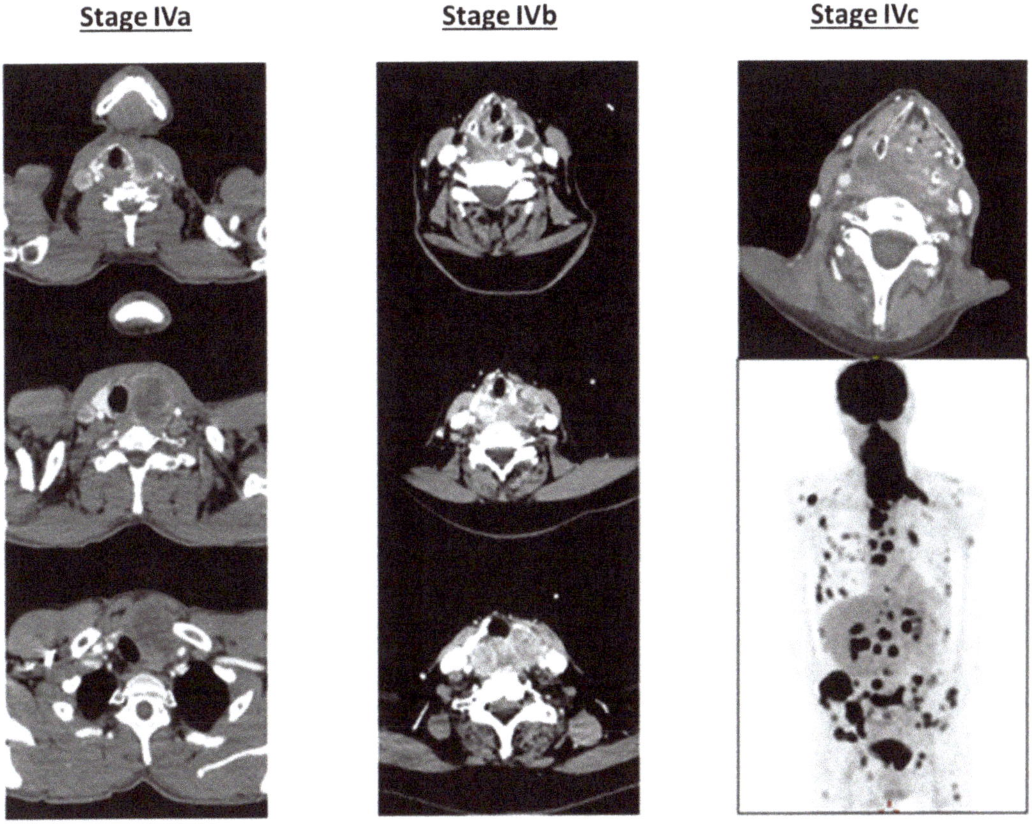

Figure 1. CT scan illustration of anaplastic thyroid carcinoma (ATC) staging.

3. Pathology and Biology: How Do We Understand the Aggressiveness of This Disease?

3.1. Pathology

ATC is defined as a highly malignant tumor composed of undifferentiated cells which retain some features of an epithelial origin on morphology and/or immunohistochemical examination [22]. Various and heterogeneous histologic features can be seen in ATC samples including epithelioid and squamous morphology, giant cells, pleomorphic morphology, osteoclast giant cell-rich morphology, and spindle cell morphology which is the most common histotype [23]. The most recent series from the Memorial Sloan Kettering Cancer Center (MKKCC) has examined the clinic–pathologic features of 360 cases from two institutions over a 34-year period. In this study, the most common histological subtypes were spindle cell (26%), pleomorphic (23%) and squamous (21% of the cases) [7]. Tumor necrosis was found in 77% of the cases, atypical mitosis in 77% and a neutrophilic infiltrate was noted in 71% of the cases. Interestingly, the mitotic index was >20 mitoses per 10 high-power fields in only 15% of the cases, and Ki67 was not reported. This study confirmed that thyroglobulin and TTF1 immunohistochemistry is almost always negative (96 and 70% of the cases, respectively), whereas cytokeratins AE1/AE3 are present in 67% of the cases and PAX 8 in up to 70% (with anti-PAX8 antibody 10336-1-AP). A recent immunohistochemical study, with the most commonly used monoclonal anti-PAX8 antibody (MRQ-50), showed lower PAX8 expression in 54.4% of the ATC cases [24]. Therefore, performing PAX8 immunohistochemistry in all samples of thyroid undifferentiated tumors suspicious for ATC, and in particular in squamous subtypes, allows for support of a differential diagnosis with squamous cell carcinoma of the head and neck which is always negative for PAX8 [25].

ATC tumorigenesis may be a multistep process with a biological transformation (synchronous or metachronous) from differentiated thyroid cancer (DTC) to ATC. This assumption is suggested by the common recognition of a concomitant DTC tumor component or a history of DTC observed in 58 to up to 90% of cases [7,26]. Poorly differentiated DTC (PDTC) and the tall cell variant of papillary DTC were the most common subtypes found associated to these transformed ATC subtypes in the MSKCC series [7]. From a molecular point of view the association of additional *TP53* and/or *TERT* promoter mutations is found in up to 80% of ATC cases harboring typical DTC molecular alteration in the *BRAF* and *RAS* genes [27–30]. These data have suggested that additional mutations in *TP53* and *TERT* may drive the tumor progression from DTC to ATC [1] in these transformed ATC subtypes. This transformation process of ATC may occur differently according to the genetic mutation background. Indeed, in *RAS* mutant ATC, a history or concomitant DTC is observed in 38% of cases and it is observed in 75% of cases with *BRAF* mutations ($p = 0.001$) [7]. A whole-exome sequencing analysis of the two tumor components (DTC and ATC) of three mixed ATC tumor samples revealed that most of the somatic mutations identified in the ATC component differed from the ones in papillary DTC. This led to the conclusion of there being very few common mutations and a large genomic divergence between the two components challenging the concept of tumor progression from DTC to ATC [31]. From the clinical point of view, a recent retrospective multicenter and SEER database study on 642 primary (i.e., tumors with no DTC component at diagnosis) and 47 secondary ATC (i.e., tumors with a DTC component at diagnosis), found no statistical differences in terms of demographic, clinical manifestations and patient survival and a more frequent *BRAF* mutation as compared with *RAS* mutation in secondary tumors [32]. However, it must be pointed out that identification of "transformed" ATC requires the knowledge of the detailed clinical history of the patient as well as the detailed pathology assessment of the tumor which may not be optimal in a very large database. Therefore, it is still not known whether primary or "pure" ATC carries a different prognosis as compared with secondary or "transformed" ATC.

3.2. Molecular Biology

In a recent series of 126 samples of ATC analyzed by Next Generation Sequencing (NGS), the most common molecular alterations were found in *TERT* promoter (75%), *TP53* (63%), *BRAF* (45%), *RAS* (22%), *PIK3CA* (18%), *EIF1AX* (14%) and *PTEN* (14%) with the first two being more frequent in ATC than the others, which can be seen in either DTC or PDTC [7,28]. Strikingly, *BRAF* mutation frequency in ATC seems to differ between recent series for US and Europe. Indeed, *BRAF* mutations are found in 40–45% of cases in US studies [7,14] whereas they are found in 14–37% of cases in European studies [27,30,33]; furthermore, data from south Korea reported a rate of 41% *BRAF* alterations in a series of 13 ATC cases [34]. Whether these discrepancies are linked to various sequencing techniques and/or to geographical differences in pathophysiology remains an open question. Recent results have revealed that *NTRK* and *RET* fusion can be detected in 2–3% of ATC cases [7,35–37] which is of utmost importance for the few patients who may be offered highly specific targeted therapies. If regulation of cell cycle has a crucial role in oncogenesis and particularly in ATC, protein metabolism control is also involved in tumorigenesis. For example, about 10% of patients with ATC harbor *EIF1AX* mutations, which has recently been involved in deregulating protein synthesis [36]. Interestingly, *EIF1AX* mutations could co-occur with *RAS* mutations in ATC with a positive feedback relationship between RAS and EIF1AX proteins, which reinforces *c-MYC* gene expression [28,38]. Molecular alteration of the Wnt signaling pathway could also be observed, notably with β-catenin gene (*CTNNB1*), *AXIN1* and *APC mutations* [36]. Although increased levels of cytoplasmic β-catenin are observed in most thyroid cancer cells, mutations of β-catenin that lead to nuclear localization of the protein are limited to PDTC and ATC, suggesting a role in tumor progression [39]. Alterations of epigenetic-related genes such as the chromatin remodeling SWI/SNF complex (*ARID1A, SMARCB1, PBRM1*, etc.) and histone methyltransferases (*KMT2A, KMT2C, KMT2D* and *SETD2*) have been found in 36% and 24% of ATC samples, respectively. The DNA Mismatch repair (MMR) pathway may be altered in 10–15% of cases [7,28,29,40–43].

Knowledge of the molecular alterations in ATC patients has been more and more prominently important in the clinics recently, with the advent of targeted therapies. This growing importance has been recognized in the recent ATA and ESMO guidelines which recommends offering molecular testing to all ATC patients with unresectable disease [2,3].

3.3. Immune Infiltrate of ATC

ATC tumors are characterized by an important infiltration of Tumor-Associated Macrophages (TAMs) which can represent 40 to 70% of the total tumor mass and could play some role as an immunosuppressive tumor stroma, in treatment resistance and in the poor prognosis of the disease [44–47]. ATCs display a very dense network of interconnected "ramified" TAMs which may have metabolic and trophic functions via direct contact with intermingled cancer cells [44]. This macrophage infiltration is composed of M2 pro-tumorigenic tumor-associated macrophages as demonstrated by the identification of the M2-TAMs transcriptomic signature of 78 genes identified in ATC samples, which is able to discriminate them from DTC samples [28]. The co-culture of thyroid cancer cell lines with M2-like TAMs facilitates dedifferentiation, proliferation, migration and invasion in thyroid cancer cells through the Wnt/ß-catenin pathway activation by Wnt1 and Wnt3a secretion [48] but also through insulin-like growth factor (IGF) secretion which promotes thyroid cancer stemness and metastasis by activating the PI3K/AKT/mTOR pathway [48]. A study of 19 ATC samples evaluated by automated digital quantification of CD68 and CD163 immunohistochemistry positivity confirmed the putative importance of macrophage infiltration. The mean macrophage infiltration rate was 17% and 23% for these two markers, respectively, and most of the ATC samples displayed a low to moderate level of the CD47 "don't eat me signal" which physiologically binds to signal regulatory protein α (SIRPα) on macrophages and inhibits phagocytosis of tumor cells. With an anti-CD47 antibody, phagocytosis of ATC cell lines by macrophages could be induced in vitro and in a xenotransplant model [49].

In ATC, this high macrophage infiltration in ATC tumor samples results in an altered-immunosuppressed immune microenvironment in 50% of cases and a hot immune environment in 34%, with a high expression of several inhibitory immune checkpoint mediators such as anti-cytotoxic T-lymphocyte-associated protein 4 (CTLA-4), programmed death-ligand 1–2 (PD-L1/PD-L2), TIGIT, etc., known to inhibit cytotoxic CD8+ T-cell functions [50]. Among these inhibitory immune checkpoint molecules, PD-L1 expression has been identified in 70% of ATC samples in the pre-clinical study by Schürch et al. [49] and in the phase I study of spartalizumab [10]. PD-L1 expression based on the proportion of stained tumor cells according to Tumor Proportion Score (TPS) has been found at ≥5% in 73% of 93 samples in a recent multicenter study from Germany [51]. In the tumor microenvironment, PD-L1 can be upregulated in both tumor cells and immune-microenvironment cells, such as TAMs in ATC samples [52,53]. This dual expression of PD-L1 may have important pathophysiological implications, because although induction of PD-L1 on tumor cells is interferon gamma (IFNg)-dependent and transient, PD-L1 induction on TAMs is of greater magnitude, only partially IFNg dependent and more stable over time, and thus may account for the immunosuppressive microenvironment in ATC [54]. This PD-L1 expression on TAMs may account for the presence of exhausted T-cells in transcriptomic analysis of ATC samples [50]. Moreover, PD-L1 expression on tumor cells, although possibly predictive of a response to immunotherapy in ATC [10], can be induced by the immune microenvironment, especially T-cells and TAMs, by different signaling pathways, and thus may result in differential responses to treatment with immune checkpoint inhibitors (ICI). This PD-L1 induction through different pathways by different immune cells of the tumor microenvironment may result in either accelerated tumor growth and resistance to doxorubicin and ICI of PD-L1+ tumor cells induced by TAMs; or delayed tumor growth and greater sensitivity to both doxorubicin and ICI when induced by T-cells, as shown in a hepatocellular cell line and a mouse model of hepatoma [55]. Therefore, although PD-L1 expression is high in ATC samples, its clinical impact and the differential expression on either tumor cells and/or TAMs still remains to be refined.

4. Treatment: To Treat Aggressively or to Palliate the Symptoms?

4.1. Multimodal Therapy or Palliative Care within a Fast-Dedicated Management Track

In ATC, goals of care may be therapeutic and/or palliative depending on staging and prognosis when considered in the context of available therapies, comorbidities and the patient's wishes. Multimodal therapy refers to the combination of excisional surgery, when possible, external beam radiation therapy (EBRT), chemotherapy and/or targeted therapy (Figures 2–4). This multimodal strategy is associated with a better OS in retrospective studies. In 1990, the mean OS was about two to six months [56,57] and it seems to be nearly the same 20 years later, with a one-year OS of less than 20% [58–61]. However, in a cohort of 479 patients treated in the same institution spanning nearly 20 years, Maniakas et al. found one- and two-year OS of 35/18% in the 2000/13 era (n = 227), 47/25% in the 2014/16 era (n = 100) and 59/42% in the 2017/19 era (n = 152) which suggests an impact of multi-modal treatment strategies on survival [14].

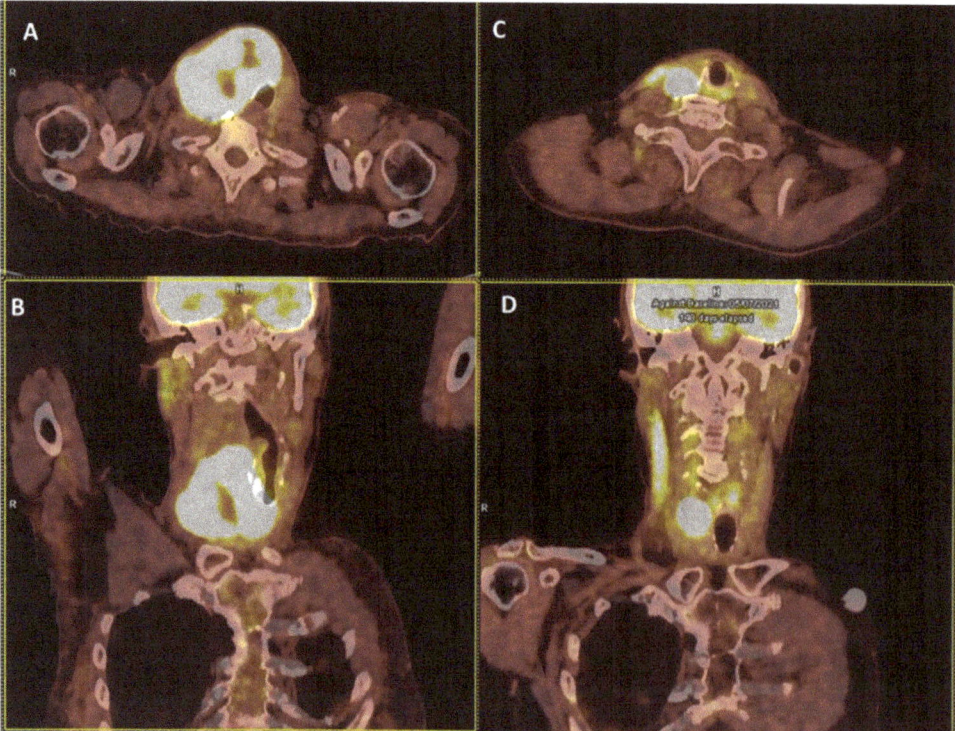

Figure 2. Illustration of ^{18}FDG PET/CT anaplastic thyroid carcinoma (ATC) response to chemotherapy and radiotherapy before surgery. The figure represents axial (**A**) and coronal (**B**) slices of the neck region with an ATC volume of 230 mL before initiating treatment comprising chemotherapy (Cisplatin-Doxorubicin, 2 cures) and radiotherapy (IMRT, 50 Gy. (**C**,**D**) represent axial (**C**) and coronal slices (**D**) of the neck region with an ATC volume of 15 mL.

Dedicated fast-track management of these patients may offer a better chance of tumor control, as early management is key according to good practice guidance for fast-growing cancers [2,62]. Although feasible in highly specialized tertiary centers, the applicability of this fast-track management approach in multiple tertiary centers at a whole-country level remains to be demonstrated, as exemplified by the huge differences in reported survival between nationwide ATC database analysis [4,5,16] in comparison with tertiary-center database analysis [14,62–64].

Although effective in providing better OS, multimodal treatment is, in most cases, a palliative aggressive approach with risks of side effects and complications which may hamper the quality of life of the patients. Indeed, in large national series, the proportion of patients unfit for combined treatments varies from 4% ($n = 4/100$) [5] to 15% in the French network on refractory thyroid cancer (ENDOCAN-TUTHYREF) experience (unpublished data). Therefore, a review of the treatment options, risks, benefits and outcomes has to be submitted to a multidisciplinary team (including palliative caregivers and geriatric oncologist) and presented to the patient to create a shared decision-making process about a realistic treatment plan [2]. One critical issue is to clarify with the patient and his family whether tracheostomy should be performed in case of acute respiratory failure versus palliative sedation, because such a procedure would profoundly impact their ability to communicate and their quality of life until death.

Whenever possible, surgery must be performed as it can provide prolonged survival and even a cure in the 10% patients with stage IVa disease, in association with chemo-radiotherapy and surgery [63,65]. It should also be performed in patients with advanced disease who may respond to initial medical/radiation treatment [2,14] (Figures 2 and 3).

4.2. Radiation Therapy: Still the Mainstem of ATC Treatment

The aggressive nature of the disease results in a high rate of local progression and recurrence [66,67] which require achieving local control with surgery, when feasible, and, more often, with EBRT. There has been a high heterogeneity of EBRT reports in the last 25 years in terms of dose administration, fractionation, techniques and combinations [26].

Since the first result from a retrospective study by Aldinger et al. in 1978 [26], and despite the absence of prospective trials, EBRT is recommended because it has been shown to improve median OS in retrospective studies, including reports from large nationwide databases such as SEER [5,19,68–76]. Moreover, this improved prognosis with EBRT is obtained through a multimodal treatment as shown, for example, in the SEER database analysis by Song et al. which reported EBRT, surgery and chemotherapy as prognostic factors on OS in multivariate analysis in 433 stage IVc patients (hazard ratio (HR): 0.562, $p \leq 0.001$) [76].

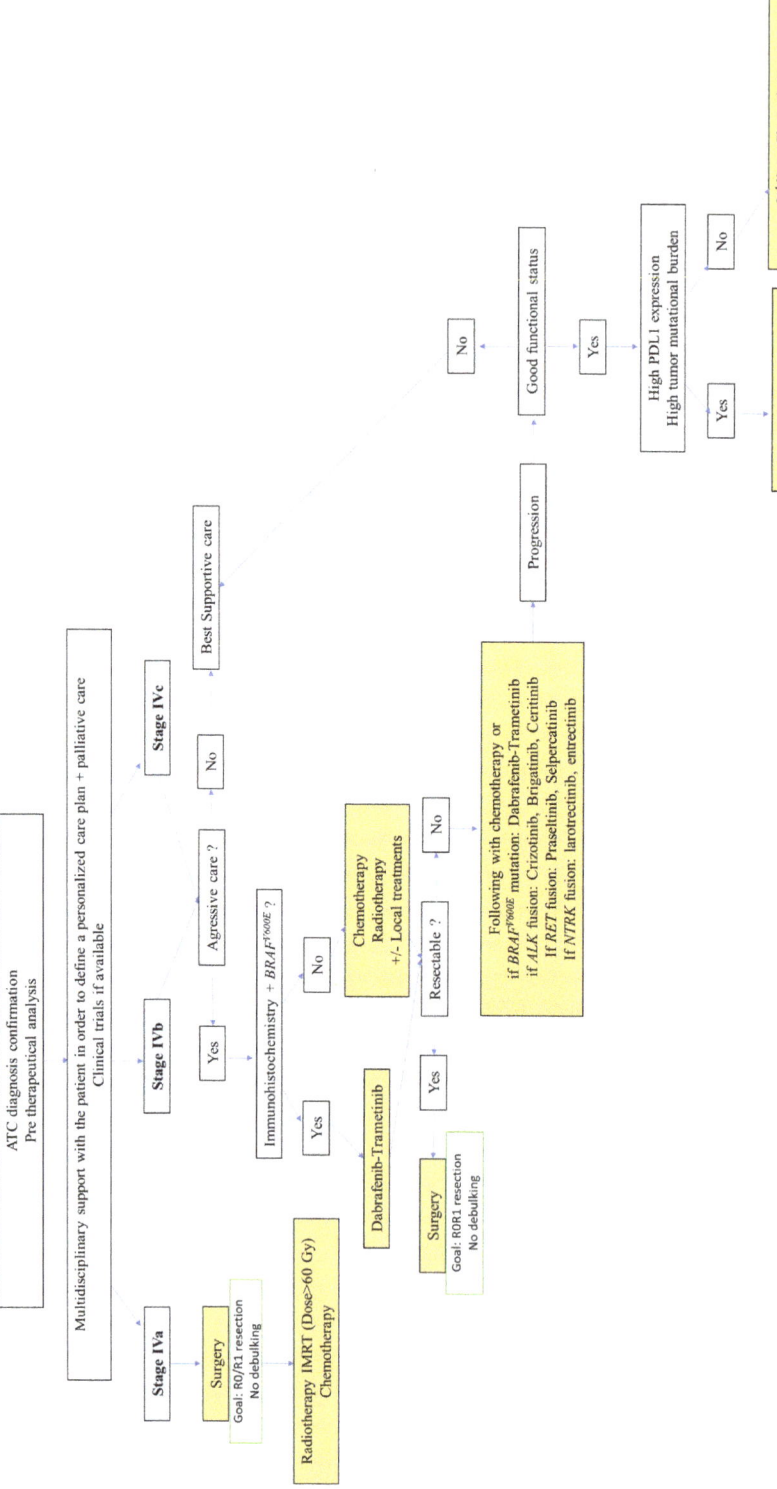

Figure 3. Initial treatment of stages IVa, IVb and IVc ATC, adapted from [2].

In order to provide the best survival benefit to the patients, EBRT dose matters. Indeed, the total dose delivered seems to be predictive of survival and local control in most of the studies, with 45–60 Gy providing an optimal control, whatever the type of fractionation, across different studies [5,59,60,77,78]. In a report of 31 patients with no distant disease at presentation who were treated by chemoradiotherapy (2 Gy daily fraction) +/− surgery, a total dose >50 Gy was associated with a significantly better median OS (9.3 vs. 1.6 months, $p = 0.019$) [79]. In the National Cancer Database (NCDB) analysis on 1288 patients with non-resected ATC, Pezzi et al. reported an improved one-year OS rate for Stage IVb and IVc patients who received 60 to 75 Gy as compared with patients treated with less than 60 Gy (31% versus 16%, $p = 0.019$) [73]. To better define the optimal dose, Nachalon et al. analyzed the total EBRT dose to the gross tumor in three different groups of 26 patients, using full dose (70 Gy), high palliative dose (50 Gy) and palliative dose (maximum 30 Gy), and found an association between dose and improved survival ($p < 0.001$) [80]. Following R0 or R1 resection, guidelines recommend that good-performance status patients with no evidence of metastatic disease who opt for aggressive management should be offered standard fractionation IMRT with concurrent systemic therapy [2].

Besides dose, fractionation modalities have been investigated for optimal tumor control in ATC patients. Bi-fractionation radiotherapy schedules can be either hyper-fractionated (multiple daily doses not exceeding 1.5 Gy) or accelerated (twice-a-day dose of 1.8–2 Gy). These schedules have been used in an attempt to overcome fast progression and radioresistance of ATC [81]. However, there have been no randomized studies to compare standard with altered fractionation; such studies may not be feasible given the rarity of this disease. In 2002, Tennvall et al. published prospective results for patients treated by association of chemotherapy and hyper-fractionated EBRT (30 Gy before surgery and 16 Gy after, twice daily either as 2 × 1 Gy or 2 × 1.3 Gy per day or 46 Gy after, twice daily as 2 × 1.6 Gy) and debulking surgery. They found a trend for hyper-fractionated radiotherapy with a better OS outcome (9% of patients (5/55) always alive after two years) and 60% (33/55) of local control [82]. In 2006, Wang Y et al. reported results from 23 ATC patients treated with radical EBRT (dose > 40 Gy), with once-daily ($n = 14$) or twice-daily fractionation ($n = 9$, 1.5 Gy per fraction). They found that hyper-fractionated treatment was well tolerated with a longer median OS (13.6 months for twice-daily radiotherapy versus 1.3 months for the other group; however, this was without statistical significance ($p = 0.3$). There were also no difference in terms of local control in the two groups [83]. A prospective study using accelerated radiotherapy with two daily fractions by De Crevoisier et al. provided encouraging results with 7 patients out of 30 alive after a median follow-up of 45 months and 47% local control rate [63]. Although bi-fractionation may provide better local tumor control, there is no definitive evidence and no data to suggest an improved OS with these techniques. Data on ATC are scarce but we can extrapolate from head and neck cancer data where altered fractionation increases acute but not late toxicity and improves local control [84].

Hypofractionation with dose per fraction > 5 Gy has been reported to prevent death from local recurrence ($p = 0.025$) but with grade > 3 toxicities in a series of 33 patients and no improved OS [85]. However, because hyperfractionation or accelerated regimens require more intensive resources and the data supporting their efficacy are scarce, recent studies have used regimens close to those used in EBRT of other head and neck cancers in 2 Gy per fraction [60,78,86–89]. In recent guidelines from the Italian Society of Radiation Oncology (AIRO) and Spanish Thyroid Group, bifractionation and standard fractionations are listed as two possible EBRT options, whereas hyperfractionation is discouraged in ESMO guidelines [3,90,91]. ATA guidelines recommend standard fractionation but do not discourage hyperfractionation [2].

Although different fractionation techniques do not seem to have a major impact in management, high-accuracy radiotherapy techniques such as intensity-modulated radiation therapy (IMRT) should also be used for decreasing toxicities [92,93]. Indeed, IMRT can achieve a better target coverage and reduced dose to the spinal cord [92]. In a monocentric retrospective analysis of 28 ATC patients treated with IMRT and 13 treated with three-dimensional conformal radiotherapy (3D-CRT), a better progression-free survival (PFS) (median 5.1 vs. 2.6 months, $p = 0.049$) and OS ($p = 0.005$ for both) were found in multivariate analysis, possibly related to an improved total dose ($p = 0.005$) without increased toxicity [94]. This lower toxicity rate was not found in all reports of IMRT [79]. This IMRT technique is important to deliver the optimal dose to the different treatment volumes which most often include the operative bed, the thyroid, and lymph node areas I to VI with the upper mediastinum up to the carina [63,78,79,89,95]. Few relapses at the edge of the radiotherapy field (less than 10% marginal relapses) have been reported [96,97]. The rate of loco-regional failure rate may relate to the extent of the EBRT field, as reported by Kim et al., with a five-year local control rate of 40% in ATC patients treated with a large extended field ($n = 12$) (such as described before) vs. 9% in case of limited field EBRT ($n = 11$) to involved site (tumor and node) ($p = 0.04$). [98]. We proposed EBRT by IMRT with a total dose of 66–70 Gy into the tumor volume with a 5 mm margin and 50 Gy to the bilateral level II–VI cervical nodes, and upper mediastinal nodes to the carina +/− area I, with an element of compromise therefore required in efforts to achieve acceptable toxicity.

The optimal timing of EBRT in the patient's treatment schedule with respect to surgery and chemotherapy/systemic treatment has not been defined. In patients with resectable stage IVa disease, adjuvant EBRT is recommended [2]. However, it is possible that preoperative radiotherapy can enable surgery (example in Figure 2). In a monocentric report of 79 patients treated between 1972 and 1998, Besic et al. found that the 12 patients treated by neoadjuvant chemo-radiotherapy, surgery and additional adjuvant EBRT (total dose of 45 to 64 Gy) had a better median OS (14.5 months as compared with the 26 patients treated with primary surgery followed by EBRT (7 months)) [99]. Although interesting, these results may reflect a selection bias with neoadjuvant treatment allowing for the selection of patients without primary refractoriness and thus, better prognosis. Indeed, Arora et al. found a longer cause-specific survival in cases of postoperative EBRT versus preoperative EBRT ($p < 0.0001$) in an analysis of PDTC and ATC patients from the SEER database [100]. Data are still needed to confirm the best timing for EBRT in patients with resectable disease.

Beside surgery, the other major question is the optimal systemic treatment to combine with EBRT and especially chemotherapy. Since the 1970s, several authors have described the results of combinations, and there are a large number of different protocols. One of the most recent analyses of the SEER database, which included an inverse probability weighting (IPW) to balance variables between groups, reported that radio-chemotherapy was associated with improved OS (adjusted HR = 0.69, 95% CI: 0.56–0.85, $p < 0.001$) versus EBRT alone; this difference remained significant within each subgroup stratified by surgical resection and distant metastasis [101]. The most recent and only randomized study in this setting is the RTOG 0912 trial which randomized 99 patients (56% Stage IVb) undergoing 2–3 weeks of weekly paclitaxel 80 mg/m^2 with placebo or pazopanib 400 mg/day followed by concomitant 66 Gy EBRT and weekly 50 mg/m^2 paclitaxel with placebo or pazopanib 300 mg/day [102]. The one-year OS rate was 29% in the placebo group and 37.1% in the pazopanib group ($p = 0.283$) in the 80% of patients who were randomized and eligible for this treatment. This randomized trial provides the prospective results of chemo-radiation therapy in ATC patients which are in line with those of the different retrospective studies which reported one-year OS rates between 30 and 50% with either doxorubicin or paclitaxel/docetaxel-based chemotherapy, with or without platin [63,65,74,103] (Table 1). No chemotherapy regimen has been shown to have a better impact on OS in the different retrospective studies published to date (Table 1). In the late 1990s and early 2000s, bi-fractionated radiotherapy (46 Gy, 1.6 Gy per fraction) associated with doxorubicin (10–20 mg/m^2 weekly) was widely considered as the standard of care but at least 10 different chemotherapy regimens were found in different series or even in single-institution cohorts [57,67,79] (Table 1). De Crevoisier et al. have studied the association of doxorubicin (60 mg/m^2) and cisplatin (120 mg/m^2) with radiotherapy (40 Gy in 1.23 Gy per fraction twice a day) within a prospective cohort. They reported a three-year OS of 27% (95% CI: 10–44%) and a median OS of 10 months [63]. In a German multicenter study, Wendler et al. found that any kind of systemic treatment (doxorubicin weekly, paclitaxel, paclitaxel and pemetrexed, paclitaxel and carboplatin, doxorubicin and cisplatin and tyrosin kinase inhibitor) was associated with a longer OS for IVc patients (HR: 0.23, 95% CI: 0.08–0.64, p = 0.005), and combined paclitaxel and pemetrexed was associated with a statistically significant likelihood of longer OS compared with other regimens (p < 0.0001) [5]. To summarize, most guidelines recommend, in eligible patients without targetable molecular alteration, the administration of chemo-radiation with either doxorubicin or paclitaxel/docetaxel +/− platin. This chemo-radiotherapy constitutes the standard induction treatment for fit stage IVb-IVc patients and has been referred to as "bridging therapy" in the recent ATA guidelines: a therapy that helps to stop the fast progression of the disease while all molecular explorations are undertaken and accessibility to targeted therapy/immunotherapy is evaluated [2]. Finally, for patients with *BRAF* mutations who are eligible for the dabrafenib/trametinib combination, the question of when to perform radiation therapy remains open as it is usually indicated to halt treatment during EBRT. However, a phase I/II trial in melanoma has shown that concurrent radiation could be feasible [104] and a phase I trial in ATC patients to evaluate the feasibility of concurrent EBRT and dabrafenib/trametinib combination (NCT03975231) is ongoing (Table 2).

Table 1. Outcome of multimodal treatment in ATC.

Authors, References	Study	Number of Patients (Total and According to the Stage)	Surgery	Radiotherapy (Dose)	Chemotherapy Protocol (n = Number of Patients)	Outcomes (ORR (n and %), Median OS (Months) and PFS (Months) Local and Distant Control at 1 Year (%))
[105]	Retrospective	n = 19 metastatic: n = 9	12	30	Bleomycin + Cyclophosphamide + 5-FU	OS: 7–12 months; ORR, PFS, local control: ND; Distant control: 16%
[106]	Prospective, randomized,	n = 39	ND	ND	Doxorubicin (n = 21); Doxorubicin + Cisplatin (n = 18)	ORR: 1/21 (4.8%); OS: ND; PFS: ND; ORR: 6/18 (22.2%); OS: ND; PFS: ND
[107]	Retrospective	n = 34	15	30	Bleomycin + Cyclophosphamide + 5-FU	ORR: 22/34 (64%); OS: 4 months; PFS: ND
[108]	Prospective, no randomization, non-controlled	n = 19 (limited to the neck)	10	19 (57.6 Gy)	Doxorubicin per week (n = 19)	OS: 12 months; Local control: 68%; Distant control: 21%
[109]	Prospective randomized but non-controlled	n = 20 metastatic: n = 6 metastatic: n = 3	12 –9 –3	20	Doxorubicin + Cisplatin (n = 12); Mitoxantrone (n = 8)	OS: 2–6 months; PFS: 6.5 months; Local control: 9/12 (75%); Distant control: 4/12 (33.3%); Local control: 3/8 (37.5%); Distant control: 0/12 (0%); PFS: 4 months
[110]	Prospective, no randomization, non-controlled	n = 32 Stage IVb: n = 23 Stage IVc: n = 9	0/32	32 (30–45 Gy)	Doxorubicin (n = 14/32)	OS: 6 months; PFS: ND; Local control: 7/32 (21.9%); Distant control: ND
[111]	Retrospective	n = 89	10	ND	Vinblastine or Cisplatin or Doxorubicin or Novantrone	ND
[56]	Retrospective	n = 121 Stage IVc: n = 64	106	58	n = 64	OS: 6 months (mean OS: 7.2 +/− 10 months); ORR, PFS, local or distant control: ND
[21]	Retrospective	n = 17	17	12	ND	OS: 12 months
[82]	Prospective study, randomized but non-controlled	n = 55 Stage IVc: n = 17	40	55 (46 Gy)	Doxorubicin (n = 55)	OS: 2–4.5 months; ORR local: 60%; ORR distant: 22%; PFS: ND
[63]	Prospective, no randomization, non-controlled	n = 30 Stage IVa: n = 4 Stage IVb: n = 20 Stage IVc: n = 6	7	30 (40 Gy)	Doxorubicin + Cisplatin	OS: 10 months; Local control: 47%; Distant control: 37%
[60]	Retrospective	n = 37	19	37 (57.6 Gy)	Doxorubicin (n = 37)	OS: 6 months Median Loco-regional-PFS: 10.1 months Local control: 45%
[112]	Retrospective	n = 44 Local: n = 12 Regional: n = 12 Distant: n = 20	44	39 (46–50 Gy)	Doxorubicin + Cisplatin (n = 33); Doxorubicin + Carboplatin (n = 3); Doxorubicin (n = 1); Paclitaxel (n = 1)	OS: 8.5 months; ORR: 22/44 (50%); PFS: 6.5 months
[113]	Retrospective	n = 13 Stage IVc: n = 6	8	5 (45–65 Gy)	Doxorubicin (n = 5)	OS: 3.8 months; ORR: ND; PFS: 2.8 months

Table 1. *Cont.*

Authors, References	Study	Number of Patients (Total and According to the Stage)	Surgery	Radiotherapy (Dose)	Chemotherapy Protocol (n = Number of Patients)	Outcomes (ORR (n and %), Median OS (Months) and PFS (Months) Local and Distant Control at 1 Year (%))
[6]	Retrospective	n = 547 Stage IVa: n = 69 Stage IVb: n = 242 Stage IVc: n = 233	n = 301	319	n = 255 Etoposide + Cisplatin (EP) Etoposide + Cisplatin + Doxorubicin 5FU + Cisplatin + Doxorubicin Paclitaxel	Stage-dependent OS: Stage IVa: 7.8 months Stage IVb: 4.8 months Stage IVc: 2.7 months PFS/ORR: ND
[114]	Phase 3	n = 80 Stage IVa: n = 1 Stage IVb: n = 6 Stage IVc: n = 72 ND: n = 1	44/80	n = 28	Fosbretabulin + Carboplatin + Paclitaxel Control: Carboplatin + Paclitaxel	OS: 8.2 months if surgery versus 4.0 months on the control arm OS: 4.0 months if no surgery and 4.6 months on the control arm
[115]	Prospective, controlled, non-randomized	n = 13 Stage IVb: n = 9 Stage IVc, n = 4	4	ND	Paclitaxel	OS and PFS: ND ORR Stage IVb: 33% ORR Stage IVc: 25%
[64]	Retrospective	n = 92 Stage IVa: n = 6 Stage IVb: n = 22 Stage IVc: n = 61 ND: n = 3	35	56 (55 Gy)	59 Doxorubicin + Cisplatin (n = 56) Carboplatin + Paclitaxel (n = 3)	OS: 7 months; PFS: 5 months Local control: 75%; Distant control: 63%
[116]	Retrospective	n = 8 Stage IVb: n = 2 Stage IVc: n = 4 ND: n = 2	6	5 (40–60 Gy)	Docetaxel + Cisplatin	OS: 30.4 months ORR: 3/8 (37.5%) PFS: 5.5 months
[73]	Retrospective	n = 1288 Stage IVc: n = 608	0	613	471 (treatment not available)	OS: 2.27 months
[5]	Retrospective	n = 100 Stage IVa: n = 9 Stage IVb: n = 32 Stage IVc: n = 54 ND: n = 5	83	81 (57.6 Gy)	Doxorubicin weekly (n = 25) Paclitaxel weekly (n = 9) Paclitaxel + Pemetrexed (n = 8) Doxorubicin + Cisplatin (n = 8) Carboplatin + Paclitaxel (n = 14) Tyrosine kinase inhibitors (n = 10) Other (n = 10)	Median OS: 5.7 months Stage-dependent OS (months and % at 1 year): Stage IVa: 26 months (66%) Stage IVb: 11 months (39%) Stage IVc: 3 months (13%) ORR and PFS: ND
[74]	Retrospective	n = 30 Stage IVa: n = 2 Stage IVb: n = 22 Stage IVc: n = 6 ND: n = 5	27	30 (66 Gy)	Doxorubicin + Docetaxel (n = 19) Carboplatin + Paclitaxel (n = 5) Doxorubicin only (n = 4) Cisplatin only (n = 2)	Median OS: 21 months Median PFS: 8.3 months ORR: 19/30 (63.3%) Local control: 93% Distant control: 22%
[65]	Retrospective	n = 44 Stage IVa: n = 10 Stage IVb: n = 17 Stage IVc: n = 27	23	29	platinum or taxane based agents (n = 46)	OS: 11.9 months (total cohort) and 22.1 months in patients treated with chemotherapy and EBRT TTF: 3.8 months

OS: Overall survival, PFS: Progression-free survival, ORR: Objective response rate, ND: Non-determinated, TTF: Time to treatment failure, EBRT: External beam radiation, ATC: Anaplastic thyroid carcinoma, IMRT: Intensity-Modulated Radiation Therapy, NA: non-applicable. Advanced ATCs, understanding advanced ATCs locally and/or at distant sites.

Table 2. Ongoing clinical trials in ATC patients.

Clinical Trials Gov. Identifier	Treatments/Interventions (Settings)	Phase	Status
NCT03565536	Sorafenib (Neoadjuvant treatment of ATC)	Phase 2	Unknown
NCT03085056	Trametinib + Paclitaxel (Advanced ATC)	Early Phase 1	Recruiting
NCT02688608	Pembrolizumab (Advanced ATC)	Phase 2	Unknown
NCT02244463	MLN0128 (Advanced ATC)	Phase 2	Active, not recruiting
NCT04739566	Dabrafenib + Trametinib (Neoadjuvant Strategy in ATC with *BRAF* mutation)	Phase 2	Recruiting
NCT03122496	Durvalumab + Tremelimumab + Stereotactic Body Radiotherapy (Advanced ATC)	Phase 1	Active, not recruiting
NCT01236547	IMRT + Paclitaxel with or without Pazopanib Hydrochloride (Advanced ATC)	Phase 2	Active, not recruiting
NCT05102292	HLX208 (Advanced ATC with *BRAF*^{V600} mutation)	Phase 1b/2	Recruiting
NCT02152137	Efatutazone + Paclitaxel (Advanced ATC)	Phase 2	Active, not recruiting
NCT04552769	Abemaciclib (CDK4 + CDK6 inhibitor) (Advanced ATC)	Phase 2	Recruiting
NCT04675710	Pembrolizumab + Dabrafenib + Trametinib (Neoadjuvant *BRAF*-Mutated ATC)	Phase 2	Recruiting
NCT04238624	Cemiplimab + Dabrafenib + Trametinib (Advanced ATC)	Phase 2	Recruiting
NCT04420754	AIC100 Chimeric Antigen Receptor T-cells (Relapsed/Refractory Thyroid Cancer)	Phase 1	Recruiting
NCT03975231	Dabrafenib + Trametinib + IMRT in (Advanced *BRAF* Mutated ATC)	Phase 1	Recruiting
NCT03449108	LN-145/LN-145-S1 (Autologous Centrally Manufactured Tumor Infiltrating Lymphocytes) (Advanced ATC)	Phase 2	Recruiting
NCT04592484	CDK-002 (exoSTING) (Advanced/Metastatic, Recurrent, Injectable ATC)	Phase 1	Recruiting
NCT03181100	Cohort I (*BRAF* mutation): Vemurafenib + Cobimetinib + Atezolizumab. Cohort II (*RAS*, *NF1* or *NF2* mutations): Cobimetinib + Atezolizumab Cohort III (non *BRAF* or *RAS* mutation): Bevacizumab + Atezolizumab Cohort IV: Nab-paclitaxel + Atezolizumab	Phase 2	Recruiting
NCT03246958	Nivolumab + Ipilimumab (Advanced ATC)	Phase 2	Active non-recruiting
NCT04400474	Cabozantinib + Atezolizumab (Advanced ATC)	Phase 2	Recruiting
NCT04579757	Surufatinib + Tislelizumab (Advanced ATC)	Phase 1/2	Recruiting
NCT04759911	Selpercatinib (Neoadjuvant ATC with RET alterations)	Phase 2	Recruiting

ATC: Anaplastic thyroid carcinoma, IMRT: Intensity-modulated radiation therapy, NA: non-applicable. Advanced ATCs, understanding advanced ATCs locally and/or at distant sites.

4.3. Systemic Therapies: Failure of Chemotherapies, Success of Targeted Therapies and the Promises of Immunotherapy

Chemotherapy and EBRT are independent prognostic factors that are associated with improved survival [4–6,14,16,117,118]. However, clinical trials comparing different chemotherapy regimens in ATC patients are scarce because of the disease's low incidence and aggressiveness limiting enrollment in clinical trials, leading to poor statistical power and a limited treatment time-frame. In the absence of molecular abnormalities, the most recent ATA Guidelines recommend starting with systemic therapy with genotoxic drugs such as paclitaxel and carboplatin combinations, cisplatin and doxorubicin combinations, docetaxel and doxorubicin combinations, paclitaxel alone, or doxorubicin alone [2,3,119,120]. Table 1 summarizes the studies on the different chemotherapy protocols in ATCs. Given the estimated doubling time of ATC is only 3–12 days, the interval between the administrations of the chemotherapeutic agent has to be short [63]. In this objective, some authors recommend using chemotherapeutic regimens at relatively short intervals (such as weekly administration compared with 3–4-week intervals). The poor prognosis of ATCs is often associated with primary chemoresistance which results in an average PFS of less than three months (Table 2). Indeed, though paclitaxel seems the most effective chemotherapeutic drug, chemo-resistance is common, which may be related to TAMs infiltration. TAMs occupy 50% of the tumor volume and provides paracrine signals via the CSF-1/CSF-1R axis, which promotes tumor progression and therapy resistance. Thus, targeting the CSF-1/CSF-1R pathway in TAMs was shown to restore the sensitivity of thyroid cancer cells to paclitaxel [121].

Due to this primary chemoresistance, other therapeutic strategies have been developed. High-throughput sequencing investigations have unveiled the molecular alterations of ATC opening the way to targeted therapies [7,14,28,29,61]. The recent approval of a combination therapy with the BRAF inhibitor dabrafenib and the MEK inhibitor trametinib for patients with unresectable or metastatic $BRAF^{V600E}$-positive ATC has generated enthusiasm in the field. Indeed, a phase II basket trial describing the efficacy and safety of dabrafenib plus trametinib has enrolled 36 ATC patients, the median age of whom was 71 years; 30/36 (83%) patients had undergone prior tumor radiation. The ORR was 56% (95% CI: 38.1–72.1%), including three complete responses and a median PFS and OS of 6.7 and 14.5 months, respectively, without new safety signals identified with this additional follow-up confirming the results of previous studies [8,9,122]. These results have led to approval by the FDA but not by the EMA. Unfortunately, this combination can only be offered to the 20–50% of ATC patients with $BRAF^{V600E}$ mutation and acquired resistance to BRAF inhibitors may develop via secondary mutations in the MAPK pathway or via the PI3K/AKT/mTOR pathway, or Hgf/Met activation, underlining the need for additional rationally designed approaches [123–125]. Much rarer than $BRAF^{V600E}$ mutations are *NTRK*, *ALK* and *RET* fusions which can be found in 2–3% of ATC patients. However, finding one of these alterations might greatly impact the prognosis of the few mutated patients given the very high response rates observed with their corresponding highly specific inhibitors in different basket trials. A pooled subgroup analysis of the larotrectinib trials (NCT02122913 and NCT02576431) reported a 29% response rate in two out of seven ATC patients; responses lasted for 3.7 and 10.2 months and the median OS was 14.1 months (95% CI: 2.6–NE) [126]. A long-lasting, dramatic response to the RET-specific inhibitor selpercatinib has been reported in a 73 year old patient with *CCD6-RET* fusion ATC [127]. Lasting responses to ALK inhibitor in patients with ALK fusions have also been reported [128]. Although these targeted therapies have demonstrated impressive activity, availability is a major issue in most countries except in the US, where approval has been obtained from the FDA. On 31 July 2020, a conditional marketing authorization valid throughout the European Union (EU) was issued for entrectinib for the treatment of adults with NTRK fusion-positive solid tumors that are locally advanced, metastatic or where surgical resection is likely to result in severe morbidity. To the best of our knowledge, no approvals have been obtained in ATC for RET inhibitors. All protocol regimens are presented in Table 3.

Inhibitors targeting the PI3K/AKT/mTOR pathway, such as everolimus, have been tested but the results were disappointing, with none of the seven patients included in a phase II study benefiting from treatment [129]. A multicenter, phase II trial of everolimus in locally advanced or metastatic thyroid cancer of all histologic subtypes included six ATC cases with only one response, and the others had progressive disease with a median PFS of 10 weeks [130]. Another phase II study evaluated the combination of sorafenib and temsirolimus in two patients with ATC, of which only one had an objective response [131]. To our knowledge, no trials have looked at mTOR inhibitors in the context of ATC with mutation in the PI3K/AKT/mTOR pathway. Antiangiogenic treatments such as lenvatinib [132], a multikinase inhibitor approved in differentiated thyroid cancers, have shown initially encouraging results but limited activity in subsequent studies, with a risk of bleeding and fistula as this disease often invades the trachea, esophagus and vessels, and are thus not recommended [2,77,133]. A recent prospective phase II trial was halted for futility as the minimum ORR threshold of 15% was not met upon interim analysis with a 2.9% response rate, a median PFS of 2.6 months and a median OS of 3.2 months [134].

Over the past few years, immuno-oncologic treatments, especially ICI (e.g., anti-PD-1, anti-PD-L1 and anti-CTLA-4) have revolutionized the field of anti-cancer therapies in many entities. PD-L1 has been suggested as a predictive biomarker of response to ICI in several cancers although its robustness has been questioned. As described above, PD-L1 is often expressed on ATC tumor cells, suggesting new treatment opportunities for ATC with immunotherapy [10,51]. Indeed, spartalizumab, an anti-PD-1 antibody, has been studied in ATC [10]. The response rate was 19% (five PR and three CR observed). The median OS in the entire cohort was 5.9 months, with 40% of patients alive at one year. The median PFS was 1.7 months. Interestingly, those patients with PD-L1 expression of <1% had a median OS of 1.6 months and there were no responses in this group; however, those with PD-L1 expression of 1–49% and ≥50% had a median OS that had not been reached and an overall response rate of 18% (2/11) and 35% (6/17), respectively. The highest rate of response was observed in the subset of patients with PD-L1 > 50% (6/17; 35%). It should be noted that spartalizumab is not FDA- or EMA-approved and is not commercially available. The ACSé basket trial evaluated pembrolizumab in rare cancers in France and included a cohort of 16 ATC patients. The response rate was 25% with a median duration of response of 7.3 ymonths in responder patients [13]. These results differ from those of a phase II study of pembrolizumab combined with chemoradiotherapy as initial treatment which enrolled only three patients, because all three patients died within six months [53]. One might hypothesize that ICI would be more effective without concurrent radiation therapy but further data will be needed to evaluate the best timing for ICI initiation and its clinical efficacy, and clinical trials are ongoing (Table 2). Although effective, ICI will only benefit a small group of patients. Therefore, combination strategies have been developed. In a phase II umbrella study, anti PD-L1 atezolizumab has been studied in combination with either vemurafenib or cobimetinib for *BRAF*-mutated patients (cohort 1), cobimetinib alone for *RAS*- and *NF1*-mutated patients (cohort 2) and bevacizumab for patients with no mutation (cohort 3) in a prospective multi-arm trial [135]. Median OSs were not reached in cohort 1; these were 18.23 months in cohort 2 and 6.21 months in cohort 3. The response rate was 71% in cohort 1 and 7% in cohort 2. Therefore, combination of ICI with targeted therapies in ATC patients with molecular alterations is very promising. In a retrospective study, Diercks et al. analyzed six patients with metastatic ATC treated with multikinase inhibitors (lenvatinib) and ICI (pembrolizumab) and showed 66% with complete remissions (4/6), 16% with stable disease (1/6), and 16% with progressive disease (1/6). The median PFS was 16.8 months and the median OS was 17.3 months [11].

These optimistic data may lead to a systematic screening of PD-L1 and/or MMR status. However, it will first be necessary to define a specific expression score for PD-L1 expression in ATCs and to correlate it with the clinical benefit. Because the ATC immune microenvironment is an immunosuppressive medium, the development of immunotherapy combinations to improve these results will also be required. Clinical trials using immunotherapy in combination with other systemic agents are underway (Table 2).

Table 3. Treatment protocols in Anaplastic Thyroid Carcinoma.

Treatment	Protocols and Dose
Chemotherapy	Every 3 or 4 weeks Doxorubicin (60 mg/m^2) + Cisplatin (120 mg/m^2) every 4 weeks Paclitaxel (175 mg/m^2) + Carboplatin (AUC 5) every 3 weeks Docetaxel (60 mg/m^2) + Doxorubicin (60 mg/m^2) every 3–4 weeks Paclitaxel (135–200 mg/m^2) every 3–4 weeks Doxorubicin (60–75 mg/m^2) every 3 weeks Every week Paclitaxel 50–100 mg/m^2 + Carboplatin AUC2 Docetaxel (20 mg/m^2) + Doxorubicin (20 mg/m^2) Paclitaxel (30–60 mg/m^2) Docetaxel (20 mg/m^2)
BRAF and MEK inhibitors	Dabrafenib 150 mg twice daily + Trametinib 2 mg once daily
RET inhibitor	Selpercatinib 160 mg twice daily, reduced to 120 mg twice daily in patients weighing less than 50 kg Praseltinib 400 mg per day
NTRK inhibitor	Larotrectinib 100 mg twice daily Entrectinib 600 mg once daily
ALK inhibitor	Crizotinib 250 mg twice daily Larotrectinib 100 mg twice daily

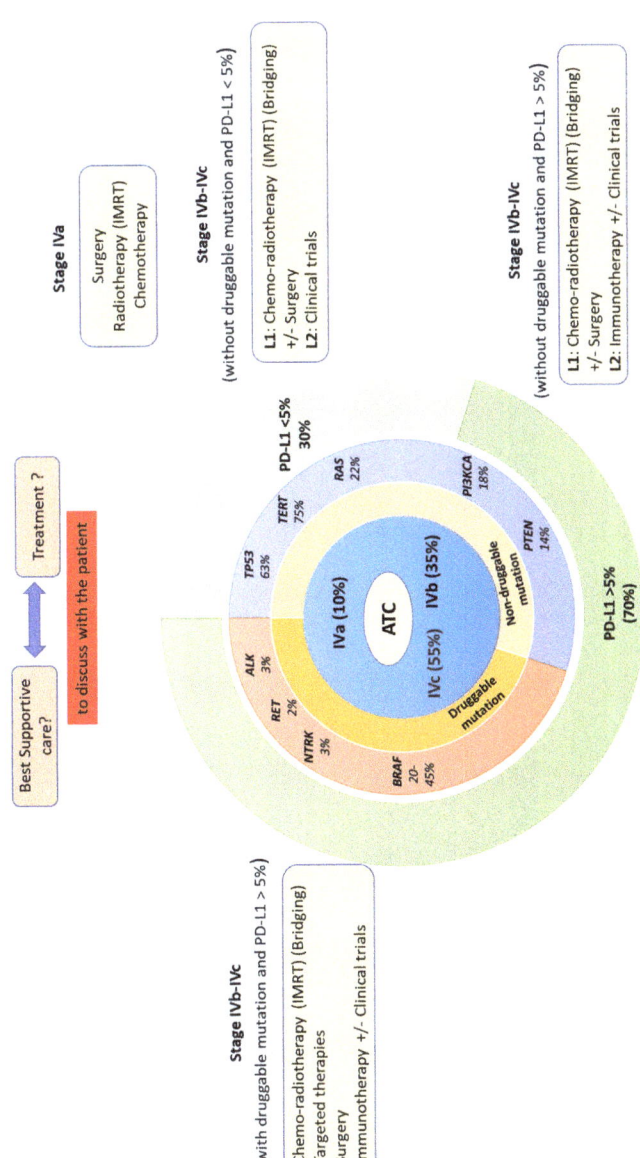

Figure 4. Molecular and treatment landscape of ATC (based on [2]). ATC: Anaplastic Thyroid Carcinoma, L1 and L2: Line of treatment one or two, IMRT: Intensity-Modulated Radiation Therapy, PD-L1: Programmed Death-Ligand 1.

4.4. Reappraisal of Surgery in the Era of Targeted Therapies

There has been substantial debate about the appropriate role for surgery in the management of locally advanced and metastatic ATC. Operative treatment of local disease offers the best opportunity for prolonged survival if the neoplasm is intrathyroidal. When the neoplasm is extrathyroidal, the operative approach is controversial, as some have found that neither the extent of the operation nor the completeness of the tumor resection affects survival [63,77,136,137]. Complete resection is recommended whenever possible for patients with confined ATC (stage IVa/IVb) in whom R0/R1 resection is anticipated, if excessive morbidity can be avoided [2,3,138]. Lateral compartment lymphadenectomy should be performed only in the setting of complete macroscopic resection. Resection of the larynx, pharynx and esophagus are discouraged [56,67,139].

ATC patients present with extensively invasive primary tumors in between 85 and 95% of cases [68,140] justifying the use of neoadjuvant therapy by chemotherapy, chemoradiotherapy (Figure 3) or by targeted therapy [82,99,115,141]. In BRAF^{V600E}-mutated ATC patients, the successful use of neoadjuvant dabrafenib plus trametinib with or without immunotherapy has been described in a case series of six patients that eventually underwent surgery [142,143]. In these patients, adjuvant therapy was prescribed with the *BRAF*-directed therapy or with chemoradiation after surgery. OS at 6 and 12 months was 100% and 83%, respectively, but the locoregional control rate was 100%. These data have revigorated interest toward primary resection upfront or following initial response to treatment in ATC patients.

5. Conclusions

ATCs are aggressive tumors occurring most often in the elderly. The survival outcomes of anaplastic thyroid carcinoma remain poor. Their diagnostic and therapeutic management must be initiated quickly and has to be coordinated within an expert center network. The objectives of the treatment are to fight against the risk of suffocation, to control the tumor mass and to ensure optimal treatment of symptoms within a multidisciplinary team involving endocrinologists, medical oncologists and radiotherapists, palliative care, geriatric oncologists, surgeons, and radiologists in order to offer appropriate care at each stage of the disease. Multimodal treatment combining surgery, radiotherapy, chemotherapy or targeted therapy can allow the control of the tumor. The results of immunotherapy are encouraging but its place is yet to be defined. With increasing knowledge of the tumor biology, the identification of the underlying molecular pathways, modifications of the transcriptome, proteome and associated immunomodulatory mechanisms of ATC (TAMs) on the one hand, and the emerging role of novel, molecular-based single/multi-targeted therapies on the other hand, a growing number of clinical trials can be noted. Prioritizing clinical trial enrollment will be a key factor in advancing care for patients with ATC.

Author Contributions: Conceptualization, A.J. and J.H.; methodology, A.J., A.E., J.H. and C.D.C.; data curation, A.E., A.A.G. and B.C.; writing—original draft preparation, A.J., A.E., J.H. and C.D.C.; writing—review and editing, A.J., J.H., C.D.C., A.A.G., B.C., F.D., P.B., D.H., L.L. (Livia Lamartina), E.B., L.L. (Ludovic Lacroix) and C.D. All authors have read and agreed to the published version of the manuscript.

Funding: This research received no external funding.

Acknowledgments: We would like to thank Clio Baillet for providing the images in Figure 2.

Conflicts of Interest: The authors declare no conflict of interest.

References

1. Molinaro, E.; Romei, C.; Biagini, A.; Sabini, E.; Agate, L.; Mazzeo, S.; Materazzi, G.; Sellari-Franceschini, S.; Ribechini, A.; Torregrossa, L.; et al. Anaplastic Thyroid Carcinoma: From Clinicopathology to Genetics and Advanced Therapies. *Nat. Rev. Endocrinol.* **2017**, *13*, 644–660. [CrossRef] [PubMed]
2. Bible, K.C.; Kebebew, E.; Brierley, J.; Brito, J.P.; Cabanillas, M.E.; Clark, T.J.; Di Cristofano, A.; Foote, R.; Giordano, T.; Kasperbauer, J.; et al. 2021 American Thyroid Association Guidelines for Management of Patients with Anaplastic Thyroid Cancer. *Thyroid* **2021**, *31*, 337–386. [CrossRef] [PubMed]
3. Filetti, S.; Durante, C.; Hartl, D.; Leboulleux, S.; Locati, L.D.; Newbold, K.; Papotti, M.G.; Berruti, A. Thyroid Cancer: ESMO Clinical Practice Guidelines for Diagnosis, Treatment and Follow-Up. *Ann. Oncol.* **2019**, *30*, 1856–1883. [CrossRef] [PubMed]
4. Hvilsom, G.B.; Londero, S.C.; Hahn, C.H.; Schytte, S.; Pedersen, H.B.; Christiansen, P.; Kiss, K.; Larsen, S.R.; Jespersen, M.L.; Lelkaitis, G.; et al. Anaplastic Thyroid Carcinoma in Denmark 1996-2012: A National Prospective Study of 219 Patients. *Cancer Epidemiol.* **2018**, *53*, 65–71. [CrossRef] [PubMed]
5. Wendler, J.; Kroiss, M.; Gast, K.; Kreissl, M.C.; Allelein, S.; Lichtenauer, U.; Blaser, R.; Spitzweg, C.; Fassnacht, M.; Schott, M.; et al. Clinical Presentation, Treatment and Outcome of Anaplastic Thyroid Carcinoma: Results of a Multicenter Study in Germany. *Eur. J. Endocrinol.* **2016**, *175*, 521–529. [CrossRef] [PubMed]
6. Sugitani, I.; Miyauchi, A.; Sugino, K.; Okamoto, T.; Yoshida, A.; Suzuki, S. Prognostic Factors and Treatment Outcomes for Anaplastic Thyroid Carcinoma: ATC Research Consortium of Japan Cohort Study of 677 Patients. *World J. Surg.* **2012**, *36*, 1247–1254. [CrossRef] [PubMed]
7. Xu, B.; Fuchs, T.; Dogan, S.; Landa, I.; Katabi, N.; Fagin, J.A.; Tuttle, R.M.; Sherman, E.; Gill, A.J.; Ghossein, R. Dissecting Anaplastic Thyroid Carcinoma: A Comprehensive Clinical, Histologic, Immunophenotypic, and Molecular Study of 360 Cases. *Thyroid* **2020**, *30*, 1505–1517. [CrossRef]
8. Subbiah, V.; Kreitman, R.J.; Wainberg, Z.A.; Cho, J.Y.; Schellens, J.H.M.; Soria, J.C.; Wen, P.Y.; Zielinski, C.; Cabanillas, M.E.; Urbanowitz, G.; et al. Dabrafenib and Trametinib Treatment in Patients With Locally Advanced or Metastatic BRAF V600-Mutant Anaplastic Thyroid Cancer. *J. Clin. Oncol.* **2018**, *36*, 7–13. [CrossRef] [PubMed]
9. Subbiah, V.; Kreitman, R.J.; Wainberg, Z.A.; Cho, J.Y.; Schellens, J.H.M.; Soria, J.C.; Wen, P.Y.; Zielinski, C.C.; Cabanillas, M.E.; Boran, A.; et al. Dabrafenib plus Trametinib in Patients with BRAF V600E–Mutant Anaplastic Thyroid Cancer: Updated Analysis from the Phase II ROAR Basket Study. *Ann. Oncol.* **2022**. [CrossRef]
10. Capdevila, J.; Wirth, L.J.; Ernst, T.; Ponce Aix, S.; Lin, C.-C.; Ramlau, R.; Butler, M.O.; Delord, J.-P.; Gelderblom, H.; Ascierto, P.A.; et al. PD-1 Blockade in Anaplastic Thyroid Carcinoma. *J. Clin. Oncol.* **2020**, *38*, 2620–2627. [CrossRef]
11. Dierks, C.; Seufert, J.; Aumann, K.; Ruf, J.; Klein, C.; Kiefer, S.; Rassner, M.; Boerries, M.; Zielke, A.; La Rosée, P.; et al. The Lenvatinib/Pembrolizumab Combination Is an Effective Treatment Option for Anaplastic and Poorly Differentiated Thyroid Carcinoma. *Thyroid* **2021**, *31*, 1076–1085. [CrossRef] [PubMed]
12. Iyer, P.C.; Dadu, R.; Gule-Monroe, M.; Busaidy, N.L.; Ferrarotto, R.; Habra, M.A.; Zafereo, M.; Williams, M.D.; Gunn, G.B.; Grosu, H.; et al. Salvage Pembrolizumab Added to Kinase Inhibitor Therapy for the Treatment of Anaplastic Thyroid Carcinoma. *J. Immunother. Cancer* **2018**, *6*, 68. [CrossRef]
13. Leboulleux, S.; Godbert, Y.; Penel, N.; Hescot, S.; De La Fouchardiere, C.; Blonski, M.; Lamartina, L.; Cousin, S.; Do Cao, C.; Hadoux, J.; et al. Benefits of Pembrolizumab in Progressive Radioactive Iodine Refractory Thyroid Cancer: Results of the AcSé Pembrolizumab Study from Unicancer. *J. Clin. Oncol.* **2021**, *39*, 6082. [CrossRef]
14. Maniakas, A.; Dadu, R.; Busaidy, N.L.; Wang, J.R.; Ferrarotto, R.; Lu, C.; Williams, M.D.; Gunn, G.B.; Hofmann, M.-C.; Cote, G.; et al. Evaluation of Overall Survival in Patients With Anaplastic Thyroid Carcinoma, 2000–2019. *JAMA Oncol.* **2020**, *6*, 1397. [CrossRef] [PubMed]
15. Casali, P.G.; Trama, A. Rationale of the Rare Cancer List: A Consensus Paper from the Joint Action on Rare Cancers (JARC) of the European Union (EU). *ESMO Open* **2020**, *5*, e000666. [CrossRef] [PubMed]
16. Janz, T.A.; Neskey, D.M.; Nguyen, S.A.; Lentsch, E.J. Is the Incidence of Anaplastic Thyroid Cancer Increasing: A Population Based Epidemiology Study. *World J. Otorhinolaryngol. Head Neck Surg.* **2019**, *5*, 34–40. [CrossRef]
17. Amphlett, B.; Lawson, Z.; Abdulrahman, G.O.; White, C.; Bailey, R.; Premawardhana, L.D.; Okosieme, O.E. Recent Trends in the Incidence, Geographical Distribution, and Survival from Thyroid Cancer in Wales, 1985–2010. *Thyroid* **2013**, *23*, 1470–1478. [CrossRef]
18. de Ridder, M.; Nieveen van Dijkum, E.; Engelsman, A.; Kapiteijn, E.; Klümpen, H.-J.; Rasch, C.R.N. Anaplastic Thyroid Carcinoma: A Nationwide Cohort Study on Incidence, Treatment and Survival in the Netherlands over 3 Decades. *Eur. J. Endocrinol.* **2020**, *183*, 203–209. [CrossRef]
19. Kebebew, E.; Greenspan, F.S.; Clark, O.H.; Woeber, K.A.; McMillan, A. Anaplastic Thyroid Carcinoma. Treatment Outcome and Prognostic Factors. *Cancer* **2005**, *103*, 1330–1335. [CrossRef]
20. Onoda, N.; Sugitani, I.; Ito, K.; Suzuki, A.; Higashiyama, T.; Fukumori, T.; Suganuma, N.; Masudo, K.; Nakayama, H.; Uno, A.; et al. Evaluation of the 8th Edition TNM Classification for Anaplastic Thyroid Carcinoma. *Cancers* **2020**, *12*, 552. [CrossRef]
21. Demeter, J.G.; De Jong, S.A.; Lawrence, A.M.; Paloyan, E. Anaplastic Thyroid Carcinoma: Risk Factors and Outcome. *Surgery* **1991**, *110*, 956–961, discussion 961–963. [PubMed]
22. Loyd, R.; Osamura, R.; Klöppel, G.; Rosai, J. *WHO Classification of Tumours of Endocrine Organs*, 4th ed.; IARC Publications; WHO Press: Geneve, Switzerland, 2017; Volume 10, ISBN 978-92-832-4493-6.

23. Ragazzi, M.; Ciarrocchi, A.; Sancisi, V.; Gandolfi, G.; Bisagni, A.; Piana, S. Update on Anaplastic Thyroid Carcinoma: Morphological, Molecular, and Genetic Features of the Most Aggressive Thyroid Cancer. *Int. J. Endocrinol.* **2014**, *2014*, 790834. [CrossRef] [PubMed]
24. Lai, W.-A.; Hang, J.-F.; Liu, C.-Y.; Bai, Y.; Liu, Z.; Gu, H.; Hong, S.; Pyo, J.Y.; Jung, C.K.; Kakudo, K.; et al. PAX8 Expression in Anaplastic Thyroid Carcinoma Is Less than Those Reported in Early Studies: A Multi-Institutional Study of 182 Cases Using the Monoclonal Antibody MRQ-50. *Virchows Arch. Int. J. Pathol.* **2020**, *476*, 431–437. [CrossRef]
25. Bishop, J.A.; Sharma, R.; Westra, W.H. PAX8 Immunostaining of Anaplastic Thyroid Carcinoma: A Reliable Means of Discerning Thyroid Origin for Undifferentiated Tumors of the Head and Neck. *Hum. Pathol.* **2011**, *42*, 1873–1877. [CrossRef] [PubMed]
26. Aldinger, K.A.; Samaan, N.A.; Ibanez, M.; Hill, C.S. Anaplastic Carcinoma of the Thyroid: A Review of 84 Cases of Spindle and Giant Cell Carcinoma of the Thyroid. *Cancer* **1978**, *41*, 2267–2275. [CrossRef]
27. Bonhomme, B.; Godbert, Y.; Perot, G.; Al Ghuzlan, A.; Bardet, S.; Belleannée, G.; Crinière, L.; Do Cao, C.; Fouilloux, G.; Guyetant, S.; et al. Molecular Pathology of Anaplastic Thyroid Carcinomas: A Retrospective Study of 144 Cases. *Thyroid* **2017**, *27*, 682–692. [CrossRef]
28. Landa, I.; Ibrahimpasic, T.; Boucai, L.; Sinha, R.; Knauf, J.A.; Shah, R.H.; Dogan, S.; Ricarte-Filho, J.C.; Krishnamoorthy, G.P.; Xu, B.; et al. Genomic and Transcriptomic Hallmarks of Poorly Differentiated and Anaplastic Thyroid Cancers. *J. Clin. Invest.* **2016**, *126*, 1052–1066. [CrossRef]
29. Pozdeyev, N.; Gay, L.M.; Sokol, E.S.; Hartmaier, R.; Deaver, K.E.; Davis, S.; French, J.D.; Borre, P.V.; LaBarbera, D.V.; Tan, A.-C.; et al. Genetic Analysis of 779 Advanced Differentiated and Anaplastic Thyroid Cancers. *Clin. Cancer Res.* **2018**, *24*, 3059–3068. [CrossRef]
30. Romei, C.; Tacito, A.; Molinaro, E.; Piaggi, P.; Cappagli, V.; Pieruzzi, L.; Matrone, A.; Viola, D.; Agate, L.; Torregrossa, L.; et al. Clinical, Pathological and Genetic Features of Anaplastic and Poorly Differentiated Thyroid Cancer: A Single Institute Experience. *Oncol. Lett.* **2018**, *15*, 9174–9182. [CrossRef]
31. Capdevila, J.; Mayor, R.; Mancuso, F.M.; Iglesias, C.; Caratù, G.; Matos, I.; Zafón, C.; Hernando, J.; Petit, A.; Nuciforo, P.; et al. Early Evolutionary Divergence between Papillary and Anaplastic Thyroid Cancers. *Ann. Oncol.* **2018**, *29*, 1454–1460. [CrossRef]
32. Ngo, T.N.M.; Le, T.T.B.; Le, T.; Bychkov, A.; Oishi, N.; Jung, C.K.; Hassell, L.; Kakudo, K.; Vuong, H.G. Primary Versus Secondary Anaplastic Thyroid Carcinoma: Perspectives from Multi-Institutional and Population-Level Data. *Endocr. Pathol.* **2021**, *32*, 489–500. [CrossRef] [PubMed]
33. Kunstman, J.W.; Juhlin, C.C.; Goh, G.; Brown, T.C.; Stenman, A.; Healy, J.M.; Rubinstein, J.C.; Choi, M.; Kiss, N.; Nelson-Williams, C.; et al. Characterization of the Mutational Landscape of Anaplastic Thyroid Cancer via Whole-Exome Sequencing. *Hum. Mol. Genet.* **2015**, *24*, 2318–2329. [CrossRef] [PubMed]
34. Yoo, S.-K.; Song, Y.S.; Lee, E.K.; Hwang, J.; Kim, H.H.; Jung, G.; Kim, Y.A.; Kim, S.; Cho, S.W.; Won, J.-K.; et al. Integrative Analysis of Genomic and Transcriptomic Characteristics Associated with Progression of Aggressive Thyroid Cancer. *Nat. Commun.* **2019**, *10*, 2764. [CrossRef] [PubMed]
35. Chu, Y.-H.; Wirth, L.J.; Farahani, A.A.; Nosé, V.; Faquin, W.C.; Dias-Santagata, D.; Sadow, P.M. Clinicopathologic Features of Kinase Fusion-Related Thyroid Carcinomas: An Integrative Analysis with Molecular Characterization. *Mod. Pathol.* **2020**, *33*, 2458–2472. [CrossRef]
36. Prete, A.; Matrone, A.; Gambale, C.; Torregrossa, L.; Minaldi, E.; Romei, C.; Ciampi, R.; Molinaro, E.; Elisei, R. Poorly Differentiated and Anaplastic Thyroid Cancer: Insights into Genomics, Microenvironment and New Drugs. *Cancers* **2021**, *13*, 3200. [CrossRef]
37. Yakushina, V.D.; Lerner, L.V.; Lavrov, A.V. Gene Fusions in Thyroid Cancer. *Thyroid* **2018**, *28*, 158–167. [CrossRef]
38. Krishnamoorthy, G.P.; Davidson, N.R.; Leach, S.D.; Zhao, Z.; Lowe, S.W.; Lee, G.; Landa, I.; Nagarajah, J.; Saqcena, M.; Singh, K.; et al. EIF1AX and RAS Mutations Cooperate to Drive Thyroid Tumorigenesis through ATF4 and C-MYC. *Cancer Discov.* **2019**, *9*, 264–281. [CrossRef]
39. Garcia-Rostan, G.; Camp, R.L.; Herrero, A.; Carcangiu, M.L.; Rimm, D.L.; Tallini, G. β-Catenin Dysregulation in Thyroid Neoplasms. *Am. J. Pathol.* **2001**, *158*, 987–996. [CrossRef]
40. Lazzereschi, D.; Palmirotta, R.; Ranieri, A.; Ottini, L.; Verì, M.C.; Cama, A.; Cetta, F.; Nardi, F.; Colletta, G.; Mariani-Costantini, R. Microsatellite Instability in Thyroid Tumours and Tumour-like Lesions. *Br. J. Cancer* **1999**, *79*, 340–345. [CrossRef]
41. Ravi, N.; Yang, M.; Gretarsson, S.; Jansson, C.; Mylona, N.; Sydow, S.R.; Woodward, E.L.; Ekblad, L.; Wennerberg, J.; Paulsson, K. Identification of Targetable Lesions in Anaplastic Thyroid Cancer by Genome Profiling. *Cancers* **2019**, *11*, 402. [CrossRef]
42. Rocha, M.L.; Schmid, K.W.; Czapiewski, P. The Prevalence of DNA Microsatellite Instability in Anaplastic Thyroid Carcinoma–Systematic Review and Discussion of Current Therapeutic Options. *Contemp. Oncol.* **2021**, *25*, 213–223. [CrossRef]
43. Wong, K.S.; Lorch, J.H.; Alexander, E.K.; Nehs, M.A.; Nowak, J.A.; Hornick, J.L.; Barletta, J.A. Clinicopathologic Features of Mismatch Repair-Deficient Anaplastic Thyroid Carcinomas. *Thyroid* **2019**, *29*, 666–673. [CrossRef] [PubMed]
44. Caillou, B.; Talbot, M.; Weyemi, U.; Pioche-Durieu, C.; Al Ghuzlan, A.; Bidart, J.M.; Chouaib, S.; Schlumberger, M.; Dupuy, C. Tumor-Associated Macrophages (TAMs) Form an Interconnected Cellular Supportive Network in Anaplastic Thyroid Carcinoma. *PLoS ONE* **2011**, *6*, e22567. [CrossRef] [PubMed]
45. Jung, K.Y.; Cho, S.W.; Kim, Y.A.; Kim, D.; Oh, B.-C.; Park, D.J.; Park, Y.J. Cancers with Higher Density of Tumor-Associated Macrophages Were Associated with Poor Survival Rates. *J. Pathol. Transl. Med.* **2015**, *49*, 318–324. [CrossRef]
46. Kim, H.; Park, Y.W.; Oh, Y.-H.; Sim, J.; Ro, J.Y.; Pyo, J.Y. Anaplastic Transformation of Papillary Thyroid Carcinoma Only Seen in Pleural Metastasis: A Case Report with Review of the Literature. *Head Neck Pathol.* **2016**, *11*, 162–167. [CrossRef]

47. Ryder, M.; Ghossein, R.A.; Ricarte-Filho, J.C.M.; Knauf, J.A.; Fagin, J.A. Increased Density of Tumor-Associated Macrophages Is Associated with Decreased Survival in Advanced Thyroid Cancer. *Endocr. Relat. Cancer* **2008**, *15*, 1069–1074. [CrossRef]
48. Lv, J.; Feng, Z.-P.; Chen, F.-K.; Liu, C.; Jia, L.; Liu, P.-J.; Yang, C.-Z.; Hou, F.; Deng, Z.-Y. M2-like Tumor-Associated Macrophages-Secreted Wnt1 and Wnt3a Promotes Dedifferentiation and Metastasis via Activating β-Catenin Pathway in Thyroid Cancer. *Mol. Carcinog.* **2021**, *60*, 25–37. [CrossRef]
49. Schürch, C.M.; Roelli, M.A.; Forster, S.; Wasmer, M.-H.; Brühl, F.; Maire, R.S.; Di Pancrazio, S.; Ruepp, M.-D.; Giger, R.; Perren, A.; et al. Targeting CD47 in Anaplastic Thyroid Carcinoma Enhances Tumor Phagocytosis by Macrophages and Is a Promising Therapeutic Strategy. *Thyroid* **2019**, *29*, 979–992. [CrossRef]
50. Giannini, R.; Moretti, S.; Ugolini, C.; Macerola, E.; Menicali, E.; Nucci, N.; Morelli, S.; Colella, R.; Mandarano, M.; Sidoni, A.; et al. Immune Profiling of Thyroid Carcinomas Suggests the Existence of Two Major Phenotypes: An ATC-like and a PDTC-Like. *J. Clin. Endocrinol. Metab.* **2019**, *104*, 3557–3575. [CrossRef]
51. Adam, P.; Kircher, S.; Sbiera, I.; Koehler, V.F.; Berg, E.; Knösel, T.; Sandner, B.; Fenske, W.K.; Bläker, H.; Smaxwil, C.; et al. FGF-Receptors and PD-L1 in Anaplastic and Poorly Differentiated Thyroid Cancer: Evaluation of the Preclinical Rationale. *Front. Endocrinol.* **2021**, *12*, 712107. [CrossRef]
52. Bastman, J.J.; Serracino, H.S.; Zhu, Y.; Koenig, M.R.; Mateescu, V.; Sams, S.B.; Davies, K.D.; Raeburn, C.D.; McIntyre, R.C.; Haugen, B.R.; et al. Tumor-Infiltrating T Cells and the PD-1 Checkpoint Pathway in Advanced Differentiated and Anaplastic Thyroid Cancer. *J. Clin. Endocrinol. Metab.* **2016**, *101*, 2863–2873. [CrossRef] [PubMed]
53. Chintakuntlawar, A.V.; Rumilla, K.M.; Smith, C.Y.; Jenkins, S.M.; Foote, R.L.; Kasperbauer, J.L.; Morris, J.C.; Ryder, M.; Alsidawi, S.; Hilger, C.; et al. Expression of PD-1 and PD-L1 in Anaplastic Thyroid Cancer Patients Treated With Multimodal Therapy: Results From a Retrospective Study. *J. Clin. Endocrinol. Metab.* **2017**, *102*, 1943–1950. [CrossRef]
54. Noguchi, T.; Ward, J.P.; Gubin, M.M.; Arthur, C.D.; Lee, S.H.; Hundal, J.; Selby, M.J.; Graziano, R.F.; Mardis, E.R.; Korman, A.J.; et al. Temporally Distinct PD-L1 Expression by Tumor and Host Cells Contributes to Immune Escape. *Cancer Immunol. Res.* **2017**, *5*, 106–117. [CrossRef] [PubMed]
55. Wei, Y.; Zhao, Q.; Gao, Z.; Lao, X.-M.; Lin, W.-M.; Chen, D.-P.; Mu, M.; Huang, C.-X.; Liu, Z.-Y.; Li, B.; et al. The Local Immune Landscape Determines Tumor PD-L1 Heterogeneity and Sensitivity to Therapy. *J. Clin. Investig.* **2019**, *129*, 3347–3360. [CrossRef] [PubMed]
56. Venkatesh, Y.S.; Ordonez, N.G.; Schultz, P.N.; Hickey, R.C.; Goepfert, H.; Samaan, N.A. Anaplastic Carcinoma of the Thyroid. A Clinicopathologic Study of 121 Cases. *Cancer* **1990**, *66*, 321–330. [CrossRef]
57. Haigh, P.I. Anaplastic Thyroid Carcinoma. *Curr. Treat. Options Oncol.* **2000**, *1*, 353–357. [CrossRef] [PubMed]
58. Smallridge, R.C.; Copland, J.A. Anaplastic Thyroid Carcinoma: Pathogenesis and Emerging Therapies. *Clin. Oncol.* **2010**, *22*, 486–497. [CrossRef]
59. Akaishi, J.; Sugino, K.; Kitagawa, W.; Nagahama, M.; Kameyama, K.; Shimizu, K.; Ito, K.; Ito, K. Prognostic Factors and Treatment Outcomes of 100 Cases of Anaplastic Thyroid Carcinoma. *Thyroid* **2011**, *21*, 1183–1189. [CrossRef]
60. Sherman, E.J.; Lim, S.H.; Ho, A.L.; Ghossein, R.A.; Fury, M.G.; Shaha, A.R.; Rivera, M.; Lin, O.; Wolden, S.; Lee, N.Y.; et al. Concurrent Doxorubicin and Radiotherapy for Anaplastic Thyroid Cancer: A Critical Re-Evaluation Including Uniform Pathologic Review. *Radiother. Oncol.* **2011**, *101*, 425–430. [CrossRef]
61. Ito, K.-I.; Hanamura, T.; Murayama, K.; Okada, T.; Watanabe, T.; Harada, M.; Ito, T.; Koyama, H.; Kanai, T.; Maeno, K.; et al. Multimodality Therapeutic Outcomes in Anaplastic Thyroid Carcinoma: Improved Survival in Subgroups of Patients with Localized Primary Tumors. *Head Neck* **2012**, *34*, 230–237. [CrossRef]
62. Cabanillas, M.E.; Williams, M.D.; Gunn, G.B.; Weitzman, S.P.; Burke, L.; Busaidy, N.L.; Ying, A.K.; Yiin, Y.H.; William, W.N.; Lu, C.; et al. Facilitating Anaplastic Thyroid Cancer Specialized Treatment: A Model for Improving Access to Multidisciplinary Care for Patients with Anaplastic Thyroid Cancer. *Head Neck* **2017**, *39*, 1291–1295. [CrossRef] [PubMed]
63. De Crevoisier, R.; Baudin, E.; Bachelot, A.; Leboulleux, S.; Travagli, J.-P.; Caillou, B.; Schlumberger, M. Combined Treatment of Anaplastic Thyroid Carcinoma with Surgery, Chemotherapy, and Hyperfractionated Accelerated External Radiotherapy. *Int. J. Radiat. Oncol. Biol. Phys.* **2004**, *60*, 1137–1143. [CrossRef] [PubMed]
64. Levy, A.; Leboulleux, S.; Lepoutre-Lussey, C.; Baudin, E.; Ghuzlan, A.A.; Hartl, D.; Deutsch, E.; Deandreis, D.; Lumbroso, J.; Tao, Y.; et al. (18)F-Fluorodeoxyglucose Positron Emission Tomography to Assess Response after Radiation Therapy in Anaplastic Thyroid Cancer. *Oral Oncol.* **2015**, *51*, 370–375. [CrossRef] [PubMed]
65. Rao, S.N.; Zafereo, M.; Dadu, R.; Busaidy, N.L.; Hess, K.; Cote, G.J.; Williams, M.D.; William, W.N.; Sandulache, V.; Gross, N.; et al. Patterns of Treatment Failure in Anaplastic Thyroid Carcinoma. *Thyroid* **2017**, *27*, 672–681. [CrossRef] [PubMed]
66. Chang, H.-S.; Nam, K.-H.; Chung, W.Y.; Park, C.S. Anaplastic Thyroid Carcinoma: A Therapeutic Dilemma. *Yonsei Med. J.* **2005**, *46*, 759–764. [CrossRef] [PubMed]
67. Haigh, P.I.; Ituarte, P.H.; Wu, H.S.; Treseler, P.A.; Posner, M.D.; Quivey, J.M.; Duh, Q.Y.; Clark, O.H. Completely Resected Anaplastic Thyroid Carcinoma Combined with Adjuvant Chemotherapy and Irradiation Is Associated with Prolonged Survival. *Cancer* **2001**, *91*, 2335–2342. [CrossRef]
68. Chen, J.; Tward, J.D.; Shrieve, D.C.; Hitchcock, Y.J. Surgery and Radiotherapy Improves Survival in Patients with Anaplastic Thyroid Carcinoma: Analysis of the Surveillance, Epidemiology, and End Results 1983-2002. *Am. J. Clin. Oncol.* **2008**, *31*, 460–464. [CrossRef]

69. Haymart, M.R.; Banerjee, M.; Yin, H.; Worden, F.; Griggs, J.J. Marginal Treatment Benefit in Anaplastic Thyroid Cancer. *Cancer* **2013**, *119*, 3133–3139. [CrossRef]
70. Huang, N.-S.; Shi, X.; Lei, B.-W.; Wei, W.-J.; Lu, Z.-W.; Yu, P.-C.; Wang, Y.; Ji, Q.-H.; Wang, Y.-L. An Update of the Appropriate Treatment Strategies in Anaplastic Thyroid Cancer: A Population-Based Study of 735 Patients. *Int. J. Endocrinol.* **2019**, *2019*, 8428547. [CrossRef]
71. Kwon, J.; Kim, B.H.; Jung, H.-W.; Besic, N.; Sugitani, I.; Wu, H.-G. The Prognostic Impacts of Postoperative Radiotherapy in the Patients with Resected Anaplastic Thyroid Carcinoma: A Systematic Review and Meta-Analysis. *Eur. J. Cancer* **2016**, *59*, 34–45. [CrossRef]
72. Liu, T.-R.; Xiao, Z.-W.; Xu, H.-N.; Long, Z.; Wei, F.-Q.; Zhuang, S.-M.; Sun, X.-M.; Xie, L.-E.; Mu, J.-S.; Yang, A.-K.; et al. Treatment and Prognosis of Anaplastic Thyroid Carcinoma: A Clinical Study of 50 Cases. *PLoS ONE* **2016**, *11*, e0164840. [CrossRef]
73. Pezzi, T.A.; Mohamed, A.S.R.; Sheu, T.; Blanchard, P.; Sandulache, V.C.; Lai, S.Y.; Cabanillas, M.E.; Williams, M.D.; Pezzi, C.M.; Lu, C.; et al. Radiation Therapy Dose Is Associated with Improved Survival for Unresected Anaplastic Thyroid Carcinoma: Outcomes from the National Cancer Data Base. *Cancer* **2017**, *123*, 1653–1661. [CrossRef] [PubMed]
74. Prasongsook, N.; Kumar, A.; Chintakuntlawar, A.V.; Foote, R.L.; Kasperbauer, J.; Molina, J.; Garces, Y.; Ma, D.; Wittich, M.A.N.; Rubin, J.; et al. Survival in Response to Multimodal Therapy in Anaplastic Thyroid Cancer. *J. Clin. Endocrinol. Metab.* **2017**, *102*, 4506–4514. [CrossRef] [PubMed]
75. Smallridge, R.C. Approach to the Patient with Anaplastic Thyroid Carcinoma. *J. Clin. Endocrinol. Metab.* **2012**, *97*, 2566–2572. [CrossRef]
76. Song, T.; Chen, L.; Zhang, H.; Lu, Y.; Yu, K.; Zhan, W.; Fang, M. Multimodal Treatment Based on Thyroidectomy Improves Survival in Patients with Metastatic Anaplastic Thyroid Carcinoma: A SEER Analysis from 1998 to 2015. *Gland Surg.* **2020**, *9*, 1205–1213. [CrossRef]
77. Baek, S.-K.; Lee, M.-C.; Hah, J.H.; Ahn, S.-H.; Son, Y.-I.; Rho, Y.-S.; Chung, P.-S.; Lee, Y.-S.; Koo, B.S.; Jung, K.-Y.; et al. Role of Surgery in the Management of Anaplastic Thyroid Carcinoma: Korean Nationwide Multicenter Study of 329 Patients with Anaplastic Thyroid Carcinoma, 2000 to 2012. *Head Neck* **2017**, *39*, 133–139. [CrossRef]
78. Brierley, J.; Sherman, E. The Role of External Beam Radiation and Targeted Therapy in Thyroid Cancer. *Semin. Radiat. Oncol.* **2012**, *22*, 254–262. [CrossRef]
79. Bhatia, A.; Rao, A.; Ang, K.-K.; Garden, A.S.; Morrison, W.H.; Rosenthal, D.I.; Evans, D.B.; Clayman, G.; Sherman, S.I.; Schwartz, D.L. Anaplastic Thyroid Cancer: Clinical Outcomes with Conformal Radiotherapy. *Head Neck* **2010**, *32*, 829–836. [CrossRef]
80. Nachalon, Y.; Stern-Shavit, S.; Bachar, G.; Shvero, J.; Limon, D.; Popovtzer, A. Aggressive Palliation and Survival in Anaplastic Thyroid Carcinoma. *JAMA Otolaryngol. Neck Surg.* **2015**, *141*, 1128. [CrossRef]
81. Sun, X.S.; Sun, S.R.; Guevara, N.; Marcy, P.Y.; Peyrottes, I.; Lassalle, S.; Lacout, A.; Sadoul, J.L.; Santini, J.; Benisvy, D.; et al. Indications of External Beam Radiation Therapy in Non-Anaplastic Thyroid Cancer and Impact of Innovative Radiation Techniques. *Crit. Rev. Oncol. Hematol.* **2013**, *86*, 52–68. [CrossRef]
82. Tennvall, J.; Lundell, G.; Wahlberg, P.; Bergenfelz, A.; Grimelius, L.; Akerman, M.; Hjelm Skog, A.-L.; Wallin, G. Anaplastic Thyroid Carcinoma: Three Protocols Combining Doxorubicin, Hyperfractionated Radiotherapy and Surgery. *Br. J. Cancer* **2002**, *86*, 1848–1853. [CrossRef] [PubMed]
83. Wang, Y.; Tsang, R.; Asa, S.; Dickson, B.; Arenovich, T.; Brierley, J. Clinical Outcome of Anaplastic Thyroid Carcinoma Treated with Radiotherapy of Once- and Twice-Daily Fractionation Regimens. *Cancer* **2006**, *107*, 1786–1792. [CrossRef] [PubMed]
84. Lacas, B.; Bourhis, J.; Overgaard, J.; Zhang, Q.; Grégoire, V.; Nankivell, M.; Zackrisson, B.; Szutkowski, Z.; Suwiński, R.; Poulsen, M.; et al. Role of Radiotherapy Fractionation in Head and Neck Cancers (MARCH): An Updated Meta-Analysis. *Lancet Oncol.* **2017**, *18*, 1221–1237. [CrossRef]
85. Takahashi, N.; Matsushita, H.; Umezawa, R.; Yamamoto, T.; Ishikawa, Y.; Katagiri, Y.; Tasaka, S.; Takeda, K.; Fukui, K.; Kadoya, N.; et al. Hypofractionated Radiotherapy for Anaplastic Thyroid Carcinoma: 15 Years of Experience in a Single Institution. *Eur. Thyroid J.* **2019**, *8*, 24–30. [CrossRef]
86. Jacobsen, A.-B.; Grøholt, K.K.; Lorntzsen, B.; Osnes, T.A.; Falk, R.S.; Sigstad, E. Anaplastic Thyroid Cancer and Hyperfractionated Accelerated Radiotherapy (HART) with and without Surgery. *Eur. Arch. Oto-Rhino-Laryngol.* **2017**, *274*, 4203–4209. [CrossRef]
87. Dumke, A.-K.; Pelz, T.; Vordermark, D. Long-Term Results of Radiotherapy in Anaplastic Thyroid Cancer. *Radiat. Oncol. Lond. Engl.* **2014**, *9*, 90. [CrossRef]
88. Houlihan, O.A.; Moore, R.; Jamaluddin, M.F.; Sharifah, A.; Redmond, H.P.; O'Reilly, S.; Feeley, L.; Sheahan, P.; Rock, K. Anaplastic Thyroid Cancer: Outcomes of Trimodal Therapy. *Rep. Pract. Oncol. Radiother.* **2021**, *26*, 416–422. [CrossRef]
89. He, X.; Li, D.; Hu, C.; Wang, Z.; Ying, H.; Wu, Y. Outcome after Intensity Modulated Radiotherapy for Anaplastic Thyroid Carcinoma. *BMC Cancer* **2014**, *14*, 235. [CrossRef]
90. Jiménez-Fonseca, P.; Gómez Saez, J.M.; Santamaria Sandi, J.; Capdevila, J.; Navarro Gonzalez, E.; Zafon Llopis, C.; Ramón Y Cajal Asensio, T.; Riesco-Eizaguirre, G.; Grande, E.; Galofré, J.C. Spanish Consensus for the Management of Patients with Anaplastic Cell Thyroid Carcinoma. *Clin. Transl. Oncol.* **2017**, *19*, 12–20. [CrossRef]
91. Mangoni, M.; Gobitti, C.; Autorino, R.; Cerizza, L.; Furlan, C.; Mazzarotto, R.; Monari, F.; Simontacchi, G.; Vianello, F.; Basso, M.; et al. External Beam Radiotherapy in Thyroid Carcinoma: Clinical Review and Recommendations of the AIRO "Radioterapia Metabolica" Group. *Tumori* **2017**, *103*, 114–123. [CrossRef]

92. Nutting, C.M.; Convery, D.J.; Cosgrove, V.P.; Rowbottom, C.; Vini, L.; Harmer, C.; Dearnaley, D.P.; Webb, S. Improvements in Target Coverage and Reduced Spinal Cord Irradiation Using Intensity-Modulated Radiotherapy (IMRT) in Patients with Carcinoma of the Thyroid Gland. *Radiother. Oncol.* **2001**, *60*, 173–180. [CrossRef]
93. Posner, M.D.; Quivey, J.M.; Akazawa, P.F.; Xia, P.; Akazawa, C.; Verhey, L.J. Dose Optimization for the Treatment of Anaplastic Thyroid Carcinoma: A Comparison of Treatment Planning Techniques. *Int. J. Radiat. Oncol. Biol. Phys.* **2000**, *48*, 475–483. [CrossRef]
94. Park, J.W.; Choi, S.H.; Yoon, H.I.; Lee, J.; Kim, T.H.; Kim, J.W.; Lee, I.J. Treatment Outcomes of Radiotherapy for Anaplastic Thyroid Cancer. *Radiat. Oncol. J.* **2018**, *36*, 103–113. [CrossRef] [PubMed]
95. Swaak-Kragten, A.T.; de Wilt, J.H.W.; Schmitz, P.I.M.; Bontenbal, M.; Levendag, P.C. Multimodality Treatment for Anaplastic Thyroid Carcinoma—Treatment Outcome in 75 Patients. *Radiother. Oncol.* **2009**, *92*, 100–104. [CrossRef] [PubMed]
96. Vulpe, H.; Kwan, J.Y.Y.; McNiven, A.; Brierley, J.D.; Tsang, R.; Chan, B.; Goldstein, D.P.; Le, L.W.; Hope, A.; Giuliani, M. Patterns of Failure in Anaplastic and Differentiated Thyroid Carcinoma Treated with Intensity-Modulated Radiotherapy. *Curr. Oncol.* **2017**, *24*, e226–e232. [CrossRef] [PubMed]
97. Gao, R.W.; Foote, R.L.; Garces, Y.I.; Ma, D.J.; Neben-Wittich, M.; Routman, D.M.; Patel, S.H.; Ko, S.J.; McGee, L.A.; Bible, K.C.; et al. Outcomes and Patterns of Recurrence for Anaplastic Thyroid Cancer Treated With Comprehensive Chemoradiotherapy. *Pract. Radiat. Oncol.* **2021**. [CrossRef]
98. Kim, T.H.; Chung, K.-W.; Lee, Y.J.; Park, C.S.; Lee, E.K.; Kim, T.S.; Kim, S.K.; Jung, Y.S.; Ryu, J.S.; Kim, S.S.; et al. The Effect of External Beam Radiotherapy Volume on Locoregional Control in Patients with Locoregionally Advanced or Recurrent Nonanaplastic Thyroid Cancer. *Radiat. Oncol.* **2010**, *5*, 69. [CrossRef]
99. Besic, N.; Auersperg, M.; Us-Krasovec, M.; Golouh, R.; Frkovic-Grazio, S.; Vodnik, A. Effect of Primary Treatment on Survival in Anaplastic Thyroid Carcinoma. *Eur. J. Surg. Oncol.* **2001**, *27*, 260–264. [CrossRef]
100. Arora, S.; Christos, P.; Pham, A.; Desai, P.; Wernicke, A.G.; Nori, D.; Chao, K.S.C.; Parashar, B. Comparing Outcomes in Poorly-Differentiated versus Anaplastic Thyroid Cancers Treated with Radiation: A Surveillance, Epidemiology, and End Results Analysis. *J. Cancer Res. Ther.* **2014**, *10*, 526–530. [CrossRef]
101. Zhou, W.; Yue, Y.; Zhang, X. Radiotherapy Plus Chemotherapy Leads to Prolonged Survival in Patients With Anaplastic Thyroid Cancer Compared With Radiotherapy Alone Regardless of Surgical Resection and Distant Metastasis: A Retrospective Population Study. *Front. Endocrinol.* **2021**, *12*, 748023. [CrossRef]
102. Sherman, E.J.; Harris, J.; Bible, K.C.; Xia, P.; Ghossein, R.A.; Chung, C.H.; Riaz, N.; Gunn, B.; Foote, R.L.; Yom, S.; et al. 1914MO Randomized Phase II Study of Radiation Therapy and Paclitaxel with Pazopanib or Placebo: NRG-RTOG 0912. *Ann. Oncol.* **2020**, *31*, S1085. [CrossRef]
103. Jonker, P.K.C.; Turchini, J.; Kruijff, S.; Lin, J.F.; Gill, A.J.; Eade, T.; Aniss, A.; Clifton-Bligh, R.; Learoyd, D.; Robinson, B.; et al. Multimodality Treatment Improves Locoregional Control, Progression-Free and Overall Survival in Patients with Anaplastic Thyroid Cancer: A Retrospective Cohort Study Comparing Oncological Outcomes and Morbidity between Multimodality Treatment and Limited Treatment. *Ann. Surg. Oncol.* **2021**, *28*, 7520–7530. [CrossRef] [PubMed]
104. Wang, W.; Smith, J.L.; Carlino, M.S.; Burmeister, B.; Pinkham, M.B.; Fogarty, G.B.; Christie, D.R.H.; Estall, V.; Shackleton, M.; Clements, A.; et al. Phase I/II Trial of Concurrent Extracranial Palliative Radiation Therapy with Dabrafenib and Trametinib in Metastatic BRAF V600E/K Mutation-Positive Cutaneous Melanoma. *Clin. Transl. Radiat. Oncol.* **2021**, *30*, 95–99. [CrossRef]
105. Werner, B.; Abele, J.; Alveryd, A.; Björklund, A.; Franzén, S.; Granberg, P.O.; Landberg, T.; Lundell, G.; Löwhagen, T.; Sundblad, R. Multimodal Therapy in Anaplastic Giant Cell Thyroid Carcinoma. *World J. Surg.* **1984**, *8*, 64–70. [CrossRef] [PubMed]
106. Shimaoka, K.; Schoenfeld, D.A.; DeWys, W.D.; Creech, R.H.; DeConti, R. A Randomized Trial of Doxorubicin versus Doxorubicin plus Cisplatin in Patients with Advanced Thyroid Carcinoma. *Cancer* **1985**, *56*, 2155–2160. [CrossRef]
107. Tallroth, E.; Wallin, G.; Lundell, G.; Löwhagen, T.; Einhorn, J. Multimodality Treatment in Anaplastic Giant Cell Thyroid Carcinoma. *Cancer* **1987**, *60*, 1428–1431. [CrossRef]
108. Kim, J.H.; Leeper, R.D. Treatment of Locally Advanced Thyroid Carcinoma with Combination Doxorubicin and Radiation Therapy. *Cancer* **1987**, *60*, 2372–2375. [CrossRef]
109. Schlumberger, M.; Parmentier, C.; Delisle, M.J.; Couette, J.E.; Droz, J.P.; Sarrazin, D. Combination Therapy for Anaplastic Giant Cell Thyroid Carcinoma. *Cancer* **1991**, *67*, 564–566. [CrossRef]
110. Wong, C.S.; Van Dyk, J.; Simpson, W.J. Myelopathy Following Hyperfractionated Accelerated Radiotherapy for Anaplastic Thyroid Carcinoma. *Radiother. Oncol.* **1991**, *20*, 3–9. [CrossRef]
111. Auersperg, M.; Us-Krasovec, M.; Petric, G.; Pogacnik, A.; Besic, N. Results of Combined Modality Treatment in Poorly Differentiated and Anaplastic Thyroid Carcinoma. *Wien. Klin. Wochenschr.* **1990**, *102*, 267–270.
112. Derbel, O.; Limem, S.; Ségura-Ferlay, C.; Lifante, J.-C.; Carrie, C.; Peix, J.-L.; Borson-Chazot, F.; Bournaud, C.; Droz, J.-P.; de la Fouchardière, C. Results of Combined Treatment of Anaplastic Thyroid Carcinoma (ATC). *BMC Cancer* **2011**, *11*, 469. [CrossRef]
113. Lim, S.M.; Shin, S.-J.; Chung, W.Y.; Park, C.S.; Nam, K.-H.; Kang, S.-W.; Keum, K.C.; Kim, J.H.; Cho, J.Y.; Hong, Y.K.; et al. Treatment Outcome of Patients with Anaplastic Thyroid Cancer: A Single Center Experience. *Yonsei Med. J.* **2012**, *53*, 352–357. [CrossRef] [PubMed]
114. Sosa, J.A.; Balkissoon, J.; Lu, S.; Langecker, P.; Elisei, R.; Jarzab, B.; Bal, C.S.; Marur, S.; Gramza, A.; Ondrey, F. Thyroidectomy Followed by Fosbretabulin (CA4P) Combination Regimen Appears to Suggest Improvement in Patient Survival in Anaplastic Thyroid Cancer. *Surgery* **2012**, *152*, 1078–1087. [CrossRef] [PubMed]

115. Higashiyama, T.; Ito, Y.; Hirokawa, M.; Fukushima, M.; Uruno, T.; Miya, A.; Matsuzuka, F.; Miyauchi, A. Induction Chemotherapy with Weekly Paclitaxel Administration for Anaplastic Thyroid Carcinoma. *Thyroid* 2010, *20*, 7–14. [CrossRef] [PubMed]
116. Seto, A.; Sugitani, I.; Toda, K.; Kawabata, K.; Takahashi, S.; Saotome, T. Chemotherapy for Anaplastic Thyroid Cancer Using Docetaxel and Cisplatin: Report of Eight Cases. *Surg. Today* 2015, *45*, 221–226. [CrossRef] [PubMed]
117. Glaser, S.M.; Mandish, S.F.; Gill, B.S.; Balasubramani, G.K.; Clump, D.A.; Beriwal, S. Anaplastic Thyroid Cancer: Prognostic Factors, Patterns of Care, and Overall Survival. *Head Neck* 2016, *38* (Suppl. 1), E2083–E2090. [CrossRef]
118. Lin, B.; Ma, H.; Ma, M.; Zhang, Z.; Sun, Z.; Hsieh, I.-Y.; Okenwa, O.; Guan, H.; Li, J.; Lv, W. The Incidence and Survival Analysis for Anaplastic Thyroid Cancer: A SEER Database Analysis. *Am. J. Transl. Res.* 2019, *11*, 5888–5896. [PubMed]
119. Cabanillas, M.E.; Zafereo, M.; Gunn, G.B.; Ferrarotto, R. Anaplastic Thyroid Carcinoma: Treatment in the Age of Molecular Targeted Therapy. *J. Oncol. Pract.* 2016, *12*, 511–518. [CrossRef] [PubMed]
120. Smallridge, R.C.; Ain, K.B.; Asa, S.L.; Bible, K.C.; Brierley, J.D.; Burman, K.D.; Kebebew, E.; Lee, N.Y.; Nikiforov, Y.E.; Rosenthal, M.S.; et al. American Thyroid Association Guidelines for Management of Patients with Anaplastic Thyroid Cancer. *Thyroid* 2012, *22*, 1104–1139. [CrossRef]
121. Ryder, M.; Gild, M.; Hohl, T.M.; Pamer, E.; Knauf, J.; Ghossein, R.; Joyce, J.A.; Fagin, J.A. Genetic and Pharmacological Targeting of CSF-1/CSF-1R Inhibits Tumor-Associated Macrophages and Impairs BRAF-Induced Thyroid Cancer Progression. *PLoS ONE* 2013, *8*, e54302. [CrossRef]
122. Keam, B.; Kreitman, R.J.; Wainberg, Z.A.; Cabanillas, M.E.; Cho, D.C.; Italiano, A.; Stein, A.; Cho, J.Y.; Schellens, J.H.M.; Wen, P.Y.; et al. Updated Efficacy and Safety Data of Dabrafenib (D) and Trametinib (T) in Patients (Pts) with BRAF V600E–Mutated Anaplastic Thyroid Cancer (ATC). *Ann. Oncol.* 2018, *29*, viii645–viii646. [CrossRef]
123. Cabanillas, M.E.; Dadu, R.; Iyer, P.; Wanland, K.B.; Busaidy, N.L.; Ying, A.; Gule-Monroe, M.; Wang, J.R.; Zafereo, M.; Hofmann, M.-C. Acquired Secondary RAS Mutation in BRAFV600E-Mutated Thyroid Cancer Patients Treated with BRAF Inhibitors. *Thyroid* 2020, *30*, 1288–1296. [CrossRef] [PubMed]
124. Knauf, J.A.; Luckett, K.A.; Chen, K.-Y.; Voza, F.; Socci, N.D.; Ghossein, R.; Fagin, J.A. Hgf/Met Activation Mediates Resistance to BRAF Inhibition in Murine Anaplastic Thyroid Cancers. *J. Clin. Invest.* 2018, *128*, 4086–4097. [CrossRef] [PubMed]
125. Ofir Dovrat, T.; Sokol, E.; Frampton, G.; Shachar, E.; Pelles, S.; Geva, R.; Wolf, I. Unusually Long-Term Responses to Vemurafenib in BRAF V600E Mutated Colon and Thyroid Cancers Followed by the Development of Rare RAS Activating Mutations. *Cancer Biol. Ther.* 2018, *19*, 871–874. [CrossRef] [PubMed]
126. Cabanillas, M.E.; Drilon, A.; Farago, A.F.; Brose, M.S.; McDermott, R.; Sohal, D.; Oh, D.-Y.; Almubarak, M.; Bauman, J.; Chu, E.; et al. 1916P Larotrectinib Treatment of Advanced TRK Fusion Thyroid Cancer. *Ann. Oncol.* 2020, *31*, S1086. [CrossRef]
127. Dias-Santagata, D.; Lennerz, J.K.; Sadow, P.M.; Frazier, R.P.; Govinda Raju, S.; Henry, D.; Chung, T.; Kherani, J.; Rothenberg, S.M.; Wirth, L.J. Response to RET-Specific Therapy in RET Fusion-Positive Anaplastic Thyroid Carcinoma. *Thyroid* 2020, *30*, 1384–1389. [CrossRef]
128. Godbert, Y.; Henriques de Figueiredo, B.; Bonichon, F.; Chibon, F.; Hostein, I.; Pérot, G.; Dupin, C.; Daubech, A.; Belleannée, G.; Gros, A.; et al. Remarkable Response to Crizotinib in Woman With Anaplastic Lymphoma Kinase–Rearranged Anaplastic Thyroid Carcinoma. *J. Clin. Oncol.* 2015, *33*, e84–e87. [CrossRef]
129. Schneider, T.C.; de Wit, D.; Links, T.P.; van Erp, N.P.; van der Hoeven, J.J.M.; Gelderblom, H.; Roozen, I.C.F.M.; Bos, M.; Corver, W.E.; van Wezel, T.; et al. Everolimus in Patients With Advanced Follicular-Derived Thyroid Cancer: Results of a Phase II Clinical Trial. *J. Clin. Endocrinol. Metab.* 2017, *102*, 698–707. [CrossRef]
130. Lim, S.M.; Chang, H.; Yoon, M.J.; Hong, Y.K.; Kim, H.; Chung, W.Y.; Park, C.S.; Nam, K.H.; Kang, S.W.; Kim, M.K.; et al. A Multicenter, Phase II Trial of Everolimus in Locally Advanced or Metastatic Thyroid Cancer of All Histologic Subtypes. *Ann. Oncol.* 2013, *24*, 3089–3094. [CrossRef]
131. Sherman, E.J.; Dunn, L.A.; Ho, A.L.; Baxi, S.S.; Ghossein, R.A.; Fury, M.G.; Haque, S.; Sima, C.S.; Cullen, G.; Fagin, J.A.; et al. Phase 2 Study Evaluating the Combination of Sorafenib and Temsirolimus in the Treatment of Radioactive Iodine-Refractory Thyroid Cancer. *Cancer* 2017, *123*, 4114–4121. [CrossRef]
132. Takahashi, S.; Kiyota, N.; Yamazaki, T.; Chayahara, N.; Nakano, K.; Inagaki, L.; Toda, K.; Enokida, T.; Minami, H.; Imamura, Y.; et al. A Phase II Study of the Safety and Efficacy of Lenvatinib in Patients with Advanced Thyroid Cancer. *Future Oncol.* 2019, *15*, 717–726. [CrossRef] [PubMed]
133. Sparano, C.; Godbert, Y.; Attard, M.; Do Cao, C.; Zerdoud, S.; Roudaut, N.; Joly, C.; Berdelou, A.; Hadoux, J.; Lamartina, L.; et al. Limited Efficacy of Lenvatinib in Heavily Pretreated Anaplastic Thyroid Cancer: A French Overview. *Endocr. Relat. Cancer* 2021, *28*, 15–26. [CrossRef] [PubMed]
134. Wirth, L.J.; Brose, M.S.; Sherman, E.J.; Licitra, L.; Schlumberger, M.; Sherman, S.I.; Bible, K.C.; Robinson, B.; Rodien, P.; Godbert, Y.; et al. Open-Label, Single-Arm, Multicenter, Phase II Trial of Lenvatinib for the Treatment of Patients With Anaplastic Thyroid Cancer. *J. Clin. Oncol.* 2021, *39*, 2359–2366. [CrossRef] [PubMed]
135. Cabanillas, M.E.; Dadu, R.; Ferrarotto, R.; Liu, S.; Fellman, B.M.; Gross, N.D.; Gule-Monroe, M.; Lu, C.; Grosu, H.; Williams, M.D.; et al. Atezolizumab Combinations with Targeted Therapy for Anaplastic Thyroid Carcinoma (ATC). *J. Clin. Oncol.* 2020, *38*, 6514. [CrossRef]
136. McIver, B.; Hay, I.D.; Giuffrida, D.F.; Dvorak, C.E.; Grant, C.S.; Thompson, G.B.; van Heerden, J.A.; Goellner, J.R. Anaplastic Thyroid Carcinoma: A 50-Year Experience at a Single Institution. *Surgery* 2001, *130*, 1028–1034. [CrossRef]

137. Hu, S.; Helman, S.N.; Hanly, E.; Likhterov, I. The Role of Surgery in Anaplastic Thyroid Cancer: A Systematic Review. *Am. J. Otolaryngol.* **2017**, *38*, 337–350. [CrossRef] [PubMed]
138. Green, L.D.; Mack, L.; Pasieka, J.L. Anaplastic Thyroid Cancer and Primary Thyroid Lymphoma: A Review of These Rare Thyroid Malignancies. *J. Surg. Oncol.* **2006**, *94*, 725–736. [CrossRef]
139. Are, C.; Shaha, A.R. Anaplastic Thyroid Carcinoma: Biology, Pathogenesis, Prognostic Factors, and Treatment Approaches. *Ann. Surg. Oncol.* **2006**, *13*, 453–464. [CrossRef]
140. Brignardello, E.; Palestini, N.; Felicetti, F.; Castiglione, A.; Piovesan, A.; Gallo, M.; Freddi, M.; Ricardi, U.; Gasparri, G.; Ciccone, G.; et al. Early Surgery and Survival of Patients with Anaplastic Thyroid Carcinoma: Analysis of a Case Series Referred to a Single Institution between 1999 and 2012. *Thyroid* **2014**, *24*, 1600–1606. [CrossRef]
141. Onoda, N.; Sugino, K.; Higashiyama, T.; Kammori, M.; Toda, K.; Ito, K.-I.; Yoshida, A.; Suganuma, N.; Nakashima, N.; Suzuki, S.; et al. The Safety and Efficacy of Weekly Paclitaxel Administration for Anaplastic Thyroid Cancer Patients: A Nationwide Prospective Study. *Thyroid* **2016**, *26*, 1293–1299. [CrossRef]
142. Wang, J.R.; Zafereo, M.E.; Dadu, R.; Ferrarotto, R.; Busaidy, N.L.; Lu, C.; Ahmed, S.; Gule-Monroe, M.K.; Williams, M.D.; Sturgis, E.M.; et al. Complete Surgical Resection Following Neoadjuvant Dabrafenib Plus Trametinib in BRAFV600E-Mutated Anaplastic Thyroid Carcinoma. *Thyroid* **2019**, *29*, 1036–1043. [CrossRef] [PubMed]
143. Cabanillas, M.E.; Ferrarotto, R.; Garden, A.S.; Ahmed, S.; Busaidy, N.L.; Dadu, R.; Williams, M.D.; Skinner, H.; Gunn, G.B.; Grosu, H.; et al. Neoadjuvant BRAF- and Immune-Directed Therapy for Anaplastic Thyroid Carcinoma. *Thyroid* **2018**, *28*, 945–951. [CrossRef] [PubMed]

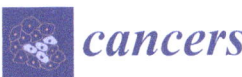

Review

Carcinoid Crisis: A Misunderstood and Unrecognized Oncological Emergency

Camilla Bardasi [1], Stefania Benatti [1], Gabriele Luppi [1], Ingrid Garajovà [2], Federico Piacentini [1], Massimo Dominici [1] and Fabio Gelsomino [1,*]

[1] Department of Oncology and Hematology, Division of Oncology, University Hospital of Modena, 41124 Modena, Italy; camilla.bardasi@gmail.com (C.B.); stefania.benatti@unimore.it (S.B.); gabriele.luppi1@gmail.com (G.L.); federico.piacentini@unimore.it (F.P.); mdominici@unimore.it (M.D.)
[2] Medical Oncology Unit, University Hospital of Parma, 43100 Parma, Italy; ingegarajova@gmail.com
* Correspondence: fabiogelsomino83@yahoo.it; Tel.: +39-059-422-4982; Fax: +39-059-422-2647

Simple Summary: In this review, the Authors are going to discuss the main highlights of the Carcinoid Crisis, an uncommon manifestation related to neuroendocrine tumors, focusing on the potential etiopathogenetic mechanisms, clinical implications, potential treatments and prophylaxis.

Abstract: Carcinoid Crisis represents a rare and extremely dangerous manifestation that can occur in patients with Neuroendocrine Tumors (NETs). It is characterized by a sudden onset of hemodynamic instability, sometimes associated with the classical symptoms of carcinoid syndrome, such as bronchospasm and flushing. Carcinoid Crisis seems to be caused by a massive release of vasoactive substances, typically produced by neuroendocrine cells, and can emerge after abdominal procedures, but also spontaneously in rare instances. To date, there are no empirically derived guidelines for the management of this cancer-related medical emergency, and the available evidence essentially comes from single-case reports or dated small retrospective series. A transfer to the Intensive Care Unit may be necessary during the acute setting, when the severe hypotension becomes unresponsive to standard practices, such as volemic filling and the infusion of vasopressor therapy. The only effective strategy is represented by prevention. The administration of octreotide, anxiolytic and antihistaminic agents represents the current treatment approach to avoid hormone release and prevent major complications. However, no standard protocols are available, resulting in great variability in terms of schedules, doses, ways of administration and timing of prophylactic treatments.

Keywords: crcinoid crisis; neuroendocrine tumors; hemodynamic instability; octreotide

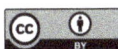

1. Introduction

Neuroendocrine Tumors (NETs) are a heterogeneous family of neoplasms that can arise from any district of the body and can occur with an extremely wide range of symptoms and clinical manifestations, due to hormonal secretion. Carcinoid Syndrome (CS) is the most typical and common clinical presentation in functional NETs and is characterized by diarrhea, gastrointestinal discomforts, such as cramps and nausea, facial flushing with apparent peripheral cyanosis, eventual right-sided valvular heart disease preceded by palpitation and dyspnea with bronchospasm. Very rarely, patients with NETs can also exhibit a life-threatening occurrence known as Carcinoid Crisis (CC), generally described as a sudden onset of hemodynamic instability (prolonged hypertension or severe hypotension, unresponsive to standard practices), sometimes accompanied by characteristics of carcinoid syndrome, such as prolonged flushing, wheezing and hyperthermia. The underlying mechanism of CC is still not well known, but some Authors first hypothesized that CC could represent an extreme complication of the Carcinoid Syndrome caused by a sudden and massive release of tumor hormones that may be triggered by tumor manipulation or anesthesia [1,2].

CC is mostly associated with foregut (respiratory tract, thymus, stomach, duodenum and pancreas) and midgut (small intestine, appendix and right colon) NETs [3]. Although theoretically every kind of tumor stress can cause CC, it typically occurs during invasive procedures, such as surgery and liver embolization [4], but it can also arise during clinical examination, biopsy, mammography [5], transesophageal echocardiography [6] or induction of anesthesia. Some cases of spontaneous onset have also been described [2,7,8]. The reported incidence of CC is about 7% in patients with NETs [9] undergoing abdominal surgery [10,11], but more recent works observed a higher number of cases, with a maximum incidence of 24–30% [12].

2. Aim

In this review, the Authors are going to discuss this uncommon manifestation, focusing on the potential etiopathogenetic mechanisms, clinical implications and potential treatments and prophylaxis.

3. Materials and Methods

The database PubMed was searched for the characteristics of CC using the term "carcinoid" combined with "crises" and "crisis" for publications with English abstracts up to September 2021. "Malignant carcinoid syndrome" was not considered. Studies included: (1) original articles, case series or case reports; (2) reporting at least one of the characteristics of Carcinoid Crisis (hemodynamic instability, continuous flushing, tachycardia predisposing to arrhythmias, bronchial wheezing, hyperthermia, peripheral cyanosis, severe diarrhea, central nervous system dysfunction with coma). In the section "Clinical Definition and Presentation", the Authors identified 12 case reports concerning CC.

4. Clinical Definition and Presentation

Carcinoid Crisis is an extremely rare life-threatening event, with little data published on this topic. The first report of CC dates back to 1964 [2], when Kahil et al. described a case of a 41-year-old woman who underwent surgical resection of a NET of the ileum and a few months later started to manifest episodes of flushing, cramps and pruritus, interpreted as malignant CS. She was treated with a peripheral serotonin antagonist, cyproheptadine and was trained to adopt a low-tryptophan diet, obtaining good control of symptoms. Thirteen days after the discontinuation of therapies, the woman manifested a sudden onset of apprehension, oppressive chest pain, abdominal cramps, frequent diarrhea, facial flushing, pruritus, paresthesia and hyperaesthesia, peripheral vascular collapse with pale cold cyanotic extremities and progressive extreme hypotension. Neither metaraminol, a potent vasoconstrictor, nor norepinephrine, was effective in blood pressure control. One hour after the onset of symptoms, a single intravenous injection of cyproheptadine was administered with a dramatic cessation of the thoracic and abdominal pain. The Authors named this an extremely dangerous condition of Carcinoid Crisis, thus suggesting for the first time that it could represent a serious complication of CS, caused by a sudden release of active substances by neuroendocrine cells, provoked by stress on tumor masses.

Table 1 summarizes published case reports of CC.

As assumed by Kahil et al., in the absence of external stress, neuroendocrine tumor cells produce a share of vasoactive peptides that provoke CS. Instead, when a greater stimulus takes place, a hormonal storm can trigger CC. As shown in Table 1, the most commonly reported primary tumor locations that can cause CC are lung and small bowel (ileum), which also represent the most common sites associated with CS, because of the overall major release of vasoactive peptides compared to other districts [3].

As previously shown in Table 1, not only direct manipulations of tumor mass, such as bronchoscopy [16,20], liver biopsy [13,16] or locoregional treatments [18,21], but also other kinds of tumor solicitations, such as the induction of anesthesia [14] or the infusion of radiotracers [17], can contribute to the rapid onset of CC. In addition, following the results of the NETTER-1 trial, the increasing use of peptide radionuclide therapy (PRRT) has led to a rise in CC due to tumor lysis [22], most frequently after the first cycle of treatment, and the main risk factors include large tumor burden, liver metastases, previous CS, carcinoid heart disease, advanced patient age, high chromogranin A levels and high 5-HIAA levels. Furthermore, in some cases, PRRT-induced CC can also occur long after therapy [24].

Table 1. Case reports of Carcinoid Crisis up to September 2021.

Authors and Date	Primary Tumor Location	Clinical Presentation	Triggering Factor	Treatment
Kahil et al., 1964 [2]	ileum	apprehension, chest pain, abdominal cramps, diarrhea, flushing, cyanotic extremities, hypotension	increased tryptophan intake in diet	metaraminol, levarterenol (ineffective), cyproheptadine
Harris AL et al., 1983 [13]	ileum	prolonged continuous flushing, confusion, hypotension, coma	ileotransverse colostomy and liver biopsy	anti-serotonin and antikinin agents (5 fluorouracil, trasylol, prednisone, cimetidine, cyproheptadine, methysergide, tryptophan, aminoplex 12)
Hughes et al., 1989 [14]	lung	hypertension, tachycardia	anesthesia induction	ketanserin, octreotide
Batchelor AM et al., 1992 [15]	lung	peripheral cyanosis, myocardial infarction, flushing	rigid bronchoscopy	adrenaline, hydrocortisone, octreotide, ketanserin
Parry R.G. et al., 1996 [16]	hepatic metastases	acute tubular necrosis oliguria, diarrhea, flushing	liver biopsy	glucocorticoids, hemodialysis, octreotide, cyproheptadine
Koopmans KP et al. 2005 [17]	ileum	hypertension, peripheral cyanosis, flushing, edema, vomiting	^{18}F-DOPA infusion during PET	antihistamine
Papadogias et al., 2007 [18]	lung	hypotension, diarrhea	radioembolization (^{111}in-octreotide infusion via intra-arterial injection)	octreotideic, alpha-interferon, glucocorticoids, and H1–H2 histamine receptor blockers
Van Diepen et al., 2013 [19]	small bowel	hypotension, fever, flushing	valve replacement	octreotide, vasopressin, norepinephrine, hydrocortisone, anti-serotonin, antihistamine, cyproheptadine
Kromas ML et al., 2017 [20]	lung	hypotension, wheezing	bronchoscopy	octreotide bolus
Maddali MV et al., 2020 [21]	ileum	initial hypertension and tachycardia, followed by shock and respiratory failure	TACE	dobutamine and vasopressin, then milrinone and nitroprusside (ineffective), octreotideic
Dhanani et al., 2020 [22]	small bowel	hypotension, loss of consciousness, cardiac arrest	Peptide Receptor Radionuclide Therapy (PRRT)	cardiopulmonary resuscitation plus adrenaline (ineffective), octreotideic
Mahdi et al., 2021 [23]	transverse colon (NEC)	abdominal pain, hypotension	not mentioned	empiric antibiotic therapy, norepinephrine ic (ineffective), octreotideic

Furthermore, clinical presentation is remarkably variable. For instance, Kromas et al., described a case of a 31-year-old woman who presented chest pain, newly onset asthma and a sudden onset of hypotension and wheezing during rigid bronchoscopy [20]. Koopmans et al. reported the case of a 61-year-old woman who developed vomiting, accompanied by flushing, edema and severe hypotension during an ^{18}F-DOPA PET scan [17]. The explanation proposed by the Canadian group of Seymour et al. is that each tumor secretes a specific cocktail of hormones, which leads to discrepancy regarding recognition and symptoms and contributes to the great clinical variety of CC [25]. To date, there has been no international consensus on the most appropriate definition of CC. Clinicians continue to identify CC as a rapid onset of hemodynamic instability, unresponsive to conventional management associated with characteristics of CS, such as continuous flushing, tachycardia and arrhythmias, bronchial wheezing, hyperthermia, peripheral cyanosis, severe diarrhea and central nervous system dysfunction. Kinney et al. first clinically termed CC as severe hypotension with the systolic blood pressure (SBP) < 80 mmHg for more than 10 min, accompanied by the presence of flushing, urticaria, ventricular dysrhythmia, bronchospasm or acidosis, and they registered 15 cases of CC among 119 patients analyzed [9]. Subsequently, Condron et al. preferred to broaden the definition to a significant hemodynamic instability (SBP < 80 or >180 mmHg, heart rate > 120 bpm) or potential end-organ dysfunction not attributable to other causes and described a much higher incidence of CC, approaching 30% in their case series [11]. Seymour et al. also included bronchoconstriction and flushing in their definition of CC [25], while Massimino et al. combined the definitions of Kinney and Condron, considering all patients with systolic blood pressure (SBP) < 80 mmHg for more than 10 min) or presentation of hemodynamic instability (including hypotension, sustained hypertension or tachycardia) [10]. As a consequence, this variability in the definition of CC leads to the impossibility of determining the real incidence and the appropriate severity of these episodes, with no conclusive studies available.

The overhang of pressure values represents a minor common denominator among all definitions. The recent study of Condron et al. tried to better characterize the underlying physiological mechanism [26]. Assuming there are three putative hormonally driven pathways of the hypotension (the reduction in cardiac output due to pulmonary artery vasoconstriction, the coronary vessels vasoconstriction resulting in cardiac failure and peripheral vasodilatation with consequent hypovolemic shock), they concluded that the pathophysiology of CC appears consistent with distributive shock. Using intraoperative, transesophageal echocardiography, pulmonary artery catheterization and intraoperative blood collection, they observed a statistically significant reduction in systemic vascular resistance among all crises. The contextual rating of hormone levels during CC exhibited markedly diverse profiles, so the Authors concluded that another carcinoid-related manifestation, such as flushing or wheezing, is not mandatory to declare a CC.

Based on the results of this study, the scientific community is now working to clarify which is the precise etiopathogenetic mechanism behind the onset of CC and which endogen molecule is the major molecule responsible for hemodynamic instability to better classify and recognize this life-threatening event and to define the best clinical approach.

5. Etiopathogenesis of Carcinoid Crisis

As previously cited, Kahil et al. were the first Authors who approached the topic of CC. At the end of their experience, they concluded that an excessive amount of serotonin in the bloodstream, the principal amine responsible for CS, could cause CC as a consequence of increased tryptophan intake in diet or, less likely, of a release after spontaneous necrosis of the tumor. The treatment consisted of anti-serotonin/histamine agents instead of epinephrine and levarterenol, to avoid catecholamines use that can worsen or elicit CC [2]. Tryptophan is an essential precursor of serotonin, which is hydroxylated by the rate-limiting enzyme tryptophan hydroxylase and subsequently decarboxylated by an aromatic acid decarboxylase to serotonin [27] (Figure 1). It has been demonstrated that increased tryptophan intake in diet promotes a rise in peripheral serotonin.

The vast majority of peripheral serotonin is produced by enterochromaffin cells, the same cells constituting NET masses. Therefore, the rise of tryptophan in blood circulation determines an upregulation in NET cells, with a massive production of serotonin. This hormone has a wide range of peripheral effects (Figure 2).

Concerning the cardiovascular system, a direct effect on the smooth muscle of blood vessels can lead to either vasoconstriction or vasodilatation, depending on the particular vessels influenced: renal, placental and umbilical vessels respond with vasoconstriction, whereas coronary vessels and vessels of the skeletal muscle respond with vasodilatation. The consequent effect on the blood pressure consists of three phases: first, there is a brief early depressor phase; then comes the pressor phase, as serotonin increases the total peripheral resistance; and finally, when serotonin dilates the vessels of the skeletal muscles, a late depressor phase is observed. Serotonin also influences respiration by stimulating the carotid and aortic chemoreceptors. The result is a short-lasting increase in respiratory minute volume by direct stimulation of the smooth muscles of the bronchi, leading to bronchoconstriction. Furthermore, serotonin stimulates the gastrointestinal tract to greater motility, with increased tone or intense spastic contractions, colics and evacuation of the bowels [28].

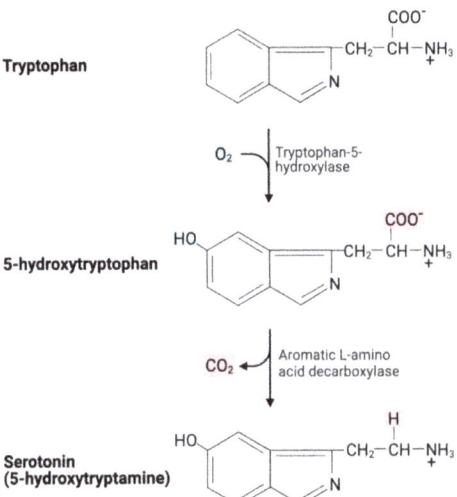

Figure 1. Tryptophan metabolic pathway.

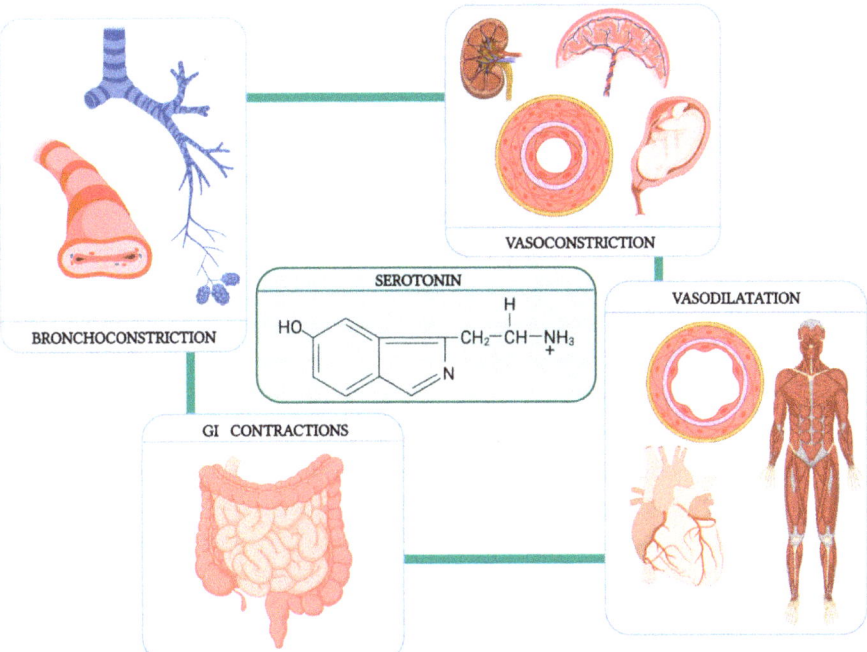

Figure 2. Peripheral effects of serotonin.

However, serotonin cannot be the unique molecule implicated in CC. Some reports denied the role of serotonin in flushing [29,30], one of the most typical symptoms associated with hemodynamic instability in CC. In addition, NETs originating from the respiratory tract and foregut do not express the aromatic acid decarboxylase, which converts 5-hydroxytryptophan to serotonin. Indeed, in this subtype of neoplasms, an atypical carcinoid syndrome can be observed characterized by patchy, sharply demarcated, serpiginous and cherry-red flushes (gastric NET) [31] or by prolonged flushing, lasting for hours or days, associated with disorientation, anxiety and tremor, lacrimation, salivation, hypotension, tachycardia, diarrhea, dyspnea, asthma and edema (Pulmonary NETs) [32]. Other potential mediators of CC are bradykinins, prostaglandins, tachykinins, substance P and histamine. Table 2 summarizes the main humoral molecules involved in the pathogenesis of CS/CC.

Table 2. Molecules implicated in CS/CC.

	Effects	Role in CC/CS
Amines		
Serotonin	vasoconstriction/vasodilatation, bronchoconstriction, fibroblastic activation	diarrhea, cramps bronchospasm carcinoid heart disease
Histamine	vasoconstriction/vasodilatation bronchoconstriction tachycardia	flushing, pruritus, edema bronchospasm
5-Hydroxytryptophan	vasodilatation	diarrhea, cramps
Norepinephrine	vasoconstriction, tachycardia, hyperglycemia, hyperlipidemia, tremor	anxiety
Dopamine	vasodilatation, GI motility block	
Polypeptides		
Kallikrein	conversion of kininogens in kinins (bradykinin and kallidin)	flushing, bronchospasm
Bradykinin	vasodilatation, bronchoconstriction, edema	flushing, bronchospasm
Somatostatin	GH, TSH, prolactin, insulin, glucagon release inhibition	diabetes, cholelithiasis, steatorrhea, hypochloridria
Motilin	GI motility stimulation	diarrhea, cramps
Pancreatic Polypeptide	pancreatic secretion regulation (inhibits the secretion of fluids, bicarbonate, and digestive enzymes)	
Vasoactive Intestinal Peptide	vasodilatation, smooth muscle relaxation induction, secretion of water into pancreatic juice, and bile stimulation	profuse diarrhea, hypokalemia, achlorhydria
Neuropeptide K (tachykinin family)	bronchoconstriction, bradycardia	
Substance P (tachykinin family)	bronchoconstriction bradycardia	
Neurokinin A (tachykinin family)	bronchoconstriction bradycardia	
Neurokinin B (tachykinin family)	bronchoconstriction bradycardia	
Corticotropin (ACTH)	cortisol release	Cushing Syndrome
Gastrin	hydrochloric acid release by the stomach	Zollinger Ellison Syndrome
Growth Hormone	cell metabolism stimulation	acromegaly
Peptide YY	anorectic effect	
Glucagon	glucose and fatty acid release	necrolytic migratory erythema, weight loss hyperglycemia
Beta-endorphin	pain relief	
Neurotensin	gastrin and motilin release inhibition, vasodilatation	
Chromogranin A	vasostatin precursor, pancreastatin, catestatin, and parastatin that inhibit hormone released by neuroendocrine cells	
Prostaglandins	vasoconstriction/vasodilatation	

In CC, the most implicated compounds seem to be vasoactive peptides, such as serotonin, histamine, bradykinin, tachykinins and kallikrein. In particular, patients with carcinoid flushing exhibit elevated levels of bradykinin and kallikrein in the bloodstream [33], which are considered the most probably responsible for flushing, rather than serotonin.

The only available data concerning the incidence and possible biological onset of CC is derived from few, small studies on intraoperative CC, such as surgical resection or locoregional treatments. When tumor manipulation occurs, the stress response triggers the release of catecholamines from the adrenals or sympathetic neurons, which in turn contribute to the release of tumor products [10]. Although CC is more typical of functional NETs, it may also occur in nonfunctional tumors. The presence of liver metastases, older age, and, for intraoperative crises, anticipated long anesthesia time, represent the most significant risk factors associated with the onset of CC, as demonstrated by Massimino et al. [10] and subsequently prospectively confirmed by Condron et al. [11]. Recently, the Research Unit of the Oregon Health and Science University has evaluated hemodynamic parameters and serum hormone levels during elective major surgery in patients with NETs [26]. Forty-six patients with a high risk of CC (older age, liver involvement, long anesthesia) were enrolled. The patients presented pulmonary artery catheters inserted to track pulmonary artery pressure, cardiac output and systemic vascular resistance, in addition to transesophageal echocardiography probes inserted to supervise cardiac function, and had serial measurements of typical hormones considered to be implicated in CC (serotonin, histamine, bradykinin and kallikrein). Seventeen patients experienced CC with prolonged hypotension. The most significant finding was that the pre-incision serotonin level was significantly higher in patients who manifested the crisis, while there were no significant changes in the mean value of any of the four hormone levels during CC. Patients manifesting CC presented an increased risk of postoperative complications, particularly if the events continued for more than 10 min. Authors concluded that elevated pre-incision serum serotonin levels represent a novel marker for increased risk of CC, as well as the severity of the crisis, and they observed no evidence of any massive release of the evaluated hormones during CC, suggesting CC may be an entirely separate pathophysiologic entity from that of CS. However, since, to date, no other study has been carried out on this topic, this hypothesis needs further confirmation.

6. Carcinoid Crisis Management

6.1. Octreotide

Assuming that CC is caused by the massive release of hormones by tumor masses, octreotide has historically represented the mainstay of its treatment. This drug is a long-acting synthetic octapeptide [34] that acts like somatostatin, a potent inhibitory peptide (Figure 3). The blockade of hormone releases, such as insulin, glucagon, gastrin and other gastrointestinal molecules, and the reduction of splanchnic and hepatic blood flow represent the mechanisms underlying the management of CC. However, the real role of octreotide in the management of CC is not well established yet, and the available data are partly contradictory.

The first report of using octreotide to treat CC dates back to 1985 [36], when Kvols et al. administered two intravenous boluses of 50 μg of this drug to a patient affected by a small bowel NET presenting life-threatening hypotension and prolonged flushing during abdominal surgery, unresponsive to intravenous fluids, intravenous calcium or intravenous conventional vasopressors. The Authors described a rapid resolution of the critical status and concluded that octreotide must be available in the operating room during surgery to rapidly manage CC. Furthermore, the same Authors conducted an explorative study on 25 patients with metastatic NET and documented CS [37] with the aim to evaluate the effect of this long-acting somatostatin analog, suggesting that this drug could be routinely safely used in the management of CS with excellent results.

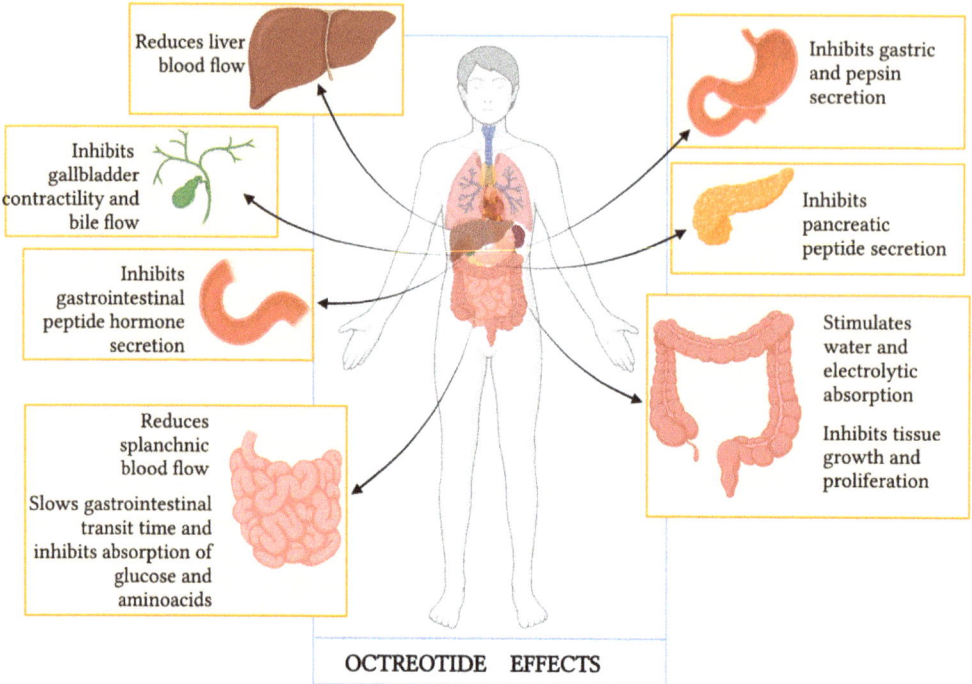

Figure 3. Octreotide clinical effects (Figure adapted by Lamberts SW, van der Lely AJ, de Herder WW, Hofland LJ. Octreotide [35]).

However, further studies have questioned the real role of octreotide in the specific treatment of CC. Considering the pharmacodynamic profile of octreotide, this drug acts as a hormone release blocker and not as a hormone receptor blocker, therefore it should not neutralize the effect of circulating vasoactive peptides [38,39]. It should possibly prevent a worsening in the CC or prevent its occurrence at all. According to the most recent analysis put forward by Wann et al. [40], the rapid resolution of the acute episode described by Kvols et al. could also be explained by a delayed effect of epinephrine or other previously administered medications.

In 2001, Kinney et al. [9] evaluated the complication rate and outcomes of a larger series of patients with metastatic NET. Among the 119 subjects undergoing abdominal surgery included, 6 received only a preoperative octreotide dose, while 45 patients received octreotide intraoperatively, and 73 patients did not receive octreotide. A total of 15 out of 119 patients experienced perioperative complications, including 3 deaths, but none of the 45 subjects who received the intraoperative drug dose had an intraoperative complication. The researchers reported a statistically significant difference in terms of intraoperative complications between the 45 patients who received intraoperative octreotide and the 73 who did not ($p = 0.023$). They concluded that patients with metastatic carcinoid tumors can undergo abdominal surgery safely with an intraoperative octreotide dose, reporting a significantly global decrease in intraoperative complications such as CC.

Based on the possible preventive role of octreotide on CC, Massimino et al. retrospectively explored the use of octreotide prophylaxis in a group of 97 patients undergoing surgery during the years 2007–2011. A total of 87 patients (90%) received prophylactic octreotide (dose range 100–1100 mg, median 500 mg), and 56% received at least one additional intraoperative dose. Despite the use of octreotide, intraoperative complications occurred in 23 (24%) patients. Therefore, the obtained data greatly diverged from the results published by Kinney et al., In their series, 18 patients (19%) experienced prolonged hypotension, while 5 (5%) were reported to have had marked hemodynamic instability consistent with a CC. Intraoperative complications occurred with the same frequency among patients with functioning (21%) and non-functioning (28%) NET, and the presence of liver metastases was found to be a predictor of intraoperative complications. These findings suggest neither outpatient octreotide LAR nor single-dose preoperative bolus octreotide prevent all intraoperative complications [10].

In 2016, Woltering et al. [41] suggested a possible solution to improve octreotide effectiveness. Their retrospective report demonstrated a reduction in CC incidence by using a continuous infusion of high-dose octreotide during surgery. As anesthetic or surgical stimuli can potentially precipitate an unpredictable release of amines, in their protocols, the researchers administered a prophylactic preoperative 500 μg bolus of octreotide acetate along with a continuous intravenous intraoperative infusion for all NET patients undergoing surgical cytoreduction, regardless of the location of their primary tumor or their functional status. The rationale behind this choice is connected to octreotide pharmacokinetics: preoperative bolus of octreotide, with a half-life of 90–120 min, might not last long enough for protection against CC during long surgery. Without a continuous infusion, blood level would fall to 50% of the original octreotide concentration after 2 h and would be only 25% of the original concentration after 4 h. As result, Woltering et al. reported an incidence of CC of only 3.6%, concluding that continuous intraoperative octreotide infusion could significantly reduce the risk of CC onset.

To demonstrate the benefits of continuous octreotide infusion on CC prevention, Condron et al. [11] prospectively enrolled 127 patients (71% with liver metastases, 74% with CS) who underwent 150 operations with continuous octreotide infusions. Contrary to what was expected, 30% of the patients manifested CC, and the crises were significantly associated with the presence of liver metastases ($p = 0.02$) or a history of CS ($p = 0.006$). The rapid use of vasopressor was effective in reducing crisis duration, with a reduction in postoperative complications. These unexpected results could be explained by analyzing CC definitions. While Woltering et al. considered only episodes of hypotension lasting $\geq$10 min [41], Condron et al. registered all cases of hemodynamic instability (systolic blood pressure < 80 or >180 mmHg, heart rate > 120 beats per minute or display of any physiology that, if sustained, would be expected to lead to end-organ dysfunction, such as ventricular arrhythmias or bronchospasm) unattributable to any other causes [11]. Considering only episodes of hypotension lasting $\geq$10 min, as Woltering et al. did, Condron et al. would have reported only 8% of CC.

Other reports on the outcome of prophylactic octreotide were published in 2018 [42] and 2019 [12]. Kinney et al. retrospectively evaluated 169 patients undergoing partial hepatic resection for metastatic NET between 1997 and 2015, and 77% (130/169) of patients preoperatively received 500 μg of subcutaneous octreotide. In their report, there were no documented cases of CC; one patient developed clinical findings of an emerging CC but was successfully treated with doses of octreotide, and findings resolved in <10 min. Of note, in this case, CC was defined as a sudden or blunt onset of at least two of the following: flushing or urticaria that are not explained by an allergic reaction; bronchospasm or bronchodilator administration; hypotension (SBP < 80 mmHg for >10 min and treated with vasopressor) not explained by volume status or hemorrhage; tachycardia $\geq$120 beats per minute [42]. Analyzing only sustained hypotension, the incidence was 5.6%, but because none of those patients exhibited any other criteria, none were considered CC.

Finally, Kwon et al. reported a retrospective series of 75 patients with metastatic well-differentiated NETs who underwent liver resection, ablation or embolotherapy from 2012 to 2016. The CC was defined subjectively by clinical documentation of occurrence by any treating physician, including the anesthesiologist, surgeon or interventional radiologist, and it had to be associated with hemodynamic instability, defined as the presence of at least one of the following events sustained for more than 10 min during the procedure: hypotension (systolic blood pressure, 80 mm Hg) or tachycardia (heart rate, >120 beats per minute). CC was identified in 32% (24) of patients. Of note, the route and dose of preprocedural octreotide administration varied widely. Neither long-acting octreotide, perioperative octreotide, intraoperative octreotide nor any combination was associated with a lower incidence of crisis. The Authors concluded that somatostatin analogs do not reliably prevent CC. One hypothesis is that CC may be a phenomenon physiologically distinct from CS, involving the release of a different distribution of vasoactive substances, against which different therapeutic agents can be used [12]. As previously mentioned, this proposal has been explored by Condron et al. [26].

Data are summarized in Table 3.

Table 3. Articles assessing the impact of octreotide in CC.

Variation	Type of Paper	Number of Patients	Number of CC	Octreotide Dose and Regimen
Kvols et al., 1986 [36]	Case report-retrospective study	25	1	a bolus of 50 μg of octreotide intraoperatively
Kinney et al. [9]	Retrospective study	119	15 (none of the pts received onctreotide intraoperatively)	- 31 pts received octreotide preoperatively (median dose 300 μg—range 50–1000 μg); 25 of these pts received additional octreotide intraoperatively. - 45 pts received octreotide intraoperatively (median dose 350 μg—range 30–4000 μg)
Massimino et al. [10]	Retrospective study	97	23	87 pts received prophylactic octreotide (median dose 500 μg—range 100–1100 μg) + intraoperative bolus if necessary (median dose 350 μg—range 100–5500 μg)
Woltering et al. [41]	Retrospective study	150	6	Continuous high-dose octreotide infusion: 500 μg/h
Condron et al. [11]	Prospective study	127	38	Continuous high-dose octreotide infusion: 100 μg/h
Kinney et al. [42]	Retrospective study	169	0	- 130 pts received 500 μg preoperatively s.c. - 39 pts received additional intravenous octreotide (median dose 500 μg—range 250–650 μg)
Kwon et al. [12]	Retrospective study	75	24	- 27 pts received preprocedure infusion (median dose 150 μg/h—range 50–300 μg/h) - 21 pts received a preprocedure i.v. or s.c. bolus (median dose 150 μg—range 100–300 μg). - 48 pts received intraprocedural infusion (median dose 150 μg/h—range 50–300 μg/h) - 20 pts receive an intraprocedural i.v or s.c. bolus (median dose 150 μg—range 20–510 μg)

As reported in the most recent guidelines referring to clinical studies discussed so far, there are no standard octreotide regimens in the management of CC; subcutaneous administration of octreotide 100–200 mcg × 2–3 daily during surgery has been suggested for a minor procedure or lower-risk patients. However, intravenous octreotide infusions should also be readily available in the operating room to be used when deemed necessary. For major surgery, perioperative prophylactic treatment with intravenous octreotide, at the starting dose of 50–100 mcg/h (mean dose 100–200 mcg/h), is the standard regimen used by most clinical centers. Although this has not been substantiated by any prospective study, most experts start treatment with intravenous octreotide 12 h before the operation and escalate the dose as necessary until symptom control is achieved. This infusion continues for at least 48 h after the operation, with dose titration as clinically required [43].

Considering the increasing use of PRRT, several studies have been conducted to estimate the impact of octreotide in PRRT-induced CC. The incidence of CC during PRRT ranges between 1 and 10%, and, as previously mentioned in this review, specific risk factors have been defined, which, if present, expose the patient to a major rate of intra-treatment complications [24]. In the clinical experience reported by de Kaizer et al., among 479 patients enrolled in the study, 7 cases of CC after the first cycle of PRRT were reported [44]. The treatment included high-dose octreotide, i.v. fluid replacement and corticosteroid. Despite additional precautions taken after their first therapy cycle (continuation of somatostatin analog, corticosteroids and reduction of administered dosage of ^{177}Lu-octreotate), 3 patients developed a second CC after the subsequent cycle of PRRT.

Analyzing the possible mechanism behind hormonal secretion during Lu-octreotate therapy (tumor lysis vs. discontinuation of short-acting somatostatin analog vs. emotional stress response to hospitalization vs. administration of arginine and lysine), the Authors concluded that hormonal crises should be managed with an infusion of somatostatin analogs i.v., fluids, corticosteroids and correction of electrolyte disturbances. More recently, Stenzel et al. came to the same conclusions [45]. Moreover, the Australian group of Tapia Rico et al. first proposed a protocol to prevent and manage severe CC and specifically defined which patients would benefit most ("high-risk patients") from premedication to PRRT therapy with corticosteroids and bolus dose of octreotide sc [46]. This work has been further enriched by De Olmo et al., who recently published the current procedure adopted for approaching patients undergoing PRRT [24]. The work of clinicians should start from the identification of risk factors for CC through:

- The evaluation of nutritional assessment with the diagnosis and correction of hydro electrolytic disorders, malnutrition and malabsorption, and the avoidance of food triggers and intensive physical exercises the previous day;
- The evaluation of NET characteristics (high tumor burden, use of somatostatin analogs to control CS).

In particular, in the case of bulky tumors, it is mandatory to consider a possible surgery or locoregional treatment before PRRT. In addition, it is essential to obtain good control of CS before the first cycle of ^{177}Lu-octreotate.

As premedication, the Authors advise the administration of corticosteroids (dexamentasone 4–8 mg), antiemetic (ondansetron 4 mg), somatostatin analog (octreotide 100 μg s.c. or 50 μg i.v. bolus), antistaminic h1 (dexchlorpheniramine 5 mg i.v. in slow infusion) and antistaminic H2 (ranitidine 50 mg i.v. in slow infusion). In the event of an outbreak of CC, the infusion of Lu-DOTATATE should immediately stop, and a bolus of octreotide (100–500 μg) should be immediately administered, followed by a maintaining dose of 50–100 μg/h infusion. In case of severe hypotension, the Authors do not exclude the use of phenylephrine or vasopressor drugs.

6.2. Vasopressors

Based on clinical experiences [2,13,14,47], sympathomimetic drugs have always been avoided in the management of CC-related hypotension, since they may worsen it by triggering further release of peptides by tumor masses. Mason et al., in 1966, first observed vascular response to systemic epinephrine injection in the forearm in 7 NET patients. The Authors noted decreased systemic blood pressure, decreased vascular resistance and an elevated bradykinin level for 5 min after injection, although the response was quite variable among the 7 patients [47]. However, data supporting a widespread concern about the abuse of beta-adrenergic agonists remain very limited [48].

More recent experiences have tried to explore the real role of this class of drugs in the management of intraoperative CC [10,26,48]. Notably, Limbach et al. retrospectively examined the use of vasoactive medications during CC to determine whether an association between induction of a secondary CC and beta-adrenergic agonist administration could be detected. They observed no close correlation between the use of sympathomimetic drugs and secondary CC and, in addition, the duration of CC did not increase with administration of beta-adrenergic agonists [48].

Based on these reports and considering the recent findings, CC-related hypotension is due to a distributive shock, as previously discussed, and the administration of vasopressors, which determine a wider systemic effect (vs. octreotide alone, which has a vasoconstrictive effect only on splanchnic vessels), should be suggested when standard measures fail [40].

7. Conclusions

The CC remains a severe, sometimes fatal, acute manifestation of NETs. The rarity and unpredictability of this event has hampered the development of randomized controlled trials to define the best clinical and therapeutical approach. Data available in the literature are mainly derived from small retrospective studies or case reports, in which the clinical definition of CC is not consistent and universally accepted. Recently, the pathophysiological mechanism has also been questioned. According to some Authors, CC should be considered a completely separate event from CS, as it can be triggered by a different cocktail of hormones.

Current guidelines, such as the European ENETS and the American NANETS, continue to recommend the administration of octreotide to prevent and manage CC onset [42,49], although without a standard scheme, duration and dose specification. Furthermore, the use of vasopressors has been recently revised, as their administration during crises could accelerate the increase in blood pressure.

Based on recent evidence, some institutes stopped using octreotide during operations altogether instead of relying on vasopressors, including beta-adrenergic agonists [50]. Their experience on 195 patients demonstrates a rate of CC not significantly higher than that reported in previous studies. The Authors conclude that perioperative octreotide use may be safely stopped, owing to inefficacy, and the treatment of crisis should be replaced with intravenous fluids and vasopressors, which address the actual pathophysiology of the crisis, without concern about increasing crisis duration or rates of major postoperative complications.

Further efforts should be directed toward the understanding of the correct pathophysiology of CC to propose more specific, effective and established treatments.

Author Contributions: Conceptualization, C.B. and F.G.; methodology, C.B.; software, C.B.; validation, C.B., S.B., G.L., I.G., F.P., M.D. and F.G.; formal analysis, C.B.; investigation, C.B.; resources, C.B.; data curation, C.B.; writing—original draft preparation, C.B.; writing—review and editing, C.B., S.B. and F.G.; visualization, C.B.; supervision, F.G.; project administration, C.B. and F.G.; funding acquisition, F.G, F.P. and M.D. All authors have read and agreed to the published version of the manuscript.

Funding: This research received no external funding.

Conflicts of Interest: F.G. received honoraria for speaker/advisory roles from Servier, Eli Lilly, Iqvia, Merck Serono, Amgen and Bristol-Myers Squibb outside the present work; the other Authors declare no conflicts of interest.

References

1. Sjoerdsma, A.; Weissbach, H.; Udenfriend, S. A clinical, physiologic and biochemical study of patients with malignant car-cinoid (argentaffinoma). *Am. J. Med.* **1956**, *20*, 520–532. [CrossRef]
2. Kahil, M.E.; Brown, H.; Fred, H.L. The carcinoid crisis. *Arch. Intern. Med.* **1964**, *114*, 26–28. [CrossRef] [PubMed]
3. Tomassetti, P.; Migliori, M.; Lalli, S.; Campana, D.; Tomassetti, V.; Corinaldesi, R. Epidemiology, clinical features and diagno-sis of gastroenteropancreatic endocrine tumours. *Ann. Oncol.* **2001**, *12*, S95–S99. [CrossRef] [PubMed]
4. Fujie, S.; Zhou, W.; Fann, P.; Yen, Y. Carcinoid crisis 24 h after bland embolization: A case report. *Biosci. Trends* **2010**, *4*, 143–144.
5. Ozgen, A.; Demirkazik, F.; Arat, A. Carcinoid crisis provoked by mammographic compression of metastatic carcinoid tu-mour of the breast. *Clin. Radiol.* **2001**, *56*, 250–251. [CrossRef]
6. Salm, E.F.; Janssen, M.; Breburda, C.S.; Van Woerkens, L.J.P.; De Herder, W.W.; Zwaan, C.V.; Roelandt, J.R.T. Carcinoid crisis during transesophageal echocardiography. *Intensiv. Care Med.* **2000**, *26*, 254. [CrossRef]
7. Morrisroe, K.; Sim, I.-W.; McLachlan, K.; Inder, W.J. Carcinoid crisis induced by repeated abdominal examination. *Intern. Med. J.* **2012**, *42*, 342–344. [CrossRef]
8. Magabe, P.C.; Bloom, A.L. Sudden death from carcinoid crisis during image-guided biopsy of a lung mass. *J. Vasc. Interv. Ra-diol.* **2014**, *25*, 484–487. [CrossRef]
9. Kinney, M.A.O.; Warner, M.E.; Nagorney, D.M.; Rubin, J.; Schroeder, D.R.; Maxson, P.M. Perianaesthetic risks and outcomes of abdominal surgery for metastatic carcinoid tumours †. *Br. J. Anaesth.* **2001**, *87*, 447–452. [CrossRef]
10. Massimino, K.; Harrskog, O.; Pommier, S.; Pommier, R. Octreotide LAR and bolus octreotide are insufficient for preventing intraoperative complications in carcinoid patients. *J. Surg. Oncol.* **2013**, *107*, 842–846. [CrossRef]
11. Condron, M.E.; Pommier, S.J.; Pommier, R.F. Continuous infusion of octreotide combined with perioperative octreotide bolus does not prevent intraoperative carcinoid crisis. *Surgery* **2016**, *159*, 358–367. [CrossRef] [PubMed]
12. Kwon, D.H.; Paciorek, A.; Mulvey, C.K.; Chan, H.; Fidelman, N.; Meng, L.; Nakakura, E.K.; Zhang, L.; Bergsland, E.K.; Van Loon, K. Periprocedural management of patients undergoing liver resection or embolotherapy for neuroendocrine tumor me-tastases. *Pancreas* **2019**, *48*, 496–503. [CrossRef] [PubMed]
13. Harris, A.L.; Smith, I.E. Tryptophan in the treatment of carcinoid crisis. *Cancer Chemother. Pharmacol.* **1983**, *10*, 137–139. [CrossRef]

14. Hughes, E.W.; Hodkinson, B.P. Carcinoid syndrome: The combined use of ketanserin and octreotide in the management of an acute crisis during anaesthesia. *Anaesth. Intensiv. Care* **1989**, *17*, 367–370. [CrossRef]
15. Batchelor, A.; Conacher, I. Anaphylactoid or carcinoid? *Br. J. Anaesth.* **1992**, *69*, 325–327. [CrossRef] [PubMed]
16. Parry, R.G.; Glover, S.; Dudley, C.R.K. Acute renal failure associated with carcinoid crisis. *Nephrol. Dial. Transplant.* **1996**, *11*, 2489–2490. [CrossRef]
17. Koopmans, K.P.; Brouwers, A.H.; De Hooge, M.N.; Van der Horst-Schrivers, A.N.; Kema, I.P.; Wolffenbuttel, B.H.; De Vries, E.G.; Jager, P.L. Carcinoid crisis after injection of 6-18F-fluorodihydroxyphenylalanine in a patient with metastatic carcinoid. *J. Nucl. Med.* **2005**, *46*, 1240–1243.
18. Papadogias, D.; Makras, P.; Kossivakis, K.; Kontogeorgos, G.; Piaditis, G.; Kaltsas, G. Carcinoid syndrome and carcinoid crisis secondary to a metastatic carcinoid tumour of the lung: A therapeutic challenge. *Eur. J. Gastroenterol. Hepatol.* **2007**, *19*, 1154–1159. [CrossRef]
19. Van Diepen, S.; Sobey, A.; Lewanczuk, R.; Singh, G.; Sidhu, S.; Zibdawi, M.; Mullen, J.C. A case of acute respiratory distress syndrome responsive to methylene blue during a carcinoid crisis. *Can. J. Anaesth.* **2013**, *60*, 1085–1088. [CrossRef]
20. Kromas, M.L.; Passi, Y.; Kuzumi, C.; Shikhar, S. Intra-operative carcinoid crisis: Revised anaesthesia management. *Indian J. Anaesth.* **2017**, *61*, 443–444. [CrossRef]
21. Maddali, M.V.; Chiu, C.; Cedarbaum, E.R.; Yogeswaran, V.; Seedahmed, M.; Smith, W.; Bergsland, E.; Fidelman, N.; Kenne-dy, J.L. Carcinoid crisis–induced acute systolic heart failure. *JACC Case Rep.* **2020**, *2*, 2068–2071. [CrossRef] [PubMed]
22. Dhanani, J.; Pattison, D.A.; Burge, M.; Williams, J.; Riedel, B.; Hicks, R.J.; Reade, M.C. Octreotide for resuscitation of cardiac arrest due to carcinoid crisis precipitated by novel peptide receptor radionuclide therapy (PRRT): A case report. *J. Crit. Care* **2020**, *60*, 319–322. [CrossRef] [PubMed]
23. Mahdi, M.; Ozer, M.; Tahseen, M. A Challenging case of carcinoid crisis in a patient with neuroendocrine tumor. *Cureus* **2021**, *13*, e15626. [CrossRef] [PubMed]
24. Del Olmo-García, M.I.; Muros, M.A.; López-De-La-Torre, M.; Agudelo, M.; Bello, P.; Soriano, J.M.; Merino-Torres, J.-F. Pre-vention and management of hormonal crisis during theragnosis with LU-DOTA-TATE in neuroendocrine tumors. A system-atic review and approach proposal. *J. Clin. Med.* **2020**, *9*, 2203. [CrossRef]
25. Seymour, N.; Sawh, S.C. Mega-dose intravenous octreotide for the treatment of carcinoid crisis: A systematic review. *Can. J. Anaesth.* **2013**, *60*, 492–499. [CrossRef] [PubMed]
26. Condron, M.E.; Jameson, N.E.; Limbach, K.E.; Bingham, A.E.; Sera, V.A.; Anderson, R.B.; Schenning, K.; Yockelson, S.; Ha-rukuni, I.; Kahl, E.A.; et al. A prospective study of the pathophysiology of carcinoid crisis. *Surgery* **2018**, *165*, 158–165. [CrossRef] [PubMed]
27. Keszthelyi, D.; Troost, F.J.; Masclee, A.A.M. Understanding the role of tryptophan and serotonin metabolism in gastrointes-tinal function. *Neurogastroenterol. Motil.* **2009**, *21*, 1239–1249. [CrossRef]
28. Sirek, A.; Sirek, O.V. Serotonin: A review. *Can. Med. Assoc. J.* **1970**, *102*, 846–849.
29. Robertson, J.I.; Peart, W.S.; Andrews, T.M. The mechanism of facial flushes in the carcinoid syndrome. *Quart. J. Med.* **1962**, *31*, 103–123.
30. Sjoerdsma, A.; Melmon, K.L. THE carcinoid spectrum. *Gastroenterology* **1964**, *47*, 104–107.
31. Borch, K.; Ahrén, B.; Ahlman, H.; Falkmer, S.; Granérus, G.; Grimelius, L. Gastric carcinoids: Biologic behavior and prognosis after differentiated treatment in relation to type. *Ann. Surg.* **2005**, *242*, 64–73. [CrossRef] [PubMed]
32. Melmon, K.L.; Sjoerdsma, A.; Mason, D.T. Distinctive clinical and therapeutic aspects of the syndrome associated with bronchial carcinoid tumors. *Am. J. Med.* **1965**, *39*, 568–581. [CrossRef]
33. Oates, J.; Sjoerdsma, K.M.A.; Gillespie, L.; Mason, D. Release of a kinin peptide in the carcinoid syndrome. *Lancet* **1964**, *1*, 514–517. [CrossRef]
34. Borna, R.M.; Jahr, J.S.; Kmiecik, S.; Mancuso, K.F.; Kaye, A.D. Pharmacology of octreotide: Clinical implications for anesthe-siologists and associated risks. *Anesthesiol. Clin.* **2017**, *35*, 327–339. [CrossRef]
35. Lamberts, S.W.; van der Lely, A.J.; de Herder, W.W.; Hofland, L.J. Octreotide. *N. Engl. J. Med.* **1996**, *334*, 246–254. [CrossRef]
36. Kvols, L.K.; Martin, J.K.; Marsh, H.M.; Moertel, C.G. Rapid reversal of carcinoid crisis with somatostatin analogue. *N. Engl. J. Med.* **1985**, *313*, 1229. [CrossRef]
37. Kvols, L.K.; Moertel, C.G.; O'Connell, M.J.; Schutt, A.J.; Rubin, J.; Hahn, R.G. Treatment of the malignant carcinoid syndrome evaluation of a long-acting somatostatin analogue. *N. Engl. J. Med.* **1986**, *315*, 663–666. [CrossRef]
38. Warner, R.R.; Mani, S.; Profeta, J.; Grunstein, E. Octreotide treatment of carcinoid hypertensive crisis. *Mt. Sinai J. Med. A J. Transl. Pers. Med.* **1994**, *61*, 349–355.
39. Veall, M.G.R.Q.; Peacock, M.J.E.; Bax, M.N.D.S.; Reilly, M.C.S. Review of the anaesthetic management of 21 patients under-going laparotomy for carcinoid syndrome. *Br. J. Anaesth.* **1994**, *72*, 335–341. [CrossRef]
40. Wonn, S.M.; Pommier, R.F. Carcinoid crisis: History, dogmas, and data. In *Neuroendocrine Tumors*; Springer: Berlin, Germany, 2021; pp. 87–103. [CrossRef]
41. Woltering, E.A.; Wright, A.E.; Stevens, M.A.; Wang, Y.-Z.; Boudreaux, J.P.; Mamikunian, G.; Riopelle, J.M.; Kaye, A.D. Develop-ment of effective prophylaxis against intraoperative carcinoid crisis. *J. Clin. Anesth.* **2016**, *32*, 189–193. [CrossRef]
42. Kinney, M.A.; Nagorney, D.M.; Clark, D.F.; O'Brien, T.D.; Turner, J.D.; Marienau, M.E.; Schroeder, D.R.; Martin, D.P. Partial hepatic resections for metastatic neuroendocrine tumors: Perioperative outcomes. *J. Clin. Anesth.* **2018**, *51*, 93–96. [CrossRef] [PubMed]

43. Kaltsas, G.; Caplin, M.; Davies, P.; Ferone, D.; Garcia-Carbonero, R.; Grozinsky-Glasberg, S.; Hörsch, D.; Janson, E.T.; Kian-manesh, R.; Kos-Kudła, B.; et al. ENETS consensus guidelines for the standards of care in neuroendocrine tumors: Pre- and perioperative therapy in patients with neuroendocrine tumors. *Neuroendocrinology* **2017**, *105*, 245–254. [CrossRef] [PubMed]
44. de Keizer, B.; Van Aken, M.; Feelders, R.A.; De Herder, W.W.; Kam, B.L.R.; Van Essen, M.; Krenning, E.; Kwekkeboom, D. Hormonal crises following receptor radionuclide therapy with the radiolabeled somatostatin analogue [177Lu-DOTA0,Tyr3]octreotate. *Eur. J. Nucl. Med. Mol. Imaging* **2008**, *35*, 749–755. [CrossRef] [PubMed]
45. Stenzel, J.; Noe, S.; Holzapfel, K.; Erlmeier, F.; Eyer, F. Fatal systemic vasoconstriction in a case of metastatic small-intestinal NET. *Rep. Gastrointest. Med.* **2017**, *2017*, 9810194. [CrossRef]
46. Rico, G.T.; Li, M.; Pavlakis, N.; Cehic, G.; Price, T.J. Prevention and management of carcinoid crises in patients with high-risk neuroendocrine tumours undergoing peptide receptor radionuclide therapy (PRRT): Literature review and case series from two Australian tertiary medical institutions. *Cancer Treat. Rev.* **2018**, *66*, 1–6. [CrossRef]
47. Mason, D.T.; Melmon, K.L. New understanding of the mechanism of the carcinoid flush. *Ann. Intern. Med.* **1966**, *65*, 1334–1339. [CrossRef]
48. Limbach, K.E.; Condron, M.E.; Bingham, A.E.; Pommier, S.J.; Pommier, R.F. B-Adrenergic agonist administration is not asso-ciated with secondary carcinoid crisis in patients with carcinoid tumor. *Am. J. Surg.* **2019**, *217*, 932–936. [CrossRef]
49. Howe, J.R.; Cardona, K.; Fraker, D.L.; Kebebew, E.; Untch, B.R.; Wang, Y.-Z.; Law, C.H.; Liu, E.H.; Kim, M.K.; Menda, Y.; et al. The surgical management of small bowel neuroendocrine tumors: Consensus guidelines of the north american neuroendo-crine tumor society. *Pancreas* **2017**, *46*, 715–731. [CrossRef]
50. Wonn, S.M.; Ratzlaff, A.N.; Pommier, S.J.; McCully, B.H.; Pommier, R.F. A prospective study of carcinoid crisis with no perioperative octreotide. *Surgery* **2021**, *171*, 88–93. [CrossRef]

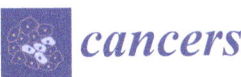

Review

Endocrine and Neuroendocrine Tumors Special Issue—Checkpoint Inhibitors for Adrenocortical Carcinoma and Metastatic Pheochromocytoma and Paraganglioma: Do They Work?

Camilo Jimenez [1,*], Gustavo Armaiz-Pena [2], Patricia L. M. Dahia [3,4], Yang Lu [5], Rodrigo A. Toledo [6], Jeena Varghese [1] and Mouhammed Amir Habra [1]

1. Department of Endocrine Neoplasia and Hormonal Disorders, The University of Texas MD Anderson Cancer Center, Houston, TX 77030, USA; jvarghese@mdanderson.org (J.V.); mahabra@mdanderson.org (M.A.H.)
2. Division of Endocrinology, Department Medicine, The University of Texas Health Science Center, San Antonio, TX 78229, USA; armaizpena@uthscsa.edu
3. Department of Medicine, University of Texas Health San Antonio, San Antonio, TX 78229, USA; dahia@uthscsa.edu
4. Mays Cancer Center, University of Texas Health San Antonio, San Antonio, TX 78229, USA
5. Department of Nuclear Medicine, The University of Texas MD Anderson Cancer Center, Houston, TX 77030, USA; ylu10@mdanderson.org
6. CIBERONC, Gastrointestinal and Endocrine Tumors, Vall d'Hebron Institute of Oncology (VHIO), Centro Cellex, 08035 Barcelona, Spain; rtoledo@vhio.net
* Correspondence: cjimenez@mdanderson.org

Simple Summary: In the past decade, the landscape of cancer treatment has radically changed after the introduction of immunotherapy. Adrenocortical carcinoma and metastatic pheochromocytoma/paraganglioma are rare cancers with limited responses to traditional cancer treatments. The use of immunotherapy against these cancers has yielded a few responses when used alone or in combination with other drugs. We reviewed the current literature to summarize the role of immunotherapy in these rare cancers.

Abstract: Adrenocortical cancers and metastatic pheochromocytomas are the most common malignancies originating in the adrenal glands. Metastatic paragangliomas are extra-adrenal tumors that share similar genetic and molecular profiles with metastatic pheochromocytomas and, subsequently, these tumors are studied together. Adrenocortical cancers and metastatic pheochromocytomas and paragangliomas are orphan diseases with limited therapeutic options worldwide. As in any other cancers, adrenocortical cancers and metastatic pheochromocytomas and paragangliomas avoid the immune system. Hypoxia-pseudohypoxia, activation of the PD-1/PD-L1 pathway, and/or microsatellite instability suggest that immunotherapy with checkpoint inhibitors could be a therapeutic option for patients with these tumors. The results of clinical trials with checkpoint inhibitors for adrenocortical carcinoma or metastatic pheochromocytoma or paraganglioma demonstrate limited benefits; nevertheless, these results also suggest interesting mechanisms that might enhance clinical responses to checkpoint inhibitors. These mechanisms include the normalization of tumor vasculature, modification of the hormonal environment, and vaccination with specific tumor antigens. Combinations of checkpoint inhibitors with classical therapies, such as chemotherapy, tyrosine kinase inhibitors, radiopharmaceuticals, and/or novel therapies, such as vaccines, should be evaluated in clinical trials.

Keywords: adrenocortical cancer; metastatic pheochromocytoma; metastatic paraganglioma; checkpoint inhibitors; avelumab; ipilimumab; nivolumab; pembrolizumab

1. Introduction

The adrenal glands are very important endocrine organs that are responsible for the regulation of many different physiological mechanisms that preserve human homeostasis and guarantee the individual's survival. These features include the modulation of the cellular responses to stress; the healing of damaged tissues; the protective responses of fighting and escape; the regulation of the corporal concentrations of acid and electrolytes; the modulation of the metabolism of glucose, fat, and proteins; and the maintenance of adequate blood pressure to satisfy metabolic needs. The adrenal glands regulate homeostasis through the synthesis and secretion of androgens, glucocorticoids, and mineralocorticoids, which are derived from the adrenal cortex, and catecholamines, which come from the adrenal medulla [1–3]. Embryologically, the adrenal cortex is derived from the intermediate mesoderm [4], and the adrenal medulla is derived from the neural crest cells close to the dorsal aorta [5]. The adrenal medulla is a modified autonomic sympathetic nervous system ganglion that, unlike other sympathetic ganglia, produces adrenaline and noradrenaline and releases these hormones directly into the bloodstream.

Primary malignant tumors may develop in the adrenal cortex or in the adrenal medulla. The most common cancers to develop in these regions are adrenocortical carcinoma (ACC), which is a tumor derived from the adrenal cortex, and metastatic pheochromocytoma, which is a tumor derived from the adrenal medulla. Similar tumors, called metastatic paragangliomas, develop in the extra-adrenal paraganglia and have genetic and molecular profiles similar to those of many metastatic pheochromocytomas [6], and current clinical trials study metastatic pheochromocytoma and metastatic paragangliomas together. For the purpose of this manuscript, we will consider metastatic pheochromocytomas and paragangliomas (MPPGL) as one tumor group.

ACCs are tumors associated with high proliferative rates and a common clinical phenotype of large, rapidly growing primary tumors that are associated with metastases in up to 80% of cases [7–9]. Conversely, pheochromocytomas and paragangliomas are usually characterized by lower proliferative rates than those observed in ACCs, and their metastatic spread is observed in up to 25% of cases [10,11]. Nevertheless, MPPGL tumors are usually large as primary tumors, and the metastases are frequently massive because the diagnosis of these tumors is frequently delayed [9,12]. Most ACCs and MPPGLs secrete excessive amounts of hormones, predisposing patients with these tumors to severe comorbidities. ACCs may secrete large amounts of glucocorticoids, mineralocorticoids, and/or androgens, which may lead to severe Cushing syndrome, hyperaldosteronism, and virilization [13,14], and MPPGLs may secrete excessive amounts of catecholamines, which may lead to severe cardiovascular and gastrointestinal diseases [15,16]. The combination of a large tumor burden, considerable tumor growth over time, and excessive hormonal secretion predisposes patients with ACC and MPPGL to a decreased quality of life and decreased overall survival rates [12–14]. In fact, only 15–44% of patients with ACC and 60% of patients with MPPGL are alive 5 years after initial diagnosis [7,17].

ACC and MPPGL are rare tumors. In the United States, approximately 200–300 new cases of ACC and 100–200 new cases of MPPGL are discovered every year [17,18]; by definition, ACC and MPPGL are orphan diseases, and, subsequently, the therapeutic options for advanced disease are limited [10,13]. ACC is mainly treated with a combination of systemic chemotherapy of cisplatin, doxorubicin, etoposide, and mitotane, and clinical responses are noted in approximately 30% of patients; ACC responses to chemotherapy usually have short duration, and treatment toxicity can be substantial [13]. Chemotherapy with cyclophosphamide, vincristine, and dacarbazine for MPPGL is widely available. However, response rates are also low, with approximately 37% of patients achieving partial response (PR), with at least a reduction of 30% of the tumor size when compared with baseline measurements, or disease stabilization; cures are exceptional, and treatment toxicity is also substantial [10,19,20]. Approximately 60–70% of MPPGLs express the noradrenaline transporter; therefore, these tumors are meta-iodine-benzyl-guanidine (MIBG)–avid [12,21]. The United States Food and Drug Administration (FDA) recently approved high-specific-activity MIBG (HSA-I-131-MIBG) for patients with MPPGL. HSA-I-131-MIBG demonstrated a clinical benefit rate (CBR), the proportion of patients who achieve a complete response or tumor disappearance, partial response, and disease stabilization as per RECIST 1.1., higher than 90%, with approximately 25% of patients exhibiting a PR and more than 60% of patients having stable disease with some degree of regression 1 year after treatment. Additionally, most patients who underwent HSA-I-131-MIBG treatment had improved blood pressure compared to baseline, and the toxicity of HSA-I-131-MIBG was acceptable [22]. This medication is only available in the United States and is not indicated for the treatment of patients with MPPGL that does not express the noradrenaline transporter [20].

Given this limited spectrum of therapeutic options, we need to identify other effective treatments for patients with ACC and MPPGL. Over the last decade, immunotherapy with checkpoint inhibitors has become one of the therapeutic pillars against cancer [23]. The results of phase 1 and 2 clinical trials with immunotherapy for ACC and MPPGL have revealed that immunotherapy is a potentially important treatment for patients with these tumors as well. In this review, we will discuss the rationale for the use of immunotherapy against ACC and MPPGL, the results of clinical trials with several checkpoint inhibitors against ACC and MPPGL, and potential mechanisms to induce or enhance an immune system response effective against ACC and MPPGL.

2. Avoidance of the Immune System as a Hallmark of Cancer

The hallmarks of cancer are the distinctive and complementary capabilities that enable tumor growth and metastatic dissemination and are the foundation for understanding the biology of any cancer. These hallmarks include the sustaining of the proliferative signaling of tumor cells, mechanisms that favor replicative immortality, genome instability and the presence of mutations, deregulation of cellular energetics and cell necrosis, tumor-promoting inflammation, the induction of abnormal vascular formation or angiogenesis, the activation of mechanisms of invasion and metastases, resistance to tumor cell death, the avoidance of growth suppressors, and the avoidance of the recognition of the cancer cell as such by the immune system [24]. Several features related to cancer cell biology theoretically lead to a destructive anti-cancer immune response. Cancer cells are characterized by the accumulation of a variable number of genetic alterations and the subsequent loss of normal cellular regulatory processes; cancer cells also accumulate neoantigens, antigens of differentiation, and cancer testis antigens, and a fraction of these antigens are bound to major histocompatibility class I molecules, allowing the immune system CD8+ T cells to recognize cancer cells [25,26].

Once the cancer cell is recognized as such, the cancer immunity cycle starts [27]. The cancer immunity cycle is a sequence of steps that must be initiated, allowed to proceed, and expanded to generate an anti-cancer immune response (Figure 1) [27]. The cycle starts with the release of antigens that are later presented to antigen-presenting cells, such as the dendritic cells, followed by the priming and activation of T cells in places, such as the lymph nodes. These T cells travel through the bloodstream, identify the location of the tumor cells, infiltrate the tumor environment, and recognize the cancer cells; the T cells then kill the cancer cells with the subsequent release of cancer antigens, enhancing and perpetuating the cancer immunity cycle [27]. The cancer immunity cycle has three important qualities: (1) adaptability, which is the capacity of the immune system to recognize the cancer cell; (2) specificity, which allows the immune system attack to be mainly focused on cancer cells, limiting toxic effects on the normal cells; and (3) memory, which guarantees that the immune system can more effectively recognize and destroy cancer cells that may develop again [27]. Tumors are, however, more than just cancer cells. Tumors are also composed of non-malignant cells that are recruited by the malignant cells to serve them. Together the malignant and non-malignant cells, the extracellular matrix and the tumor vasculature, and their complex communications create the tumor microenvironment.

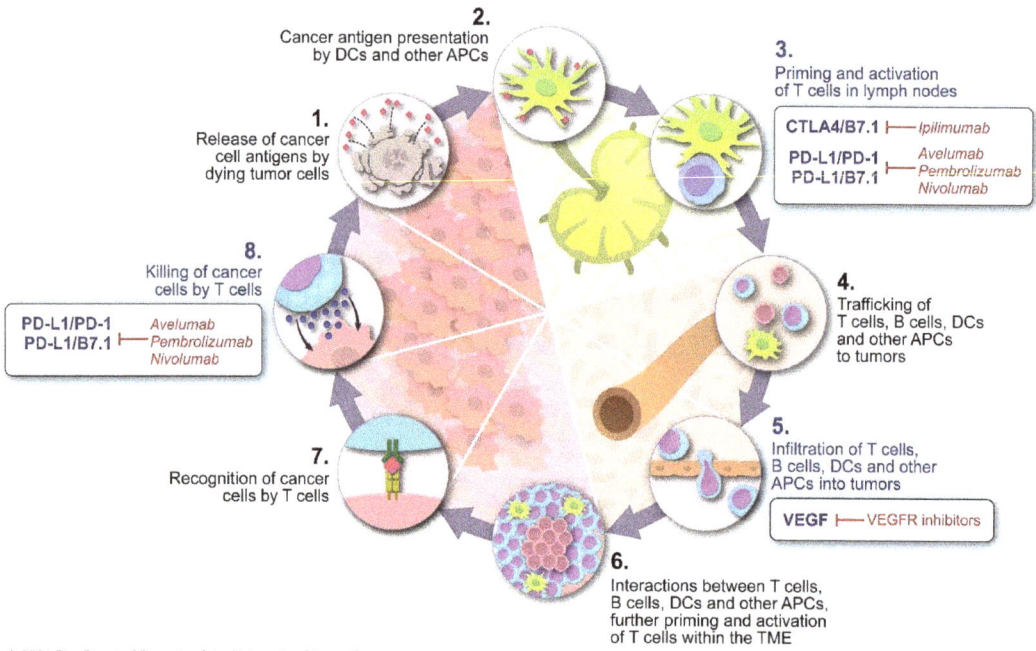

Figure 1. The cancer immunity cycle and the mechanisms of action of checkpoint inhibitors and potential therapies that enhance immune system response. Abbreviations are as follows: PD1: programmed death cell protein 1; PD-L1: programmed death-ligand 1; CTLA-4: cytotoxic T-lymphocyte antigen-4; DC: dendritic cells; APC: antigen presenting cells; VEGF: vascular endothelial growth factor; VEGFR: vascular endothelial growth factor receptor; TME: tumor microenvironment.

The cancer immunity cycle is a complex process [27] regulated by many inhibitory or stimulatory factors and pathways in the tumor microenvironment that determine the successful identification of cancer cells by the immune system. While many of these factors have been recognized, many others are unknown. Examples of inhibitory mechanisms of the cancer immunity cycle are the CTLA4 pathway, which prevents antigen-presenting cells from priming and activating T cells; the PD-L1/PD-1 pathway, which prevents the killing of cancer cells; vascular endothelial factors and the endothelin B receptor, which prevent T cells from infiltrating tumors and reduce the expression of the proteins of the major histocompatibility complex by the cancer cells (Figure 1) [27]. Subsequently, several medications that antagonize the activity of inhibitory factors and/or stimulate factors that enhance the cancer immunity cycle have been developed (Figure 1) [23]. Antibodies that block the actions of CTLA4, PD-1, and PD-L1, known as checkpoint inhibitors, such as ipilimumab (CTLA4 inhibitor), pembrolizumab (anti-PD-1 antibody), or nivolumab (anti–PD-L1 antibody), are currently indicated for the treatment of many different malignancies [23]. In some cases, checkpoint inhibitors alone have led to permanent remissions [23]. Antiangiogenic medications, such as cabozantinib, a tyrosine kinase inhibitor, may induce tumor vessel normalization, enhancing tumor infiltration and the recognition of cancer cell by immune T cells [28]. When combined with checkpoint inhibitors, antiangiogenic medications may lead to impressive clinical responses in clear cell renal cell carcinomas [29,30]. Interferon alpha or vaccines made with tumor antigens may facilitate antigen presentation [27]. Clinical trials combining checkpoint inhibitors and vaccines for different types of cancer are ongoing [31]. Chemotherapy, targeted therapies, radiation therapy, and radiopharmaceuticals may release tumor antigens that could be recognized by the immune system. Combinations of these classical systemic therapies with checkpoint inhibitors have been associated with clinical benefits in several malignancies [23,32,33].

In clinical trials, pembrolizumab demonstrated objective responses in patients with advanced clear cell renal cell carcinomas, lung adenocarcinomas, and melanomas that express PD-L1 [34]. Nevertheless, not all tumors that express PD-L1 exhibited objective responses [34]. Many tumors for which pembrolizumab is currently indicated are characterized by an inflamed tumor microenvironment and a high tumor mutation burden (TMB) [35]. ACC may exhibit an inflammatory environment and several somatic mutations [36]; nevertheless, these features are not as notable as the ones noted in the aforementioned cancers [35]. Pheochromocytomas and paragangliomas are associated with minimal or no tumor inflammation and, as such, are classified as "cold" tumors [35]. In addition, MPPGLs are mainly associated with monogenic germline and somatic mutations; in fact, up to 50% of MPPGLs are exclusively associated with germline mutations of the *SDHB* gene, and many MPPGLs have no recognized or a few additional somatic mutations [35]. These observations raise the question of whether immunotherapy with checkpoint inhibitors could be effective for ACC or MPPGL.

3. Scientific Rationale for the Potential Use of Checkpoint Inhibitors for ACC or MPPGL

Recent studies have found that some ACCs and MPPGLs express the programmed cell death ligands in tumor cell membranes or stromal cells in the tumor microenvironment [37–39]. Small immunohistochemical studies found PD-L1 expression in up to 70% of ACC samples [38] and 18% of MPPGL samples [37], suggesting that several patients with ACC and some patients with MPPGL may benefit from checkpoint inhibitors, such as avelumab, nivolumab, or pembrolizumab. In addition, it has been recognized that 3–18% of ACC cases are associated with somatic or germline mutations of DNA mismatch repair genes, such as *ML1*, *MSH2*, *MSH6*, and *PMS2* mutations (e.g., ACC-associated Lynch syndrome), and these mutations lead to microsatellite instability [40–42]. The use of checkpoint inhibitors seems to be an appealing option for this subset of ACC cases. In fact, the FDA approved the use of pembrolizumab for the treatment of any solid cancer associated with DNA mismatch repair gene mutations and microsatellite instability [43]. This approval was based on an impressive overall response rate (ORR) of pembrolizumab of approximately 40% (including some complete responses), with a duration of benefits longer than 6 months in 78% of patients treated with pembrolizumab across five clinical trials for several malignancies [43]. Nevertheless, these trials did not include ACC patients, so checkpoint inhibitors for ACC with DNA mismatch repair gene mutations and microsatellite instability must be evaluated through clinical trials. Importantly, microsatellite instability is associated with an increased TMB in approximately 4% of ACC [44].

In general, the cancer microenvironment is characterized by a rapid proliferation of the tumor cells that is unmatched by the available blood supply. To compensate, abnormal vessels develop; however, the supply of oxygen is still limited leading to hypoxia with subsequent stabilization of the inducible (alpha) subunit of hypoxia inducible factors (HIFs) [45]. HIFs activate the PD-L1 gene, which, in turn, induces tumor immune escape by suppressing the activity of cytolytic T cells [45]. Most MPPGL are characterized by an environment of pseudohypoxia [46]. Up to 50% of patients with MPPGL carry germline mutations of the subunit B of the succinate dehydrogenase gene (*SDHB*), and metastatic tumors also happen in carriers of other mutations involved in the regulation of the oxygen metabolism (e.g., *SDHA*, *SDHC*, *SDHD*, *FH*, and *VHL* genes) [46]. Furthermore, many apparently sporadic MPPGs are characterized by a microenvironment of pseudohypoxia, including those that carry activating mutations of *EPAS1*, the gene encoding for HIF2 alpha [46,47]. Therefore, it is worth exploring checkpoint inhibitors for patients with MPPGL. Of interest, there are rare cases of succinyl dehydrogenase gene mutation–associated

ACC [48]. However, because these cases are very rare, it is unlikely that pseudohypoxia is a major player determining a potential response to checkpoint inhibitors in ACC.

For a variety of reasons, checkpoint inhibitors are a potentially attractive therapy to orphan tumors [49]. Unlike other systemic therapies, immunotherapy with checkpoint inhibitors has been demonstrated as an effective treatment for many different cancers, irrespective of their embryological origin and histological characteristics [23]. In addition, clinical responses do not seem to always correlate with PD-L1 expression in the tumor cells and/or tumor microenvironment [50]. Adverse events associated with checkpoint inhibitors are, for the most part, acceptable and correctable with supportive measures [23,49,51]. Furthermore, there are no reliable preclinical models to predict the actions of immunotherapy in specific malignancies. The following sections describe the results of phase 1 and 2 clinical trials against ACC and MPPGL.

4. Clinical Trials with Immune Checkpoint Inhibitors
4.1. Clinical Trials with Immune Checkpoint Inhibitors for ACC
4.1.1. Avelumab

Avelumab, a PD-L1 inhibitor, was the first checkpoint inhibitor evaluated for ACC in clinical trials. Avelumab's pharmacokinetics, efficacy, and safety were evaluated in JAVELIN, a phase 1b international, multicenter clinical trial that included 50 patients with progressive metastatic ACC [52]. Objective responses (PR) were seen in 3 patients (6%), but the CBR was 48%. Almost half of the study participants received concomitant mitotane therapy, including two of the three patients with PR. A large majority of ACCs progressed over a short time; thus, the median progression-free survival (PFS) was only 2.6 months, and overall survival (OS) was 10.6 months [52]. Toxicity was acceptable, although 16% of patients had grade ≥3 adverse events. The study showed that 60% of tumors did not express PD-L1, and these patients exhibited shorter PFS and OS when compared with patients with PD-L1–positive tumors. Nevertheless, this difference was not statistically significant. The few PRs did not correlate with PD-L1 expression [52].

4.1.2. Nivolumab

Nivolumab is a PD-1 inhibitor that was evaluated in a phase 2 investigator-initiated, single-center clinical trial for patients with ACC [53]. The primary endpoint of this trial was ORR. This small trial included 10 patients with progressive ACC who were either previously treated with platinum-based chemotherapy and/or mitotane or who were therapy naïve. The results of the study indicated that nivolumab did not elicit a response. ACC progressed in seven patients. Two patients had stable disease, one for a very short period and the other for 48 weeks. One patient had an unconfirmed PR; however, this patient withdrew from the trial because of a severe side effect. As expected, toxicity was acceptable overall and similar to what has been observed in clinical trials for nivolumab treatment of other malignancies. Finally, the PFS was only 1.8 months [53].

4.1.3. Pembrolizumab

Like nivolumab, pembrolizumab is a PD-1 inhibitor. Pembrolizumab has been evaluated in two phase 2 clinical trials for patients with ACC. The first published phase 2 clinical trial with pembrolizumab included 16 patients with advanced ACC [54,55]. These patients previously underwent failed standard systemic therapy for ACC. The primary endpoint was the non-progression rate at 27 weeks. Two patients were not evaluable for the primary endpoint. Five patients (36%) did not have disease progression 27 weeks after treatment was initiated. The ORR was 14%, and the CBR was 57%. Tumor responses did not correlate with PD-L1 tumor expression, tumor-infiltrating lymphocytes, microsatellite instability, or tumor hormonal activity [55]. In fact, none of the patients had PD-L1 expression. Nevertheless, clinical observations suggest that clinical responses were more likely in patients with tumors that did not secrete hormones when compared with those with tumors associated with Cushing syndrome [55]. Nevertheless, tumors associated with Cushing syndrome achieved either PR or stable disease, suggesting that combining pembrolizumab with medications that lower cortisol production may lead to better responses [55]. Pembrolizumab had severe side effects, including colitis and pneumonitis.

The second trial with pembrolizumab evaluated ORR as the primary endpoint and included 39 patients [56]. The ORR was 39%, and the CBR was 52%. However, the median PFS was only 2.1 months, and the median OS was 24.9 months. Serious adverse events were noted in 13% of patients. Positive tumor responses did not correlate with PD-L1 expression or microsatellite instability. This study did not provide information on tumor hormonal activity [56].

4.1.4. Ipilimumab Plus Nivolumab

In a phase 2 clinical trial of ipilimumab plus nivolumab for patients with rare genitourinary tumors, a subset of 16 patients with advanced ACC was included. The ORR was only 6%; however, the CBR was almost 50%. The toxicity of ipilimumab plus nivolumab was acceptable [57]. The results of this study suggest that the combination of these two checkpoint inhibitors do not provide better responses than what is noticed in patients with ACC treated with single-agent pembrolizumab.

4.1.5. Does Immunotherapy with Checkpoint Inhibitors Work for ACC?

In general, the ORRs for single-agent immune checkpoint inhibitors are low; however, the CBRs for these inhibitors are more impressive. Almost half of the patients treated with these therapies have shown at least disease stabilization, which is frequently associated with some degree of tumor regression for some time; in addition, the risk for significant toxicity of these inhibitors is much lower when compared with that of platinum-based chemotherapy. Furthermore, the few patients who respond to checkpoint inhibitors often enjoy a long duration of response [55,56], and a few cases of complete responses have been seen outside the clinical trials [58]. Nevertheless, it is currently very difficult to predict which patients may benefit from immunotherapy. Clinical trials have demonstrated that the expression of PD-L1 in ACC does not necessarily predict a positive clinical outcome; in fact, there are some patients with very impressive radiographic responses with ACC samples lacking PD-L1 expression [52,55]. Conversely, there are patients with PD-L1 expression in whom antitumor responses are not observed [55]. Although the absence of PD-L1 expression could represent a mechanism of tumor resistance to checkpoint inhibitors, observations from clinical trials indicate that this process is much more complicated.

However, other mechanisms of avoidance of the immune system have been proposed [59]. These mechanisms may include, but are likely not limited to, the frequently observed inactivation of the *P53* gene pathway in ACC due to somatic and occasional germline mutations of *P53* (as are common with Li-Fraumeni syndrome) [36,60]. These mutations may lead to the decreased recruitment of natural killer and other immune cells [61–63] or the sometimes-noted upregulation of the WNT/β-catenin pathway [36,60], which may impair adequate antigen presentation, chemotaxis, and tumor infiltration by T cells [59,64]. Nevertheless, clinical trials have not explored correlations with these molecular phenotypes, and these phenotypes may not necessarily predict an immunotherapy response. Moreover, ACC linked to excessive glucocorticoid secretion is associated with worse prognosis when compared with non-hormonally active ACC [7]. The glucocorticoid-related toxicity suggests an increased risk for complications, such as osteoporosis and fractures, muscle weakness, hypertension, and especially immune suppression, which may predispose patients to systemic infections. Furthermore, ACC associated with Cushing syndrome exhibits elevated mitotic rates and, subsequently, more aggressive oncological behavior; these characteristics, together with the inherent comorbidity of Cushing syndrome, lead to lower overall survival rates compared with non-hormonally active tumors [36].

Considering the modest mutation burden of ACC, it is speculated that the effective immune targeting of ACC will require combination therapy or an engineered cellular therapy [65]. Emerging data show that checkpoint inhibitors combined with other treatments may overcome the mechanisms of avoidance or resistance to the immune system. Based on the concern that excess cortisol creates an unfavorable atmosphere for immunotherapy [63], a phase 1b study is ongoing to evaluate the effect of combining pembrolizumab with relacorilant, a glucocorticoid receptor blocker (ClinicalTrials.gov Identifier: NCT04373265). In addition, checkpoint inhibitors may be combined with inhibitors of adrenal glucocorticoid synthesis, such as metyrapone.

The combination of mitotane, as the standard of care, with immune checkpoint inhibitors has been reported with avelumab, and this combination is likely safe, considering the relatively low risk of severe adverse events in the study [52]. A recent retrospective case series of six patients treated with pembrolizumab and mitotane found durable responses in the majority of patients, including two patients with a durable response rate [66]. This combination is of great interest because it can utilize the adrenolytic and steroid reduction properties of mitotane to make the tumors more susceptible to checkpoint inhibitor therapy.

In the past few years, the use of antiangiogenic agents has transformed the management of multiple malignancies. Targeting vascular endothelial growth factor receptor signaling, in combination with checkpoint inhibitors, e.g., by combining pembrolizumab and lenvatinib in renal cell carcinoma and endometrial carcinoma, has proven beneficial in multiple malignancies and resulted in exceptionally high response rates [67,68]. It is hypothesized that combining immunotherapy with antiangiogenic drugs has synergistic effects that enhance response rates [69]. A recent cases series evaluated the combination of lenvatinib with pembrolizumab in ACC. Despite undergoing many failed lines of therapy, some patients treated with this combination had durable responses to therapy, whereas checkpoint inhibitors and antiangiogenic therapy as single-agent therapies were unsuccessful [70].

4.2. Clinical Trials with Immune Checkpoint Inhibitors for MPPGL
4.2.1. Pembrolizumab

A phase 2 clinical trial with pembrolizumab at 200 mg intravenously every 3 weeks explored the actions of PD-1 inhibition against MPPGL [71]. The primary endpoint of this trial was a non-progression rate at 27 weeks (9 cycles) greater than 20%, based on the Response Evaluation Criteria in Solid Tumors 1.1. Secondary endpoints included ORR, CBR, PFS, OS, safety, and correlations with PD-L1 expression and infiltrating mononuclear inflammatory cells in the primary tumor with disease response and genotype. The clinical trial included 11 patients with progressive MPPGL. Sixty-four percent of patients had apparently sporadic MPPGL, 18% had paraganglioma syndrome type 4 (germline *SDHB* mutations), 1 patient had paraganglioma syndrome type 1 (germline *SDHD* mutation), and 1 patient had a germline *PMS2* mutation. Sixty-four percent of patients had tumors that secreted noradrenaline. Fifty-five percent of the primary tumors were in the sympathetic extra-adrenal paraganglia, 36% of patients had pheochromocytomas, and 1 patient had a primary head and neck paraganglioma. Patients had an acceptable performance status, with an Eastern Cooperative Oncology Group performance score of ≤1. Only 28% of patients were naïve to therapy; most patients had previously undergone cyclophosphamide, vincristine, and dacarbazine chemotherapy, and treatment with HSA-I-131-MIBG, and/or tyrosine kinase inhibitors. Forty percent of patients had no evidence of disease progression at 27 weeks; however, the ORR was only 9%. The toxicity of pembrolizumab was acceptable, and there were no grade 4 or 5 side effects or cases of catecholamine crisis. The median PFS was 5.7 months, and the median OS was 19 months, with 55% of patients deceased at the time of publication of clinical trial results because of tumor progression [71]. There was no clear association between PD-L1 expression or tumor-infiltrating lymphocytes in the primary tumor with clinical response, genetic background, or hormonal activity.

A clinical assessment indicated that only two patients (18%) had an obvious benefit. One patient had a non-hormonally active tumor that achieved a confirmed immune-related partial response that persisted for longer than 2 years. The patient with the most impressive clinical response had paraganglioma syndrome type 4 metastatic paraganglioma associated with excessive noradrenaline secretion, overwhelming symptoms of catecholamine excess, and massive lymph node, lung, liver, and skeletal metastases. The patient had previously undergone cabozantinib treatment, which was complicated by severe hand and foot syndrome and a superinfection with pseudomonas aeruginosa. Cabozantinib was then discontinued, and the patient exhibited a rapid progression. Several metastases were palpable and visible on physical examination. The blood pressure was difficult to control, and the patient complained of palpitation, sweats, and headaches. The patient underwent pembrolizumab treatment. Four days after infusion, the metastases were no longer palpable or visible, the blood pressure normalized, and several antihypertensives were discontinued, as the patient complained of near syncopal episodes. Symptoms of catecholamine excess were no longer reported. Radiographic studies found a 56% tumor size reduction (Figure 2). The patient had elevated levels of liver enzymes, which delayed treatment with pembrolizumab. At the time of radiographic follow-up three months later, a new liver lesion was noted, and the patient discontinued his participation in the trial [71].

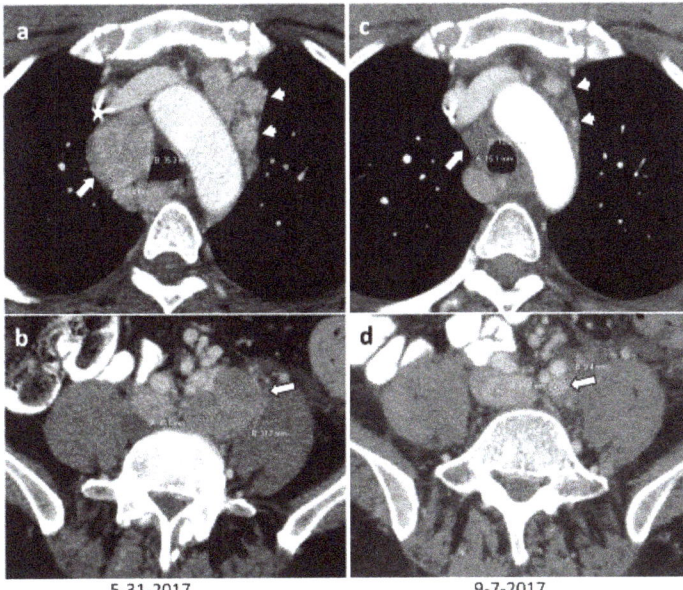

Figure 2. A 42-year-old man with metastatic paraganglioma underwent multiple surgery resection, post-surgical therapy with CVD × 6 months, cabozantinib × 8 months, then treatment with pembrolizumab. The pre-immunotherapy contrast enhanced CT (CECT) showed innumerable lymph node metastases in the chest, abdomen, and pelvis. At 2 months post initiation of immunotherapy, the lymph node metastases had significantly decreased by number and size (long and short arrows in images (a–d)). Representative axial CECT images ((**a**): pretherapy axial CECT of chest, (**b**): pretherapy axial CECT of pelvis, (**c**): post-therapy axial CECT of chest, (**d**): post-therapy axial CECT of pelvis) showed that the mediastinal (long and short arrows in (**a,c**)) and left common iliac (long arrow in (**b,d**)) lymph node metastases had significantly improved. The right paratracheal lymph node (long arrows in (**a,c**)) decreased from 4.3 × 3.5 cm to 1.5 × 1.2 cm, and the left common iliac lymph node (long arrows in (**b,d**)) decreased from 4.5 × 3.2 cm to 1.1 × 0.9 cm.

4.2.2. Ipilimumab Plus Nivolumab

This phase 2 clinical trial included two patients with progressive MPPGL [57]. One patient did not experience a response to the therapy and exhibited disease progression. The other patient had stable disease for longer than 2 years, with excellent performance status, occasional fatigue, and no symptoms of tumor burden. However, the tumor size did not decrease [57]. Whether the second patient exhibited disease stabilization because of immunotherapy or because of the nature of MPPGL tumors, which may become stable with no intervention despite initial growth, is still to be defined.

4.2.3. Does Immunotherapy with Checkpoint Inhibitors Work for MPPGL?

The authors of the manuscript and others believe that checkpoint inhibitors and other types of immunotherapy can work for patients with MPPGL [72]. However, we need to better understand the mechanisms that may successfully activate the immune system. At this time, the clinical scientific experience with checkpoint inhibitors is limited to the definitive results of the small phase 2 clinical trial with single-agent pembrolizumab and the limited results of a phase 2 clinical trial that combined nivolumab and ipilimumab [71,72]. The results of these trials indicate that checkpoint inhibitors are associated with modest responses and that pembrolizumab alone or ipilimumab combined with nivolumab should not be considered as first-line therapies for patients with MPPGL [71,72]. Combining checkpoint inhibitors with other therapeutic modalities that enhance antigen recognition and/or facilitate vascular normalization could activate the immune system more successfully. Preliminary results of a phase 2 clinical trial with cabozantinib (the most potent antiangiogenic medication available in clinical practice) seem impressive and suggest that a substantial number of patients with MPPGL may benefit from this medication [28]. Similarly, a recent report described a patient who had a positive oncological response characterized by tumor size reduction and stabilization after receiving 40 mg of cabozantinib daily for 7.5 months. The patient was then treated with pembrolizumab with no response, followed by chemotherapy, which caused substantial toxicity. The patient later underwent a combined treatment of cabozantinib with nivolumab. Combining cabozantinib with nivolumab was associated with a PR, disease stabilization, the disappearance of the symptoms of catecholamine excess, and an acceptable toxicity, and the clinical benefits of this combined therapy lasted for 22 months. This case report suggests that cabozantinib could have induced some degree of tumor vascular normalization that facilitated the activation of the immune system [73].

In the phase 2 clinical trial with pembrolizumab, one patient had an impressive clinical response, raising the question of whether previous exposure to cabozantinib and/or the introduction of foreign bacterial antigens can activate the immune system against MPPGL. Pseudomonas aeruginosa is a Gram-negative bacterium, characterized by the presence of lipopolysaccharides in the outer layer and many other components that trigger or enhance an immune response. These bacteria may become trapped in the tumor microenvironment within the abnormal vessels, inducing an immune attack against tumor cells, thus supporting bacteria-based MPPGL immunotherapy [74,75].

A recent retrospective study found that patients with MPPGL may have a higher incidence of other malignancies, such as lung, prostate, melanoma, and colorectal cancers, when compared to the general population [76]; this finding suggests that some of the MPPGL tumorigenesis pathways and mechanisms of immune resistance could be similar to the ones observed in more common tumors for which immunotherapy has been demonstrated to be effective; thus, learning from the experience with the aforementioned malignancies may provide clues on how to treat MPPGL with immunotherapies.

5. The Gut Microbiome and Peptide-Based Vaccination against ACC and MPPGL

Peptide-based vaccination delivers immunogenic peptides, corresponding to tumor-associated or tumor-specific antigens, to elicit a T-cell immune response. It is challenging to generate a strong immune response against tumor-associated antigens (TAAs), mainly because the non-mutated tumor-associated antigens are part of the repertoire of self-antigens. To circumvent this problem, the immune response should target mutated, non-self-antigens.

Sequencing of the human fecal microbiota revealed that all TAAs had a closely structurally related "mimic" in the microbiome, with higher affinities for the MHC than the corresponding TAA [77]. As these "mimics" are produced by bacteria, they have the potential to "pre-expose" any person and generate memory T-cells; the re-activation and subsequent expansion of these T cells can generate a robust response against the TAAs. The links between the microbiome, clinical response, and inhibition of cancer progression in cancer patients treated with targeted immunotherapies or with specific chemotherapeutic agents have already been emphasized [78]. The presence of commensal bacteria-specific memory T cells in the gut and in the periphery has been described as well [79]. These microbiome-derived peptides stimulate strong immune responses against TAAs and trigger in vivo tumor regression after vaccination.

The NCT04187404 trial (SPENCER Trial) is evaluating the vaccine EO2401 against ACC and MPPGL. This vaccine includes three microbiome-derived CD8+ epitopes mimicking parts of TAAs, such as the interleukin receptor alpha 2 (IL13Rα2), survivin (BIRC5), and the mammalian forkhead box M1 (FOXM1); these antigens are overexpressed and linked to clinical outcomes in ACC and MPPGL [80–87]. These antigens may induce an immune response against tumors of adrenal origin and have minimal to no expression in normal organs. The SPENCER trial is a multicenter, phase 1/2, first-in-human study to assess the safety, tolerability, immunogenicity, and preliminary efficacy of EO2401 in combination with nivolumab for patients with untreated or previously treated ACC or MPPGL. The initial data from the trial is awaited in 2022.

6. Conclusions

Immunotherapy for adrenal tumors, such as ACC and MPPGL, is at an early stage of development. Single-agent immunotherapy has led to some impressive and durable responses in patients with ACC; however, ORRs are generally low. In patients with MPPGL, responses have been uncommon, and the mechanisms of response are unclear. However, the failure of checkpoint inhibitors to elicit a response is not an indication of an absolute lack of success. Conversely, the failure of single-agent checkpoint inhibitor therapy represents an opportunity to identify the mechanisms that could lead to more successful treatment strategies. Combining checkpoint inhibitors with chemotherapy, mitotane, tyrosine kinase inhibitors, and/or vaccines for ACC or chemotherapy, tyrosine kinase inhibitors, and/or radiopharmaceuticals for MPPGL needs to be proactively explored.

Author Contributions: Conceptualization: C.J., G.A.-P., P.L.M.D., J.V. and M.A.H.; investigation: C.J. and M.A.H.; writing—original draft preparation: C.J.; writing—review and editing: C.J., G.A.-P., P.L.M.D., J.V., Y.L., R.A.T. and M.A.H.; supervision: C.J. All authors have read and agreed to the published version of the manuscript.

Funding: This research did not receive external funding.

Acknowledgments: We thank Ashli Nguyen-Villarreal, Associate Scientific Editor, and Sarah Bronson, Scientific Editor, in the Research Medical Library at The University of Texas MD Anderson Cancer Center for editing this article.

Conflicts of Interest: C.J. is scientific advisor for HRA Pharma, Lantheus Pharmaceuticals, Merck Sharp and Dohme, and Pfizer Pharmaceuticals. C.J. has received research support from Enterome, Exelixis, Lantheus Pharmaceuticals, Merck Sharp and Dohme, Pfizer Pharmaceuticals, and Progenics; G.A.-P. does not have conflicts of interest; P.L.M.D. is a recipient of funds from the NIH (GM114102 and CA264248) and the Neuroendocrine Tumor Research Foundation and is the holder of the Robert Tucker Hayes Distinguished Chair in Oncology; J.V. does not have conflicts of interest; Y.L. does not have conflicts of interest; R.A.T. holds a Miguel Servet-I research contract by Institute of Health Carlos III (ISCIII) of the Ministry of Economy [grant number CP17/00199] and Competitiveness from the Spanish government and is supported by an Olga Torres Foundation emerging researcher grant, by the Swiss Bridge Award, and received a research grant from Novartis, Astrazeneca, Beigene (all pharma grants are not related to this project); M.A.H. received research support from Corcept Therapeutics Exelixis Inc.

References

1. Miller, W.L.; Auchus, R.J. The molecular biology, biochemistry, and physiology of human steroidogenesis and its disorders. *Endocr. Rev.* **2011**, *32*, 81–151. [CrossRef] [PubMed]
2. Mesiano, S.; Jaffe, R.B. Developmental and functional biology of the primate fetal adrenal cortex. *Endocr. Rev.* **1997**, *18*, 378–403. [CrossRef] [PubMed]
3. Fung, M.M.; Viveros, O.H.; O'Connor, D.T. Diseases of the adrenal medulla. *Acta Physiol.* **2008**, *192*, 325–335. [CrossRef] [PubMed]
4. Wartenberg, H. Development of the early human ovary and role of the mesonephros in the differentiation of the cortex. *Anat. Embryol.* **1982**, *165*, 253–280. [CrossRef] [PubMed]
5. Souto, M.; Mariani, M.L. Immunochemical localization of chromaffin cells during the embryogenic migration. *Biocell* **1996**, *20*, 179–184.
6. Dahia, P.L.; Ross, K.N.; Wright, M.E.; Hayashida, C.Y.; Santagata, S.; Barontini, M.; Kung, A.L.; Sanso, G.; Powers, J.F.; Tischler, A.S.; et al. A HIF1alpha regulatory loop links hypoxia and mitochondrial signals in pheochromocytomas. *PLoS Genet.* **2005**, *1*, 72–80. [CrossRef]
7. Ayala-Ramirez, M.; Jasim, S.; Feng, L.; Ejaz, S.; Deniz, F.; Busaidy, N.; Waguespack, S.G.; Naing, A.; Sircar, K.; Wood, C.G.; et al. Adrenocortical carcinoma: Clinical outcomes and prognosis of 330 patients at a tertiary care center. *Eur. J. Endocrinol.* **2013**, *169*, 891–899. [CrossRef]
8. Fassnacht, M.; Johanssen, S.; Quinkler, M.; Bucsky, P.; Willenberg, H.S.; Beuschlein, F.; Terzolo, M.; Mueller, H.H.; Hahner, S.; Allolio, B.; et al. Limited prognostic value of the 2004 International Union Against Cancer staging classification for adrenocortical carcinoma: Proposal for a Revised TNM Classification. *Cancer* **2009**, *115*, 243–250. [CrossRef]
9. Amin, M.B.; Edge, S.B.; Greene, F.L.; Trottli, A. *AJCC Cancer Staging Manual*, 8th ed.; Springer: New York, NY, USA, 2017.
10. Fishbein, L.; Del Rivero, J.; Else, T.; Howe, J.R.; Asa, S.L.; Cohen, D.L.; Dahia, P.L.M.; Fraker, D.L.; Goodman, K.A.; Hope, T.A.; et al. The North American Neuroendocrine Tumor Society Consensus Guidelines for Surveillance and Management of Metastatic and/or Unresectable Pheochromocytoma and Paraganglioma. *Pancreas* **2021**, *50*, 469–493. [CrossRef]
11. Ayala-Ramirez, M.; Feng, L.; Johnson, M.M.; Ejaz, S.; Habra, M.A.; Rich, T.; Busaidy, N.; Cote, G.J.; Perrier, N.; Phan, A.; et al. Clinical risk factors for malignancy and overall survival in patients with pheochromocytomas and sympathetic paragangliomas: Primary tumor size and primary tumor location as prognostic indicators. *J. Clin. Endocrinol. Metab.* **2011**, *96*, 717–725. [CrossRef]
12. Jasim, S.; Jimenez, C. Metastatic pheochromocytoma and paraganglioma: Management of endocrine manifestations, surgery and ablative procedures, and systemic therapies. *Best Pract. Res. Clin. Endocrinol. Metab.* **2020**, *34*, 101354. [CrossRef] [PubMed]
13. Fassnacht, M.; Assie, G.; Baudin, E.; Eisenhofer, G.; de la Fouchardiere, C.; Haak, H.R.; de Krijger, R.; Porpiglia, F.; Terzolo, M.; Berruti, A.; et al. Adrenocortical carcinomas and malignant phaeochromocytomas: ESMO-EURACAN Clinical Practice Guidelines for diagnosis, treatment and follow-up. *Ann. Oncol.* **2020**, *31*, 1476–1490. [CrossRef] [PubMed]
14. Jasim, S.; Habra, M.A. Management of Adrenocortical Carcinoma. *Curr. Oncol. Rep.* **2019**, *21*, 20. [CrossRef] [PubMed]
15. Thosani, S.; Ayala-Ramirez, M.; Roman-Gonzalez, A.; Zhou, S.; Thosani, N.; Bisanz, A.; Jimenez, C. Constipation: An overlooked, unmanaged symptom of patients with pheochromocytoma and sympathetic paraganglioma. *Eur. J. Endocrinol.* **2015**, *173*, 377–387. [CrossRef]
16. Y-Hassan, S.; Falhammar, H. Cardiovascular Manifestations and Complications of Pheochromocytomas and Paragangliomas. *J. Clin. Med.* **2020**, *9*, 2435. [CrossRef] [PubMed]
17. Jimenez, C.; Rohren, E.; Habra, M.A.; Rich, T.; Jimenez, P.; Ayala-Ramirez, M.; Baudin, E. Current and future treatments for malignant pheochromocytoma and sympathetic paraganglioma. *Curr. Oncol. Rep.* **2013**, *15*, 356–371. [CrossRef]
18. Kebebew, E.; Reiff, E.; Duh, Q.Y.; Clark, O.H.; McMillan, A. Extent of disease at presentation and outcome for adrenocortical carcinoma: Have we made progress? *World J. Surg.* **2006**, *30*, 872–878. [CrossRef]
19. Niemeijer, N.D.; Alblas, G.; van Hulsteijn, L.T.; Dekkers, O.M.; Corssmit, E.P. Chemotherapy with cyclophosphamide, vincristine and dacarbazine for malignant paraganglioma and pheochromocytoma: Systematic review and meta-analysis. *Clin. Endocrinol.* **2014**, *81*, 642–651. [CrossRef]
20. Jimenez, C.; Erwin, W.; Chasen, B. Targeted Radionuclide Therapy for Patients with Metastatic Pheochromocytoma and Paraganglioma: From Low-Specific-Activity to High-Specific-Activity Iodine-131 Metaiodobenzylguanidine. *Cancers* **2019**, *11*, 1018. [CrossRef]
21. Jimenez, C.; Nunez, R.; Wendt, R. High-specific-activity iodine 131 metaiodobenzylguanidine for the treatment of metastatic pheochromocytoma or paraganglioma: A novel therapy for an orphan disease. *Curr. Opin. Endocrinol. Diabetes Obes.* **2020**, *27*, 162–169. [CrossRef]
22. Pryma, D.A.; Chin, B.B.; Noto, R.B.; Dillon, J.S.; Perkins, S.; Solnes, L.; Kostakoglu, L.; Serafini, A.N.; Pampaloni, M.H.; Jensen, J.; et al. Efficacy and Safety of High-Specific-Activity (131)I-MIBG Therapy in Patients with Advanced Pheochromocytoma or Paraganglioma. *J. Nucl. Med.* **2019**, *60*, 623–630. [CrossRef]
23. Vaddepally, R.K.; Kharel, P.; Pandey, R.; Garje, R.; Chandra, A.B. Review of Indications of FDA-Approved Immune Checkpoint Inhibitors per NCCN Guidelines with the Level of Evidence. *Cancers* **2020**, *12*, 738. [CrossRef] [PubMed]
24. Hanahan, D.; Weinberg, R.A. Hallmarks of cancer: The next generation. *Cell* **2011**, *144*, 646–674. [CrossRef] [PubMed]
25. Tian, T.; Olson, S.; Whitacre, J.M.; Harding, A. The origins of cancer robustness and evolvability. *Integr. Biol.* **2011**, *3*, 17–30. [CrossRef]

26. Boon, T.; Cerottini, J.C.; Van den Eynde, B.; van der Bruggen, P.; Van Pel, A. Tumor antigens recognized by T lymphocytes. *Annu. Rev. Immunol.* **1994**, *12*, 337–365. [CrossRef] [PubMed]
27. Chen, D.S.; Mellman, I. Oncology meets immunology: The cancer-immunity cycle. *Immunity* **2013**, *39*, 1–10. [CrossRef]
28. Jimenez, C.; Fazeli, S.; Roman-Gonzalez, A. Antiangiogenic therapies for pheochromocytoma and paraganglioma. *Endocr. Relat. Cancer* **2020**, *27*, R239–R254. [CrossRef]
29. Choueiri, T.K.; Powles, T.; Burotto, M.; Escudier, B.; Bourlon, M.T.; Zurawski, B.; Oyervides Juarez, V.M.; Hsieh, J.J.; Basso, U.; Shah, A.Y.; et al. Nivolumab plus Cabozantinib versus Sunitinib for Advanced Renal-Cell Carcinoma. *N. Engl. J. Med.* **2021**, *384*, 829–841. [CrossRef]
30. Bedke, J.; Albiges, L.; Capitanio, U.; Giles, R.H.; Hora, M.; Lam, T.B.; Ljungberg, B.; Marconi, L.; Klatte, T.; Volpe, A.; et al. Updated European Association of Urology Guidelines on Renal Cell Carcinoma: Nivolumab plus Cabozantinib Joins Immune Checkpoint Inhibition Combination Therapies for Treatment-naive Metastatic Clear-Cell Renal Cell Carcinoma. *Eur. Urol.* **2021**, *79*, 339–342. [CrossRef]
31. Zhao, J.; Chen, Y.; Ding, Z.Y.; Liu, J.Y. Safety and Efficacy of Therapeutic Cancer Vaccines Alone or in Combination with Immune Checkpoint Inhibitors in Cancer Treatment. *Front. Pharmacol.* **2019**, *10*, 1184. [CrossRef]
32. Gandhi, L.; Garassino, M.C. Pembrolizumab plus Chemotherapy in Lung Cancer. *N. Engl. J. Med.* **2018**, *379*, e18. [CrossRef]
33. Vacchelli, E.; Bloy, N.; Aranda, F.; Buque, A.; Cremer, I.; Demaria, S.; Eggermont, A.; Formenti, S.C.; Fridman, W.H.; Fucikova, J.; et al. Trial Watch: Immunotherapy plus radiation therapy for oncological indications. *Oncoimmunology* **2016**, *5*, e1214790. [CrossRef] [PubMed]
34. Topalian, S.L.; Hodi, F.S.; Brahmer, J.R.; Gettinger, S.N.; Smith, D.C.; McDermott, D.F.; Powderly, J.D.; Carvajal, R.D.; Sosman, J.A.; Atkins, M.B.; et al. Safety, activity, and immune correlates of anti-PD-1 antibody in cancer. *N. Engl. J. Med.* **2012**, *366*, 2443–2454. [CrossRef] [PubMed]
35. Spranger, S.; Luke, J.J.; Bao, R.; Zha, Y.; Hernandez, K.M.; Li, Y.; Gajewski, A.P.; Andrade, J.; Gajewski, T.F. Density of immunogenic antigens does not explain the presence or absence of the T-cell-inflamed tumor microenvironment in melanoma. *Proc. Natl. Acad. Sci. USA* **2016**, *113*, E7759–E7768. [CrossRef] [PubMed]
36. Zheng, S.; Cherniack, A.D.; Dewal, N.; Moffitt, R.A.; Danilova, L.; Murray, B.A.; Lerario, A.M.; Else, T.; Knijnenburg, T.A.; Ciriello, G.; et al. Comprehensive Pan-Genomic Characterization of Adrenocortical Carcinoma. *Cancer Cell* **2016**, *30*, 363. [CrossRef] [PubMed]
37. Pinato, D.J.; Black, J.R.; Trousil, S.; Dina, R.E.; Trivedi, P.; Mauri, F.A.; Sharma, R. Programmed cell death ligands expression in phaeochromocytomas and paragangliomas: Relationship with the hypoxic response, immune evasion and malignant behavior. *Oncoimmunology* **2017**, *6*, e1358332. [CrossRef] [PubMed]
38. Fay, A.P.; Signoretti, S.; Callea, M.; Telomicron, G.H.; McKay, R.R.; Song, J.; Carvo, I.; Lampron, M.E.; Kaymakcalan, M.D.; Poli-de-Figueiredo, C.E.; et al. Programmed death ligand-1 expression in adrenocortical carcinoma: An exploratory biomarker study. *J. Immunother. Cancer* **2015**, *3*, 3. [CrossRef]
39. Tierney, J.F.; Vogle, A.; Poirier, J.; Min, I.M.; Finnerty, B.; Zarnegar, R.; Pappas, S.G.; Scognamiglio, T.; Ghai, R.; Gattuso, P.; et al. Expression of programmed death ligand 1 and 2 in adrenocortical cancer tissues: An exploratory study. *Surgery* **2019**, *165*, 196–201. [CrossRef]
40. Raymond, V.M.; Everett, J.N.; Furtado, L.V.; Gustafson, S.L.; Jungbluth, C.R.; Gruber, S.B.; Hammer, G.D.; Stoffel, E.M.; Greenson, J.K.; Giordano, T.J.; et al. Adrenocortical carcinoma is a lynch syndrome-associated cancer. *J. Clin. Oncol.* **2013**, *31*, 3012–3018. [CrossRef]
41. Vatrano, S.; Volante, M.; Duregon, E.; Giorcelli, J.; Izzo, S.; Rapa, I.; Votta, A.; Germano, A.; Scagliotti, G.; Berruti, A.; et al. Detailed genomic characterization identifies high heterogeneity and histotype-specific genomic profiles in adrenocortical carcinomas. *Mod. Pathol.* **2018**, *31*, 1257–1269. [CrossRef]
42. Domenech, M.; Grau, E.; Solanes, A.; Izquierdo, A.; Del Valle, J.; Carrato, C.; Pineda, M.; Duenas, N.; Pujol, M.; Lazaro, C.; et al. Characteristics of Adrenocortical Carcinoma Associated With Lynch Syndrome. *J. Clin. Endocrinol. Metab.* **2021**, *106*, 318–325. [CrossRef]
43. Marcus, L.; Lemery, S.J.; Keegan, P.; Pazdur, R. FDA Approval Summary: Pembrolizumab for the Treatment of Microsatellite Instability-High Solid Tumors. *Clin. Cancer Res.* **2019**, *25*, 3753–3758. [CrossRef]
44. Bonneville, R.; Krook, M.A.; Kautto, E.A.; Miya, J.; Wing, M.R.; Chen, H.Z.; Reeser, J.W.; Yu, L.; Roychowdhury, S. Landscape of Microsatellite Instability Across 39 Cancer Types. *JCO Precis. Oncol.* **2017**, *2017*, PO.17.00073. [CrossRef]
45. Jiang, X.; Wang, J.; Deng, X.; Xiong, F.; Ge, J.; Xiang, B.; Wu, X.; Ma, J.; Zhou, M.; Li, X.; et al. Role of the tumor microenvironment in PD-L1/PD-1-mediated tumor immune escape. *Mol. Cancer* **2019**, *18*, 10. [CrossRef] [PubMed]
46. Dahia, P.L. Pheochromocytoma and paraganglioma pathogenesis: Learning from genetic heterogeneity. *Nat. Rev. Cancer* **2014**, *14*, 108–119. [CrossRef]
47. Dahia, P.L.M.; Toledo, R.A. Recognizing hypoxia in phaeochromocytomas and paragangliomas. *Nat. Rev. Endocrinol.* **2020**, *16*, 191–192. [CrossRef] [PubMed]
48. Else, T.; Lerario, A.M.; Everett, J.; Haymon, L.; Wham, D.; Mullane, M.; Wilson, T.L.; Rainville, I.; Rana, H.; Worth, A.J.; et al. Adrenocortical carcinoma and succinate dehydrogenase gene mutations: An observational case series. *Eur. J. Endocrinol.* **2017**, *177*, 439–444. [CrossRef] [PubMed]

49. Pegna, G.J.; Roper, N.; Kaplan, R.N.; Bergsland, E.; Kiseljak-Vassiliades, K.; Habra, M.A.; Pommier, Y.; Del Rivero, J. The Immunotherapy Landscape in Adrenocortical Cancer. *Cancers* **2021**, *13*, 2660. [CrossRef] [PubMed]
50. Patel, S.P.; Kurzrock, R. PD-L1 Expression as a Predictive Biomarker in Cancer Immunotherapy. *Mol. Cancer Ther.* **2015**, *14*, 847–856. [CrossRef] [PubMed]
51. Karwacka, I.; Obolonczyk, L.; Kaniuka-Jakubowska, S.; Sworczak, K. The Role of Immunotherapy in the Treatment of Adrenocortical Carcinoma. *Biomedicines* **2021**, *9*, 98. [CrossRef]
52. Le Tourneau, C.; Hoimes, C.; Zarwan, C.; Wong, D.J.; Bauer, S.; Claus, R.; Wermke, M.; Hariharan, S.; von Heydebreck, A.; Kasturi, V.; et al. Avelumab in patients with previously treated metastatic adrenocortical carcinoma: Phase 1b results from the JAVELIN solid tumor trial. *J. Immunother. Cancer* **2018**, *6*, 111. [CrossRef] [PubMed]
53. Carneiro, B.A.; Konda, B.; Costa, R.B.; Costa, R.L.B.; Sagar, V.; Gursel, D.B.; Kirschner, L.S.; Chae, Y.K.; Abdulkadir, S.A.; Rademaker, A.; et al. Nivolumab in Metastatic Adrenocortical Carcinoma: Results of a Phase 2 Trial. *J. Clin. Endocrinol. Metab.* **2019**, *104*, 6193–6200. [CrossRef] [PubMed]
54. Naing, A.; Meric-Bernstam, F.; Stephen, B.; Karp, D.D.; Hajjar, J.; Rodon Ahnert, J.; Piha-Paul, S.A.; Colen, R.R.; Jimenez, C.; Raghav, K.P.; et al. Phase 2 study of pembrolizumab in patients with advanced rare cancers. *J. Immunother. Cancer* **2020**, *8*, e000347. [CrossRef]
55. Habra, M.A.; Stephen, B.; Campbell, M.; Hess, K.; Tapia, C.; Xu, M.; Rodon Ahnert, J.; Jimenez, C.; Lee, J.E.; Perrier, N.D.; et al. Phase II clinical trial of pembrolizumab efficacy and safety in advanced adrenocortical carcinoma. *J. Immunother. Cancer* **2019**, *7*, 253. [CrossRef]
56. Raj, N.; Zheng, Y.; Kelly, V.; Katz, S.S.; Chou, J.; Do, R.K.G.; Capanu, M.; Zamarin, D.; Saltz, L.B.; Ariyan, C.E.; et al. PD-1 Blockade in Advanced Adrenocortical Carcinoma. *J. Clin. Oncol.* **2020**, *38*, 71–80. [CrossRef] [PubMed]
57. McGregor, B.A.; Campbell, M.T.; Xie, W.; Farah, S.; Bilen, M.A.; Schmidt, A.L.; Sonpavde, G.P.; Kilbridge, K.L.; Choudhury, A.D.; Mortazavi, A.; et al. Results of a multicenter, phase 2 study of nivolumab and ipilimumab for patients with advanced rare genitourinary malignancies. *Cancer* **2021**, *127*, 840–849. [CrossRef]
58. Mota, J.M.; Sousa, L.G.; Braghiroli, M.I.; Siqueira, L.T.; Neto, J.E.B.; Chapchap, P.; Hoff, A.A.O.; Hoff, P.M. Pembrolizumab for metastatic adrenocortical carcinoma with high mutational burden: Two case reports. *Medicine* **2018**, *97*, e13517. [CrossRef]
59. Cosentini, D.; Grisanti, S.; Dalla Volta, A.; Lagana, M.; Fiorentini, C.; Perotti, P.; Sigala, S.; Berruti, A. Immunotherapy failure in adrenocortical cancer: Where next? *Endocr. Connect.* **2018**, *7*, E5–E8. [CrossRef]
60. Fojo, T.; Huff, L.; Litman, T.; Im, K.; Edgerly, M.; Del Rivero, J.; Pittaluga, S.; Merino, M.; Bates, S.E.; Dean, M. Metastatic and recurrent adrenocortical cancer is not defined by its genomic landscape. *BMC Med. Genom.* **2020**, *13*, 165. [CrossRef]
61. Wasserman, J.D.; Zambetti, G.P.; Malkin, D. Towards an understanding of the role of p53 in adrenocortical carcinogenesis. *Mol. Cell. Endocrinol.* **2012**, *351*, 101–110. [CrossRef]
62. Mantovani, F.; Walerych, D.; Sal, G.D. Targeting mutant p53 in cancer: A long road to precision therapy. *FEBS J.* **2017**, *284*, 837–850. [CrossRef]
63. Fiorentini, C.; Grisanti, S.; Cosentini, D.; Abate, A.; Rossini, E.; Berruti, A.; Sigala, S. Molecular Drivers of Potential Immunotherapy Failure in Adrenocortical Carcinoma. *J. Oncol.* **2019**, *2019*, 6072863. [CrossRef]
64. Liu, S.; Ding, G.; Zhou, Z.; Feng, C. beta-Catenin-driven adrenocortical carcinoma is characterized with immune exclusion. *OncoTargets Ther.* **2018**, *11*, 2029–2036. [CrossRef]
65. Khalil, D.N.; Smith, E.L.; Brentjens, R.J.; Wolchok, J.D. The future of cancer treatment: Immunomodulation, CARs and combination immunotherapy. *Nat. Rev. Clin. Oncol.* **2016**, *13*, 394. [CrossRef] [PubMed]
66. Head, L.; Kiseljak-Vassiliades, K.; Clark, T.J.; Somerset, H.; King, J.; Raeburn, C.; Albuja-Cruz, M.; Weyant, M.; Cleveland, J.; Wierman, M.E.; et al. Response to Immunotherapy in Combination With Mitotane in Patients With Metastatic Adrenocortical Cancer. *J. Endocr. Soc.* **2019**, *3*, 2295–2304. [CrossRef] [PubMed]
67. Motzer, R.; Alekseev, B.; Rha, S.Y.; Porta, C.; Eto, M.; Powles, T.; Grunwald, V.; Hutson, T.E.; Kopyltsov, E.; Mendez-Vidal, M.J.; et al. Lenvatinib plus Pembrolizumab or Everolimus for Advanced Renal Cell Carcinoma. *N. Engl. J. Med.* **2021**, *384*, 1289–1300. [CrossRef] [PubMed]
68. Makker, V.; Taylor, M.H.; Aghajanian, C.; Oaknin, A.; Mier, J.; Cohn, A.L.; Romeo, M.; Bratos, R.; Brose, M.S.; DiSimone, C.; et al. Lenvatinib Plus Pembrolizumab in Patients With Advanced Endometrial Cancer. *J. Clin. Oncol.* **2020**, *38*, 2981–2992. [CrossRef] [PubMed]
69. Manegold, C.; Dingemans, A.C.; Gray, J.E.; Nakagawa, K.; Nicolson, M.; Peters, S.; Reck, M.; Wu, Y.L.; Brustugun, O.T.; Crino, L.; et al. The Potential of Combined Immunotherapy and Antiangiogenesis for the Synergistic Treatment of Advanced NSCLC. *J. Thorac. Oncol.* **2017**, *12*, 194–207. [CrossRef]
70. Bedrose, S.; Miller, K.C.; Altameemi, L.; Ali, M.S.; Nassar, S.; Garg, N.; Daher, M.; Eaton, K.D.; Yorio, J.T.; Daniel, D.B.; et al. Combined lenvatinib and pembrolizumab as salvage therapy in advanced adrenal cortical carcinoma. *J. Immunother. Cancer* **2020**, *8*, e001009. [CrossRef] [PubMed]
71. Jimenez, C.; Subbiah, V.; Stephen, B.; Ma, J.; Milton, D.; Xu, M.; Zarifa, A.; Akhmedzhanov, F.O.; Tsimberidou, A.; Habra, M.A.; et al. Phase II Clinical Trial of Pembrolizumab in Patients with Progressive Metastatic Pheochromocytomas and Paragangliomas. *Cancers* **2020**, *12*, 2307. [CrossRef]

72. Fanciulli, G.; Di Molfetta, S.; Dotto, A.; Florio, T.; Feola, T.; Rubino, M.; de Cicco, F.; Colao, A.; Faggiano, A.; Nike, G. Emerging Therapies in Pheochromocytoma and Paraganglioma: Immune Checkpoint Inhibitors in the Starting Blocks. *J. Clin. Med.* **2020**, *10*, 88. [CrossRef]
73. Economides, M.P.; Shah, A.Y.; Jimenez, C.; Habra, M.A.; Desai, M.; Campbell, M.T. A Durable Response with the Combination of Nivolumab and Cabozantinib in a Patient With Metastatic Paraganglioma: A Case Report and Review of the Current Literature. *Front. Endocrinol.* **2020**, *11*, 594264. [CrossRef] [PubMed]
74. Nejman, D.; Livyatan, I.; Fuks, G.; Gavert, N.; Zwang, Y.; Geller, L.T.; Rotter-Maskowitz, A.; Weiser, R.; Mallel, G.; Gigi, E.; et al. The human tumor microbiome is composed of tumor type-specific intracellular bacteria. *Science* **2020**, *368*, 973–980. [CrossRef] [PubMed]
75. Huang, X.; Pan, J.; Xu, F.; Shao, B.; Wang, Y.; Guo, X.; Zhou, S. Bacteria-Based Cancer Immunotherapy. *Adv. Sci.* **2021**, *8*, 2003572. [CrossRef] [PubMed]
76. Canu, L.; Puglisi, S.; Berchialla, P.; De Filpo, G.; Brignardello, F.; Schiavi, F.; Ferrara, A.M.; Zovato, S.; Luconi, M.; Pia, A.; et al. A Multicenter Epidemiological Study on Second Malignancy in Non-Syndromic Pheochromocytoma/Paraganglioma Patients in Italy. *Cancers* **2021**, *13*, 5831. [CrossRef]
77. Almeida, A.; Nayfach, S.; Boland, M.; Strozzi, F.; Beracochea, M.; Shi, Z.J.; Pollard, K.S.; Sakharova, E.; Parks, D.H.; Hugenholtz, P.; et al. A unified catalog of 204,938 reference genomes from the human gut microbiome. *Nat. Biotechnol.* **2021**, *39*, 105–114. [CrossRef] [PubMed]
78. Zitvogel, L.; Daillere, R.; Roberti, M.P.; Routy, B.; Kroemer, G. Anticancer effects of the microbiome and its products. *Nat. Rev. Microbiol.* **2017**, *15*, 465–478. [CrossRef] [PubMed]
79. Belkaid, Y.; Bouladoux, N.; Hand, T.W. Effector and memory T cell responses to commensal bacteria. *Trends Immunol.* **2013**, *34*, 299–306. [CrossRef]
80. Jain, M.; Zhang, L.; He, M.; Patterson, E.E.; Nilubol, N.; Fojo, A.T.; Joshi, B.; Puri, R.; Kebebew, E. Interleukin-13 receptor alpha2 is a novel therapeutic target for human adrenocortical carcinoma. *Cancer* **2012**, *118*, 5698–5708. [CrossRef]
81. Sbiera, S.; Kroiss, M.; Thamm, T.; Beyer, M.; Majidi, F.; Kuehner, D.; Wobser, M.; Becker, J.C.; Adam, P.; Ronchi, C.; et al. Survivin in adrenocortical tumors—Pathophysiological implications and therapeutic potential. *Horm. Metab. Res.* **2013**, *45*, 137–146. [CrossRef]
82. Koch, C.A.; Vortmeyer, A.O.; Diallo, R.; Poremba, C.; Giordano, T.J.; Sanders, D.; Bornstein, S.R.; Chrousos, G.P.; Pacak, K. Survivin: A novel neuroendocrine marker for pheochromocytoma. *Eur. J. Endocrinol.* **2002**, *146*, 381–388. [CrossRef]
83. Qin, Z.K.; Zhou, F.J.; Dai, Y.P.; Chen, W.; Hou, J.H.; Han, H.; Liu, Z.W.; Yu, S.L.; Zhang, D.Z.; Yang, J.A. Expression and clinical significance of survivin and PTEN in adrenal tumors. *Ai Zheng* **2007**, *26*, 1143–1147. [PubMed]
84. Yuan, L.; Qian, G.; Chen, L.; Wu, C.L.; Dan, H.C.; Xiao, Y.; Wang, X. Co-expression Network Analysis of Biomarkers for Adrenocortical Carcinoma. *Front. Genet.* **2018**, *9*, 328. [CrossRef] [PubMed]
85. Liao, G.B.; Li, X.Z.; Zeng, S.; Liu, C.; Yang, S.M.; Yang, L.; Hu, C.J.; Bai, J.Y. Regulation of the master regulator FOXM1 in cancer. *Cell Commun. Signal.* **2018**, *16*, 57. [CrossRef] [PubMed]
86. Lai, E.W.; Joshi, B.H.; Martiniova, L.; Dogra, R.; Fujisawa, T.; Leland, P.; de Krijger, R.R.; Lubensky, I.A.; Elkahloun, A.G.; Morris, J.C.; et al. Overexpression of interleukin-13 receptor-alpha2 in neuroendocrine malignant pheochromocytoma: A novel target for receptor directed anti-cancer therapy. *J. Clin. Endocrinol. Metab.* **2009**, *94*, 2952–2957. [CrossRef] [PubMed]
87. Fernandez-Ranvier, G.G.; Weng, J.; Yeh, R.F.; Khanafshar, E.; Suh, I.; Barker, C.; Duh, Q.Y.; Clark, O.H.; Kebebew, E. Identification of biomarkers of adrenocortical carcinoma using genomewide gene expression profiling. *Arch. Surg.* **2008**, *143*, 841–846, discussion 846. [CrossRef]

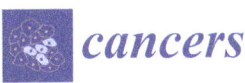

Systematic Review

Cardiovascular Toxicities Secondary to Biotherapy and Molecular Targeted Therapies in Neuroendocrine Neoplasms: A Systematic Review and Meta-Analysis of Randomized Placebo-Controlled Trials

Charalampos Aktypis [1,†], Maria-Eleni Spei [2,†], Maria Yavropoulou [2], Göran Wallin [3], Anna Koumarianou [4], Gregory Kaltsas [2], Eva Kassi [2,5] and Kosmas Daskalakis [2,3,*]

[1] Department of Gastroenterology, Laiko General Hospital, Medical School of National & Kapodistrian University, 11527 Athens, Greece; aktypischar@live.com

[2] 1st Department of Propaedeutic Internal Medicine, Endocrine Unit, National and Kapodistrian University of Athens, 11527 Athens, Greece; marilena_0108@hotmail.com (M.-E.S.); maria.yavropoulou.my@gmail.com (M.Y.); gkaltsas@endo.gr (G.K.); evakassis@gmail.com (E.K.)

[3] Department of Surgery, Faculty of Medicine and Health, Örebro University, 701 85 Örebro, Sweden; goran.wallin@regionorebrolan.se

[4] Hematology-Oncology Unit, Fourth Department of Internal Medicine, Attikon Hospital, Medical School, National and Kapodistrian University of Athens, 124 62 Athens, Greece; akoumari@yahoo.com

[5] Department of Biological Chemistry, Medical School, National and Kapodistrian University of Athens, 11527 Athens, Greece

* Correspondence: kosmas.daskalakis@oru.se; Tel.: +46-737510629

† These authors contributed equally to this work.

Simple Summary: Recent innovations in molecular pathogenesis of neuroendocrine neoplasms (NEN) and improvements in their multidisciplinary management, including the introduction of novel targeted therapies have contributed to favorable patient outcomes. Compared with traditional chemotherapy, targeted therapies have fewer toxicities and a more distinct safety profile. However, treatment-induced cardiovascular toxicities are occasionally critical issues in NEN management. Herein, we present a comprehensive summary of high quality randomized evidence with the methodology of a systematic review and quantitative meta-analysis on the safety profile of biotherapy and molecular targeted therapies in advanced and/or metastatic NEN with a special focus on cardiovascular toxicities in order to promote a patient-tailored approach and assist clinicians involved in the management of NEN patients.

Abstract: A broad spectrum of novel targeted therapies with prime antitumor activity and/or ample control of hormonal symptoms together with an overall acceptable safety profile have emerged for patients with metastatic neuroendocrine neoplasms (NENs). In this systematic review and quantitative meta-analysis, the PubMed, EMBASE, Cochrane Central Register of Controlled Trials and clinicaltrials.gov databases were searched to assess and compare the safety profile of NEN treatments with special focus on the cardiovascular adverse effects of biotherapy and molecular targeted therapies (MTTs). Quality/risk of bias were assessed using GRADE criteria. Placebo-controlled randomized clinical trials (RCTs) in patients with metastatic NENs, including medullary thyroid cancer (MTC) were included. A total of 3695 articles and 122 clinical trials registered in clinicaltrials.gov were screened. We included sixteen relevant RCTs comprising 3408 unique patients assigned to different treatments compared with placebo. All the included studies had a low risk of bias. We identified four drug therapies for NENs with eligible placebo-controlled RCTs: somatostatin analogs (SSAs), tryptophan hydroxylase (TPH) inhibitors, mTOR inhibitors and tyrosine kinase inhibitors (TKI). Grade 3 and 4 adverse effects (AE) were more often encountered in patients treated with mTOR inhibitors and TKI (odds ratio [OR]: 2.42, 95% CI: 1.87–3.12 and OR: 3.41, 95% CI: 1.46–7.96, respectively) as compared to SSAs (OR:0.77, 95% CI: 0.47–1.27) and TPH inhibitors (OR:0.77, 95% CI: 0.35–1.69). MTOR inhibitors had the highest risk for serious cardiac AE (OR:3.28, 95% CI: 1.66–6.48) followed by TKIs (OR:1.51, 95% CI: 0.59–3.83). Serious vascular

AE were more often encountered in NEN patients treated with mTOR inhibitors (OR: 1.72, 95% CI: 0.64–4.64) and TKIs (OR:1.64, 95% CI: 0.35–7.78). Finally, patients on TKIs were at higher risk for new-onset or exacerbation of pre-existing hypertension (OR:3.31, 95% CI: 1.87–5.86). In conclusion, SSAs and TPH inhibitors appear to be safer as compared to mTOR inhibitors and TKIs with regards to their overall toxicity profile, and cardiovascular toxicities in particular. Special consideration should be given to a patient-tailored approach with anticipated toxicities of targeted NEN treatments together with assessment of cardiovascular comorbidities, assisting clinicians in treatment selection and early recognition/management of cardiovascular toxicities. This approach could improve patient compliance and preserve cardiovascular health and overall quality of life.

Keywords: neuroendocrine neoplasms; molecular targeted therapies; mTOR inhibitors; somatostatin analogs; TPH inhibitors; meta-analysis

1. Introduction

Neuroendocrine neoplasms (NENs) comprise a group of diverse histopathological entities across different organs and systems, including the gastrointestinal system, the lungs, the adrenals and the thyroid. Although the majority of NENs are well differentiated (WD) and may exhibit a prolonged indolent course, some patients categories, e.g., the ones with medullary thyroid cancer (MTC), atypical lung carcinoids (LCs) and pancreatic NENs of higher proliferation may exhibit a more aggressive course [1,2]. Many NEN patients are diagnosed with established distant metastases or exhibit progress to stage IV under disease surveillance [3]. Systemic cytotoxic chemotherapy has a generally low response rate in patients with metastatic WD NENs of lower proliferation and MTC and is nevertheless associated with serious toxicities. On the other hand, prime anti-tumor activity and/or control of hormonal excess syndromes has been demonstrated for targeted agents in NENs, resulting in the approval of somatostatin analogs (SSAs) and tryptophan hydroxylase (TPH) inhibitors for gastroenteropancreatic NENs, also referred to as biotherapy, as well as novel molecular targeted therapies (MTTs), such as the mTOR inhibitor everolimus and a number of tyrosine kinase inhibitors (TKIs) with the latter being approved across a diverse spectrum of NEN primaries, including pancreatic NENs and MTC [4,5].

In the last decades, an increment in the prevalence of NENs along with a prolongation in life expectancy of these patients has been observed despite a rising prevalence of cardiovascular diseases in the elderly [1]. On the other hand, carcinoid heart disease, a rare cardiac manifestation involving the right-sided heart valves, constitutes a well-recognized sequela in patients with small intestinal neuroendocrine neoplasms (SI-NENs) often complicating the disease clinical course and eventually leading to right heart failure [6]. Finally, NEN metastases to the heart are rare, with associated clinical features ranging from asymptomatic patients to heart failure [7]. All these factors taken together with the cardiovascular side effects of different agents in the therapeutic NEN armamentarium may have a negative impact on patient outcomes, including quality of life and possibly survival outcomes. Nevertheless, the continual and occasionally prolonged nature of the administration of targeted agents leads to new challenges in their application with respect to the management of anticipated cardiovascular toxicities [5,8].

The most frequent side effects of SSAs consist mainly of gastrointestinal toxicities, with potentially a beneficial effect on cardiac parameters in the setting of acromegalic heart disease, a constellation of cardiac complications associated with acromegaly that involves nearly all aspects of the cardiovascular system [9]. In addition, SSAs and TPH inhibitors inhibit serotonin secretion from the tumor and subsequently lower 5-HIAA levels, relieving carcinoid syndrome, a rare secretory syndrome mainly associated with small intestinal and bronchial NENs that becomes manifest when serotonin and other vasoactive substances from the tumor enter the systemic circulation escaping hepatic degradation [4]. However, SSAs do not unequivocally reverse the progression of the carcinoid cardiac involvement nor improve survival in the setting of carcinoid heart disease [10]. The role of the recently introduced telotristat ethyl for prevention or control of carcinoid heart disease remains largely unknown, but could be elucidated in the near future as we obtain further evidence from clinical trials.

With regards to pathophysiology, MTTs may induce cardiovascular adverse effects (AEs) as a result of "on-target" and "off-target" mechanisms [11,12]. The on-target toxicity mechanism implicates mainly the mTOR complex 1 pathway with the target of MTT playing a crucial role in oncogenesis and angiogenesis, but also in hypertrophic response and survival of cardiomyocytes [12]. Off-target toxicity on the other hand, implicates an unintentional inhibition of a kinase that is also important for cardiac cell survival or function. For example certain TKIs induce a cardiomyocyte damage-related lactate dehydrogenase (LDH) release, that is in turn associated with the binding specificity of TKIs to their molecular target [13].

The placebo-controlled RCTs on biotherapy and MTTs for NENs and MTC report treatment-related toxicities according to the National Cancer Institute Common Terminology Criteria for Adverse Events, and therefore constitute a complete resource of treatment-related toxicities [14–16]. The present overview provides a comprehensive summary of high quality randomized evidence with the methodology of a systematic review and quantitative meta-analysis on the distinct safety profile of biotherapy and MTTs in advanced and/or metastatic NEN with a special focus on cardiovascular toxicities in order to assist clinicians involved in the management of NEN patients.

2. Results

2.1. Study Selection

We screened 3695 titles and abstracts from PubMed, Excerpta Medica database (EMBASE), Cochrane Central Register of Controlled Trials and additional 122 clinical trials in clinicaltrials.gov and identified 202 potentially eligible RCT reports (Figure 1). Some of the RCTs were reported in multiple publications or were posthoc analysis of the initial RCT; thus, they were excluded. After full article assessment, we included a total of 16 placebo-controlled RCTs reporting cardiovascular toxicities in the quantitative meta-analysis. Only patients with metastatic NET or MTC were included. The results on the safety profile of most RCTs were available from the published article or abstract and clinicaltrials.gov. A total of 3408 unique patients were recruited; four different categories of targeted agents were evaluated: SSAs, the TPH inhibitor telotrist etiprate, the mTOR inhibir everolimus and different TKIs. In particular, six RCTs addressed biotherapy (three RCTs on SSAs and three RCTs on telotrist etiprate) and ten RCTs addressed MTTs (the RADIANT-2, 3 and 4 trials on everolimus and seven RCTs on TKIs). All RCTs in the quantitative meta-analysis were industry sponsored. Study and patient characteristics are provided in Table 1 and Table S1, respectively.

Table 1. Characteristics of placebo-controlled randomized controlled trials included in the meta-analysis.

Study	Drug	Origin	Type of Treatment	Median Treatment Duration	Median Follow-Up [Months]	Complete Follow-Up [%]	Sample Size Calculation	N Participants Randomized	Included in Enets, ATA/ETA Guidelines	Industry Sponsorship
SSAs										
Caplin et al., 2014 [17] (CLARINET)	Lanreotide	14 countries	Lanreotide 120 mg/28 d Placebo	24.0 15.0	n.a n.a.	100	Yes	101 103	Yes	Yes
Rinke et al., 2009 [18] (PROMID)	Octreotide LAR	Germany	Octreotide LAR 30 mg/28 d Placebo	n.d n.d.	n.a. n.a.	99	Yes	42 43	Yes	Yes
Vinik et al., 2016 [19] (ELECT)	Lanreotide	11 countries	Lanreotide 120 mg/4weeks Placebo	4.6 3.7	n.a. n.a.	99	Yes	86 85	Yes	Yes

Table 1. Cont.

Study	Drug	Origin	Type of Treatment	Median Treatment Duration	Median Follow-Up [Months]	Complete Follow-Up [%]	Sample Size Calculation	N Participants Randomized	Included in Enets, ATA/ETA Guidelines	Industry Sponsorship
TPH Inhibitors										
Kulke et al., 2017 [20] (TELESTAR).	Telotristat etiprate	12 countries	Telotristat ethyl 250 mg or 500 mg three times per day or placebo three times per day	12.0 12.0	n.a. n.a.	100	Yes	45 45 45	No	Yes
Pavel et al., 2018 [21] (TELECAST).	Telotristat ethyl	11 counties	Telotristat ethyl 250 mg tid or 500 mg tid or placebo	12.0 12.0	36	89	Yes	26 25 25	No	Yes
Kulke et al., 2014 [22]	Telotristat etiprate	USA	telotristat etiprate 150 mg or 250 mg or 350 mg or 500 mg tid or placebo	4.0 4.0 4.0 4.0 4.0	n.a. n.a.	95	Yes	5 3 3 3 9	No	Yes
mTOR Inhibitors										
Pavel et al., 2017 [23] (RADIANT-2).	Everolimus + octreotide	16 countries	Everolimus 10 mg/d + octreotide LAR 30 mg/28 d Placebo + octreotide LAR 30 mg/28 d	9.3 9.2	n.a. n.a.	100	Yes	216 213	Yes	Yes
Yao et al., 2011 [24] (RADIANT-3).	Everolimus	18 countries	Everolimus 10 mg/d Placebo	8.8 3.7	17 17	62	Yes	207 203	Yes	Yes
Yao et al., 2016 [25] (RADIANT-4).	Everolimus	25 countries	Everolimus 10 mg/d Placebo	9.3 4.5	21 21	Above 80	Yes	205 97	Yes	Yes
TKI										
Raymond et al., 2011 [26]	Sunitinib	11 countries	Sunitinib 37.5 mg/d Placebo	4.6 3.7	n.a. n.a.	99	Yes	86 85	Yes	Yes
Wells et al., 2012 [27] (ZETA)	Vandetanib	3 countries	Vandetanib 300 mg vs. placebo	n.a. n.a.	24	100	Yes	330	Yes	Yes
Schlumberger et al., 2017 [28] (EXAM).	Cabozatinib	Germany	Cabozantinib vs. placebo	n.a. n.a.	n.a. n.a.	99.7	Yes	330	No	Yes
Xu et al., 2020 [29] (SANET-p)	Surufatinib	China	Surufatinib 300 mg vs. placebo	7.6 4.1	19.3 11.1	n.a	Yes	172	No	Yes
Carbonero et al., 2021 [30] (AXINET)	Axinitib	NA	Axitinib 5 mg BID + Sandostatin LAR 30 mg/28 days	n.a. n.a.	n.a. n.a.	n.a.	Yes	126 130	No	Yes
Bergland et al. [31] 2019	Pazopanib Hydrochloride		Pazopanib 800 mg PO QD on days 1–28 vs. placebo	60 60	60 60	100	Yes	97 74	No	Yes
Xu et al., 2020 [32] (SANET-ep).	Surufatinib	China	Surufatinib 300 mg vs. placebo	7.1 4.8	13.8 16.6	100	Yes	88 53	No	Yes

Abbreviations. ATA: American Thyroid Association; ENETS: European Neuroendocrine Tumor Society; ETA: European Thyroid Association; mTOR: Mechanistic target of rapamycin; n.a.: Non available; SSAs: Somatostatin analogs; TKI: Tyrosine kinase inhibitor; TPH: Tryptophan hydroxylase.

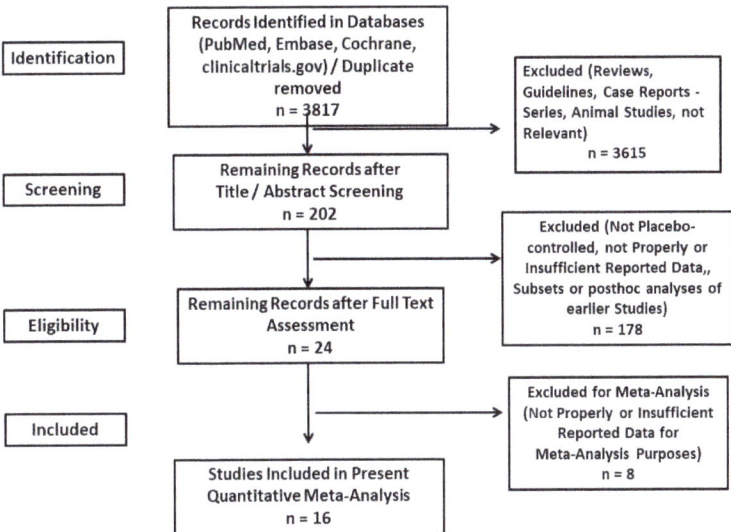

Figure 1. PRISMA flowchart of search results.

2.2. Representation in International Guidelines

Among the sixteen RCTs included in the present meta-analysis, six out of 14 RCTs on WD-NENs are included in the latest 2017 European Neuroendocrine Tumor Society (ENETS) [4], whereas one study on MTC, the ZETA trial, is included in both the 2015 Society American Thyroid Association (ATA) consensus guidelines [15] and the 2012 European Thyroid Association (ETA) guidelines for MTC (Table 1) [16].

2.3. Risk of Bias Assessment

In none of the included studies did we encounter high risk for bias in random sequence generation (selection bias), allocation concealment (selection bias), blinding participants and personnel (performance bias), blinding the outcome assessment (detection bias), incomplete outcome data (attrition bias), and selective reporting (reporting bias) (Table 2).

Table 2. Risk of bias summary: Authors' judgments about each risk of bias item for each included study following the Grading of Recommendations Assessment, Development and Evaluation (GRADE) Approach.

Study	Random Sequence Generation	Allocation Concealment	Blinding of Participants and Personnel	Blinding of Outcome Assessment	Incomplete Outcome Data	Selective Reporting	Other Bias
Caplin et al., 2014 [17] (CLARINET).	(-)	(-)	(-)	(-)	(-)	(-)	?
Rinke et al., 2009 [18] (PROMID)	(-)	(-)	(-)	(-)	(-)	(-)	?
Vinik et al., 2016 [19] (ELECT).	(-)	(-)	(-)	?	(-)	(-)	(-)
Kulke et al., 2017 [20] (TELESTAR).	?	?	?	?	(-)	(-)	(-)
Pavel et al., 2018 [21] (TELECAST).	(-)	(-)	(+)	(+)	(-)	(-)	(-)
Kulke et al., 2014 [22]	?	?	?	?	(-)	(-)	(-)
Pavel et al., 2017 [23] (RADIANT-2).	?	(-)	(-)	(-)	(-)	(-)	?
Yao et al., 2011 (RADIANT-3) [24].	(-)	(-)	(-)	(-)	(-)	(-)	?
Yao et al., 2016 (RADIANT-4) [25].	(-)	(-)	?	?	(-)	(-)	?

Table 2. Cont.

Study	Random Sequence Generation	Allocation Concealment	Blinding of Participants and Personnel	Blinding of Outcome Assessment	Incomplete Outcome Data	Selective Reporting	Other Bias
Raymond et al., 2011 [26]	?	?	(-)	(-)	?	(-)	?
Wells et al., 2012 [27] (ZETA).	?	?	(-)	(-)	(-)	(-)	?
Schlumberger et al. [28] 2017 (EXAM).	?	?	(-)	(-)	(-)	(-)	?
Xu et al., 2020 [29] (SANET-p).	(+)	(+)	(+)	(+)	(+)	(-)	?
Carbonero et al., 2021 [30] (AXINET)	(+)	?	(+)	(+)	?	(-)	(-)
Bergsland et al. [31] 2019	(+)	?	(+)	?	(-)	(-)	?
Xu et al., 2020 [32] (SANET-ep).	(+)	(+)	(+)	(+)	(+)	(-)	(-)

Each domain was judged as 'low risk of bias' (-), 'high risk of bias' (+), or 'unclear risk of bias' (?) in each study according to the Cochrane Handbook for Systematic Reviews of Interventions 1.

2.4. Serious Toxicities' Profile

Sixteen placebo-controlled RCTs compared grade 3 and 4 AE for four different categories of targeted agents in WD-NENs and MTC (Figure 2). TKIs exhibited a pooled odds ratio (OR) for serious AE of 3.41 (95% CI: 1.46–7.96). For surafatinib AE_OR in pancreatic NENs was as high as 23.46 (95% CI: 9.99–55.09), whereas for sunitinib in the same subset of patients AE_OR was 0.52 (95% CI: 0.27–0.99), as compared to placebo. In addition, the recently tested in phase III NEN trials axitinib and pazopanib demontrated a relatively high AE_OR (axitinib AE_OR: 7.08; 95% CI: 3.83–13.14 and pazopanib AE_OR: 4.67; 95% CI: 1.31–16.71, respectively). For MTC, the effect estimates were AE_OR: 2.97 (95% CI, 1.56–5.67) for vandetanib and 2.40 (95% CI: 1.43–4.04) for cabozatinib, as compared to placebo (Figure 2).The mTOR inhibitor everolimus exhibited a pooled OR for serious AE of 2.42 (95% CI: 1.87–3.12). With regards to biotherapy, SSAs demonstrated a pooled OR for serious AE as low as 0.77 (95% CI: 0.47–1.27), which was comparable to that of the TPH inhibitor telotristat etiprate (AE_OR: 0.77; 95% CI: 0.35–1.69; Figure 2). Significant heterogeneity was observed across the subset of studies on TKI (I^2 = 89.8%, p-value < 0.0001; Figure 2). A funnel plot was also produced demonstrating asymmetry (Figure S1A), that was mainly attributed to the recent studies on novel TKIs by Xu et al. on surufatinib in pancreatic NENs and by Carbonero et al. on axitinib in extra-pancreatic NENs (Galbraith's plot; Figure S1B) [29,30]. Egger's test showed no indication of publication bias across the included studies (p-value > 0.05). In the subset of studies on SSAs, TPH inhibitors and everolimus, we did not observe inter-study heterogeneity or publication bias (Figure 2 and Figure S1A–C).

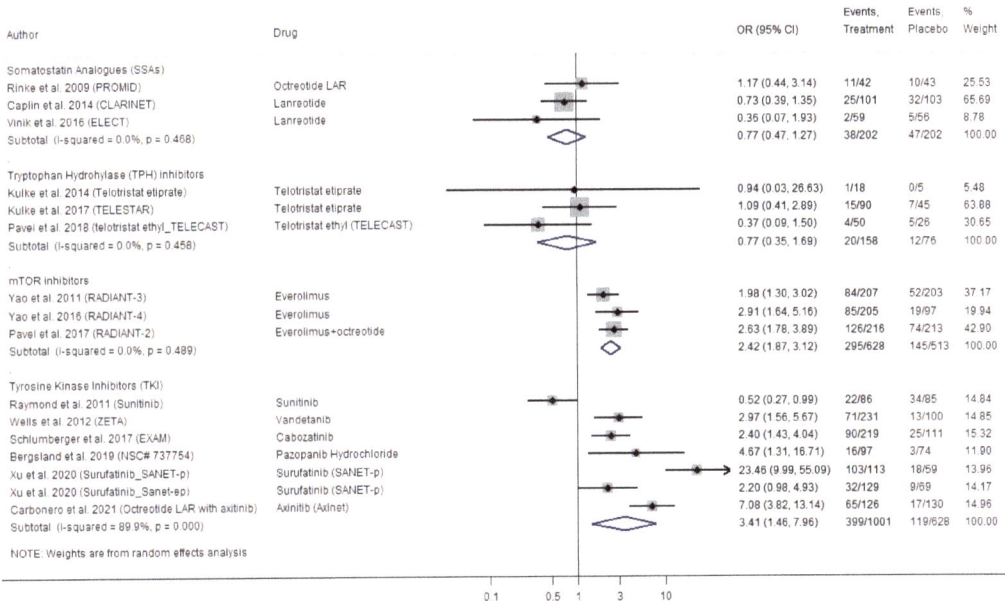

Figure 2. Targeted Agents' Serious Toxicities profile per drug category in patients with Metastatic Well-Differentiated Neuroendocrine Neoplasms or Medullary Thyroid Cancer (Odds Ratios [OR] with 95% Confidence Intervals). Tyrosine kinase inhibitors exhibited the highest pooled OR: 3.41 (95% CI: 1.46–7.96) followed by everolimus (pooled OR: 2.42 [95% CI: 1.87–3.12]). Somatostatin analogues pooled OR was relatively low(0.77 [95% CI: 0.47–1.27], same as that of telotristat etiprate (OR: 0.77 [95% CI: 0.35–1.69]).

2.5. All Grade Toxicities' Profile

We conducted a meta-analysis of AE of all grades reported in the included RCTs (Figure 3). Our findings showed comparable figures compared to serious toxicities analysis with TKIs and everolimus demonstrating the highest risk of all grade toxicity (pooled TKI AE_OR: 3.78; 95% CI: 1.35–10.56 across both WD-NEN and MTC diagnoses; and pooled everolimus AE_OR: 3.91, 95% CI: 1.88–8.11). SSAs appeared to have the safest all grade toxicity profile (AE_OR: 1.08, 95% CI: 0.52–2.23; Figure 3).

Significant heterogeneity was evident across the subset of studies on TKI ($I^2 = 77.7\%$, p-value < 0.0001; Figure 3). A funnel plot was demonstrated signs of asymmetry (Figure S2A), that was mainly attributed to the study by Wells et al. on vandetanib in MTC and Xu et al. on surufatinib in pancreatic NENs (Galbraith's plot; Figure S2B). Egger's test showed no indication of publication bias across the included studies (p-value > 0.05). With regards to SSA, TPH inhibitors and everolimus, we did not observe inter-study heterogeneity or publication bias (Figure 3 and Figure S2A–C).

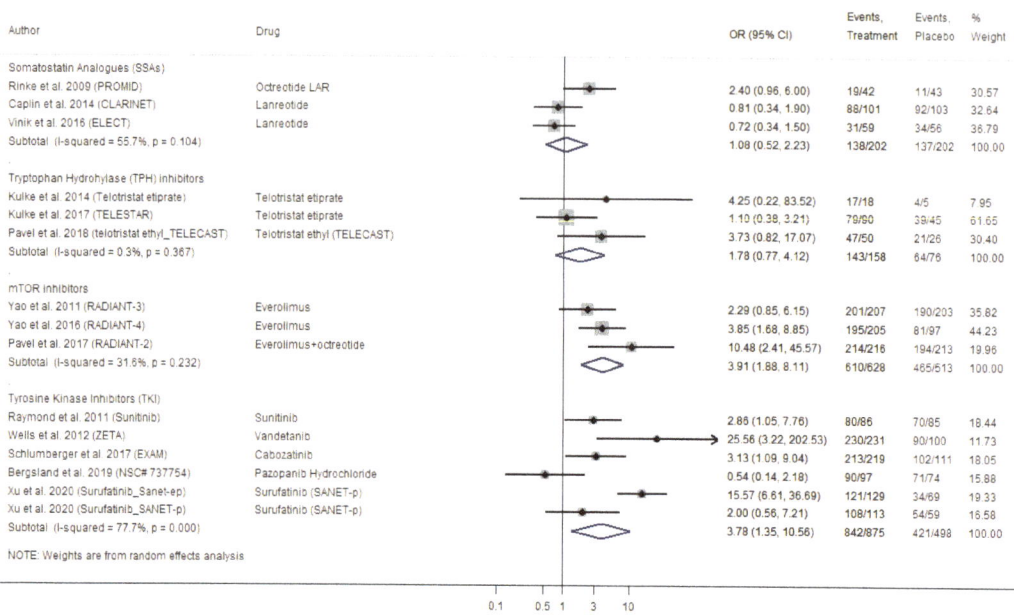

Figure 3. Targeted Agents' All Grade Toxicities profile per drug category in patients with Metastatic Well-Differentiated Neuroendocrine Neoplasms or Medullary Thyroid Cancer (Odds Ratios with 95% Confidence Intervals). Tyrosine kinase inhibitors (TKI) and everolimus demonstrated the highest risk of all grade toxicity (pooled OR: 3.78 [95% CI: 1.35–10.56] and OR: 3.91 [95% CI: 1.88–8.11], respectively).

2.6. Serious Cardiac Toxicities' Profile

Eleven placebo-controlled RCTs compared grade 3 and 4 cardiac AE for all four different categories of targeted agents in WD-NENs and MTC, investigated in our meta-analysis (Figure 4). Everolimus exhibited a pooled OR for serious cardiac AE of 3.28 (95% CI: 1.66–6.48) followed by TKIs with a pooled AE_OR of 1.51 (95% CI: 0.59–3.83). Within TKI analysis, sunitinib demonstrated the highest cardiac AE_OR in pancreatic NEN patients with OR figures as high as 7.17 (95% CI: 0.36–140.90), as compared to placebo. Surufatinib in pancreatic NENs, as well as vandetanib and cabozatinib in MTC do not appear to confer a risk for serious cardiac AE in the included RCTs (Figure 4).

With regards to biotherapy, SSAs demonstrated a potential prophylactic effect with respect to serious cardiac AE with an OR as low as 0.07 (95% CI: 0.0–1.33), which was comparable to that of telotristat etiprate (AE_OR: 0.21; 95% CI: 0.03–1.48; Figure 4).

Grade 3 and 4 cardiac AE in the 628 WD-NEN patients recieving everolimus in the intervention arm of the RADIANT trials included acute coronary syndrome (two patients), angina pectoris (two patients), cardiac arrest (two patients), cardiac failure (seven patients), congestive cardiac failure (six patients), cardio-respiratory arrest (two patients), left ventricular dysfunction/failure (two patients), right ventricular dysfunction (one patient), myocardial dysfunction (one patient), myocarditis (one patient), palpitations (one patient), tachycardia (one patient), pericardial efusion (two patients), tricuspid valve incompetence (one patient), mitral valve incompetence (one patient), pulmonary valve stenosis (one patient).

In patients receiving TKIs, Grade 3 and 4 cardiac AE included atrial flutter (one patient), atrial fibrillation (two patients), cardiac failure (three patients), cardiopulmonary failure (one patient), left ventricular dysfunction (one patient), supraventricular tachycardia (one patient), right ventricular dysfunction (one patient), bradycardia (one patient), arrhythmia (one patient), and pericarditis (one patient). Finally, we did not observe any inter-study heterogeneity or publication bias within the different pooled analyses across different targeted NEN treatments (Figure 4 and Figure S3A–C).

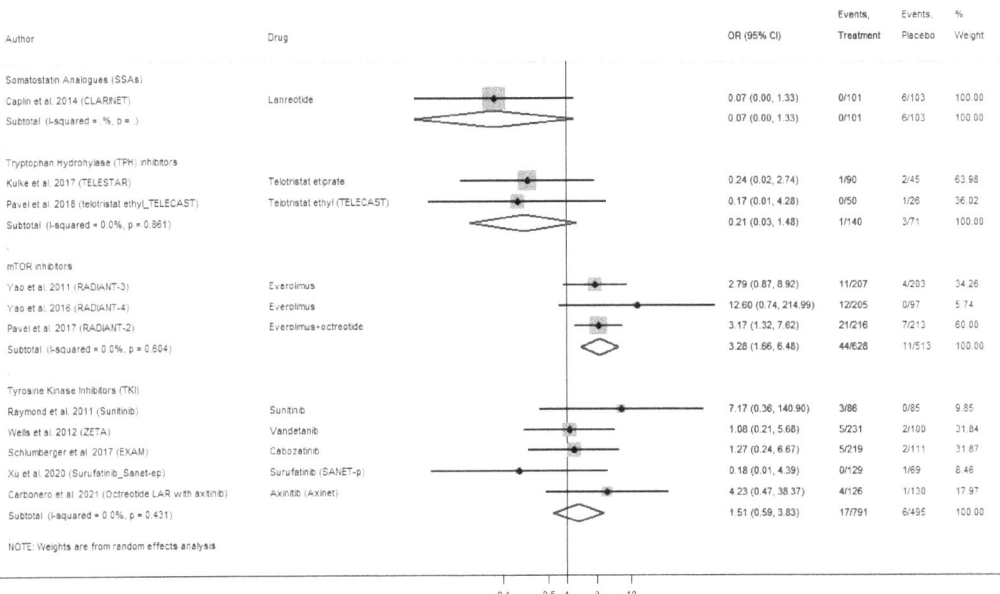

Figure 4. Targeted Agents' Serious Cardiac Toxicities profile per drug category in patients with Metastatic Well-Differentiated Neuroendocrine Neoplasms or Medullary Thyroid Cancer (Odds Ratios [OR] with 95% Confidence Intervals). Everolimus exhibited the highest pooled OR: 3.28 (95% CI: 1.66–6.48) followed by tyrosine kinase inhibitors with a pooled OR: 1.51 (95% CI: 0.59–3.83). Somatostatin analogs and telotristat etiprate demonstrated a potential prophylactic effect with with an OR: 0.07 (95% CI: 0.0–1.33) and OR: 0.21 (95% CI: 0.03–1.48), respectively.

2.7. Serious Vascular Toxicities' Profile

Nine placebo-controlled RCTs reported grade 3 and 4 vascular AE for WD-NENs treated with SSAs, everolimus or TKI and MTC treated with TKIs (Figure 5). Everolimus exhibited a pooled OR for serious vascular AE of 1.72 (95% CI: 0.64–4.64) followed by TKIs with a comparable pooled AE_OR of 1.64 (95% CI: 0.35–7.78). Within TKI analysis, vandetanib and cabozatinib, the two TKIs approved for MTC demonstrated the highest vascular AE_OR as high as 9.53 (95% CI: 0.55–164.60) for vandetanib and 5.82 (95% CI: 0.74–45.65) for cabozatinib, respectively when compared to placebo (Figure 5). With regards to biotherapy, SSAs in the CLARINET trial were not linked to a higher risk for serious vascular AE with an OR of 1.02 (95% CI: 0.14–7.39). The included placebo-controlled RCTs on telotristat etiprate did not report any serious vascular AEs.

The grade 3 and 4 vascular toxicities that were reported in the RADIANT trials included hypertension (two patients), hypotension (four patients), deep vein thrombosis (three patients), phlebitis, i.e., inflammation of the walls of a vein (one patient) and hematoma, i.e., a collection of blood outside of a blood vessel (one patient). Finally, the TKI trials reported the following serious vascular toxicities: hypertension (83 patients), hypertensive crisis (four patients), deep vein thrombosis (three patients) and hypotesion (one patient).

As in cardiac AEs' pooled analyses, we did not observe any inter-study heterogeneity or publication bias (Figure 5 and Figure S4A–C).

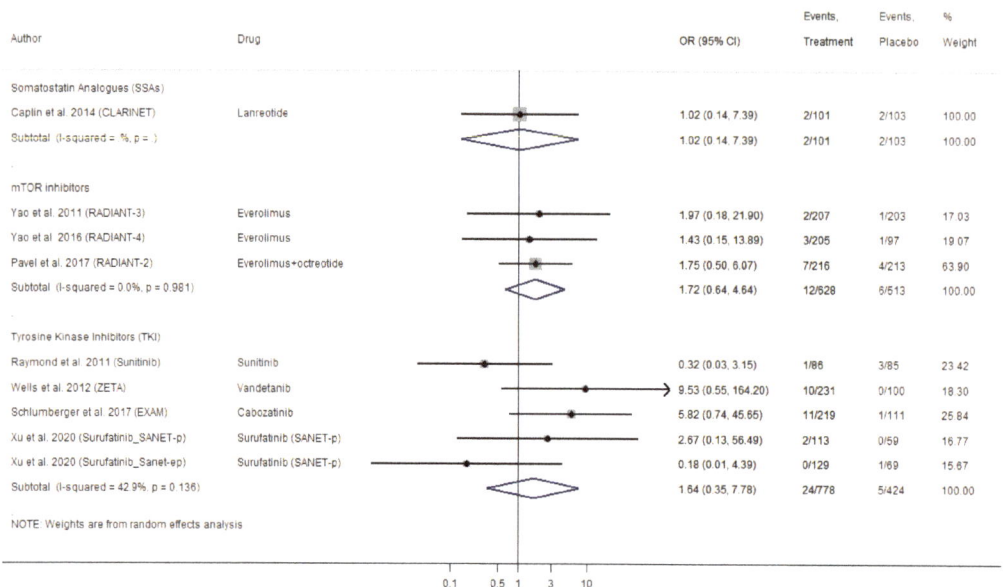

Figure 5. Targeted Agents' Serious Vascular Toxicities profile per drug category in patients with Metastatic Well-Differentiated Neuroendocrine Neoplasms or Medullary Thyroid Cancer (Odds Ratio [OR] with 95% Confidence Intervals). Molecular targeted therapies were linked with higher risk for Serious Vascular Toxicities (Everolimus pooled OR: 1.72 [95% CI: 0.64–4.64]; Tyrosine kinase inhibitorsTKIs pooled OR of 1.64 [95% CI: 0.35–7.78]).

2.8. Hypertension Secondary to Molecular Targeted Therapies

Nine placebo-controlled RCTs reported treatment-related hypertension, in particular new-onset or excarbation of pre-existing hyperension, in WD-NEN patients treated with everolimus or TKI and also MTC patients treated with TKIs (Figure 6). Everolimus was not linked to a significantly higher risk for treatment-related hypertension, as a pooled OR of 1.16 (95% CI: 0.14–9.45) was evident in RADIANT-2 and RADIANT-4 trials with only two cases of hypertension among 421 patients in the intervention arm. TKIs on the other hand exhibited a pooled OR for hypertension of 3.31 (95% CI: 1.87–5.86) with 193 patients with treatment-related hypertension among the 1021 patients in the intervention arm of these trials (Figure 6). Within TKI analysis, surufatinib in patients with pancreatic and extra-pancreatic NENs and cabozatinib in patients with MTC, demonstrated the highest ORs for treatment-related hypertension (SANET-p OR: 8.45; 95% CI: 2.86–24.96; SANET-ep OR: 3.82; 95% CI: 1.74–8.39; EXAM OR: 5.22; 95% CI: 0.31–104.34, respectively; Figure 6). The included placebo-controlled RCTs on biotherapy (SSAs and telotristat etiprate) did not report any treatment-related hypertension. Pooled analyses for hypertension were only available for everolimus and TKI, and did not reveal any inter-study heterogeneity or publication bias (Figure 6 and Figure S5A–C).

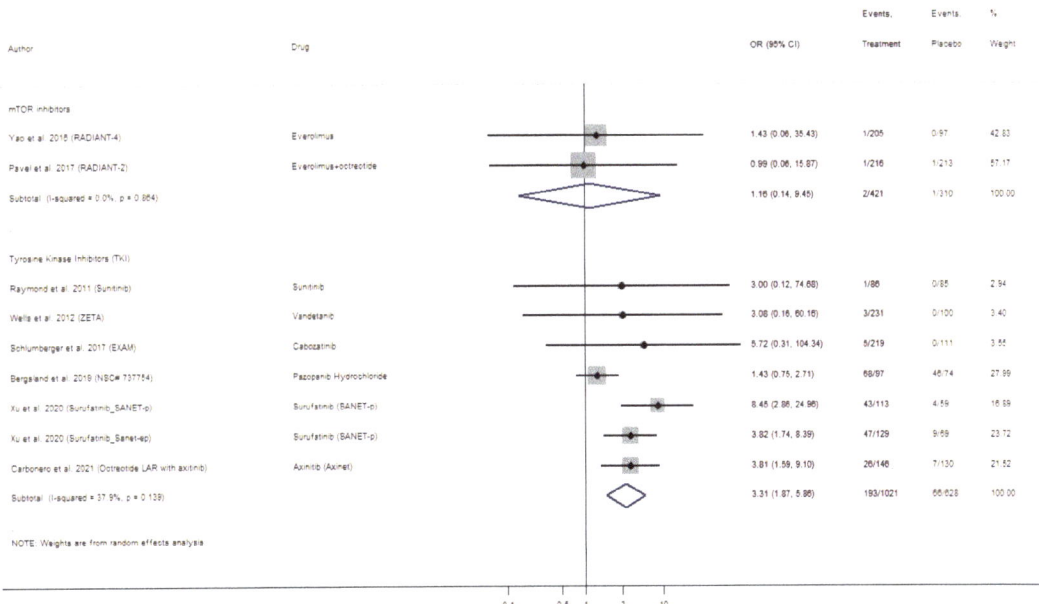

Figure 6. Targeted Agents' Risk Assessment for new-onset or exacerbation of pre-existing Hypertension per drug category in patients with Metastatic Well-Differentiated Neuroendocrine Neoplasms or Medullary Thyroid Cancer (Odds Ratios with 95% Confidence Intervals). Tyrosine kinsae inhibitors exhibited a pooled OR for hypertension of 3.31 (95% CI: 1.87–5.86).

3. Discussion

In this systematic review and quantitative meta-analysis, we present all the available placebo-controlled randomized trials evaluating the safety profile of targeted therapies for metastatic WD-NEN and MTC with special focus on cardiovascular treatment-related toxicities. We identified sixteen RCTs that randomized 3408 patients with WD-NEN or MTC to biotherapy or MTTs. In general, the investigated targeted therapies exhibit a broad range of overall and grade 3 and 4 AE with regards to each drug' distinct safety profile. In particular, analysis of grade 3 and 4 AE across both WD-NEN and MTC diagnoses, showed that there is evidence of a higher risk for serious toxicities in patients receiving the mTOR inhibitor everolimus and different TKIs and involved more commonly cardiovascular disorders for these agents, as compared to SSAs and telotristat etiprate. Furthermore, new onset or exacerbation of pre-existing hypertension was often encountered in patients that received TKI; with the highest risk being evident among patients that were administered the recently tested TKIs surufatinib and axitinib.

We applied the GRADE system to assess the risk of bias of the included placebo-controlled RCTs and were able to present high quality randomized evidence with a low risk of bias in most of the categories assessed (Table 2). However, inter-study heterogeneity was observed in the TKI subgroup meta-analysis for grade 3 and 4 as well as for all grade toxicities' analyses. Complementary testing confirmed between study heterogeneity in our meta-analysis with respect to the aforementioned analyses. The studies that apparently contributed mostly to inter-study heterogeneity were the ones by Wells et al. on vandetanib for MTC (ZETA trial) and by Xu et al. on surufatinib far pancreatic NENs (SANET-p) [27,29]. Nevertheless, the studies included in our meta-analysis lacked the granularity to identify certain subsets of patients who may derive the most benefit from the administered treatments both in terms of therapeutic efficacy but also in terms of drug safety. For example, data on cardiovascular comorbidities, carcinoid heart disease, as well as detailed data on prior systemic therapies and potential additive toxicities were not available in the included studies.

Targeted NEN agents have indeed been associated with a wide range of toxicities that may have an impact on the patients' quality of life. Therefore, determining the timing and appropriate selection of the right agent to initiate the targeted treatment represents one of the most important future tasks, as for example the somatostatin receptor avidity per se is not sufficient to determine if a NEN patient is a good candidate for TPH inhibitors and MTT; and the currently available biomarkers, chromogranin A and 5-hydroxy indoloaceatic acid lack a predictive value with regards to treatment selection and monitoring response to biotherapy and MTTs [33,34]. In addition, the clinical efficacy of the investigated targeted therapies in WD-NEN and MTC have not been clearly associated with specific mutations, apart from cabozatinib for MTC in the EXAM trial, where a higher treatment effect was evident in patients with RET M918T mutant tumors [28]. Finally, it remains to be determined the exact sequencing of lines of treatments upon disease progression since there are many treatments not yet tested in trials with a head-to-head comparison or even placebo-controlled RCT of targeted agents, including immunotherapy, novel inhibitors of specific molecular targets, such as novel multikinases, MEK kinases and checkpoint immune factors.

In general, patients who could be candidates for biotherapy and MTTs should be counseled on the potential risks and benefits of this specificic therapy, as these drugs are linked with a disctinct safety profile, more commonly involving gastrointestinal AE and depression for biotherapy and a more diverse spectrum of AE also including cardiovascular AE for everolimus and TKIs. These AE have indeed a certain probability of negatively affecting patient compliance as well as cardiovascular health and overall quality of life, often necessitating dosage adaptations or therapy discontinuation. In our meta-analysis, NEN patients receiving the mTOR inhibitor everolimus or different TKIs exhibited a higher risk of developing serious (grade 3 and 4) or any other toxicities, lending further support to the notion that biotherapy appears to be a safer therapeutic approach with the least risk for treatment-related AE. Further analysis with a focus on cardiovascular health of NEN patients revealed that the placebo treatment has a similar or lower toxicity as compared to biotherapy (SSA and telotristat etiprate arms) pointing out the importance of recognizing the true causality of cardiovascular morbidity and the need to assess the potential prophylactic effect of biotherapy in cardiovascular health, for example in the context of carcinoid heart disease secondary to carcinoid syndrome in well-designed studies. Currently, the recommended monitoring for TKIs in context of renal cell carcinoma is mainly focused on blood pressure in agreement with the finding of our meta-analysis on higher risk for new onset or exacerbation of pre-existing hypertension following the administration of TKIs [35]. In addition, in patients receiving TKI therapy, cardiovascular events, including QTc prolongation, left ventricular HF, myocardial infarction (MI), hypertension, pulmonary hypertension, and stroke, were commonly reported by investigators [36]. For patients on sunitinib therapy in particular, baseline and periodic electrocardiograms are recommended [37].

However, besides therapy-induced cardiotoxicity, there are several other plausible interactions between cardiovascular health and NENs that still need to be determined as implicated above, with modulation of the immune system being an important player, but also the effect of serotonin, vasoactive substances and growth factors in cases of the carcinoid heart disease. For instance, the management of patients with poorly controlled hypertension or patients with a right heart failure due to fibrosis of right-sided valves may indeed be challenging and raise issues concerning treatment with targeted agents that could have an impact in patients' already compromised cardiovascular health. Overall, despite their anti-tumor benefits, the use of MTTs and TKIs in particular has been hampered by potent cardiovascular toxicities, including hypertension. In addition, there is a paucity of real-world data on cardiovascular AEs caused by novel targeted agents in NENs and also a lack of studies on the pathophysiological mechanisms implicated in cardiovascular toxicity related to MTTs in this setting. As new cardiovascular AEs related to novel agents have emerged, clinicians managing NENs are now compelled to respond despite the lack of evidence regarding optimal management. Generally, routine monitoring of heart function and blood pressure during therapy with TKIs and identification of at risk patients before therapy seem to be the key steps in preventing cardiovascular events, regardless of the agent used. For patients on TKIs, baseline and periodic electrocardiograms are recommended. However, further studies are warranted to identify which of several targeted agents is at fault, acquire a complete understanding of the mechanisms of cardiovascular toxicity and provide follow-up guidelines specifically focusing on cardiovascular health with suggestions on modality and timing of toxicity prevention and management.

Our meta-analysis has some limitations. Some trials did not report on cardiovascular treatment-related AE and had an unclear risk of bias due to insufficiently reported data on random sequence generation, allocation concealment and blinding of outcome assessment. Due to the rather low number of studies included in the subgroup analysis of each drug category, the assessment of inter-study heterogeneity was limited. In addition, in the subset of MTC, tumors of more aggressive behavior might have been included. Furthermore, MTC patients were only eligible for treatment with two of the TKIs investigated in our study (vandetanib and cabozatinib); hence, the MTC trials have probably contributed to the heterogeneity of the included studies. Nevertheless, our study is also subject to confounding encountered in the original trials; thus, our results are only generalizable to patient groups that could be eligible for the original RCTs. Another limitation of our study, was the lack of detailed data on the number of new-onset and exacerbation of pre-existing hypertension, when assessing the safety profiles of TKIs for NEN patients. However, the strengths of our study was that it clearly provided its aim, as we applied a comprehensive search strategy, obtaining data also from unpublished placebo-controlled RCTs including all available randomized evidence according to Cochrane guidelines on the safety profile of targeted NEN therapies with a special focus on cardiovascular health, that could constitute a reference standard for clinicians in the future.

4. Materials and Methods

We followed the Cochrane Guidelines for Systematic Reviews and Meta-analyses of Interventions for the design and conduct of the present systematic review and quantitative meta-analysis and the Preferred Reporting Items for Systematic Reviews and Meta-Analyses (PRISMA) guidelines for reporting the study results [38,39].

4.1. Search Strategy and Study Selection

We aimed to identify all potentially eligible placebo-controlled RCTs comparing targeted therapies (biotherapy and MTTs) in metastatic WD-NEN or MTC. We developed a comprehensive search algorithm using MeSH terms and text words in the title or the abstract in combination with a systemic treatment, and a RCT study design filter. The search strategy for each database and the applied filters regarding treatment selection and study design are presented in Table S2. Only placebo-controlled RCTs on targeted therapies for NENs reporting data on safety were included. A study protocol for this systematic review was not registered in PROSPERO at the stage of inception owing to feasibility issues with respect to the specific nature of our study hypothesis and the pausity of potentially eligible NEN studies addressing cardiovascular toxicities. Importantly, a search was conducted to ensure that no similar systematic review had been previously published.

The PubMed, Embase, the Cochrane Central Register of Controlled Trials and the website of ClinicalTrials.gov were searched through until 1 December 2020. We did not apply any language or date restrictions. Key search terms included neuroendocrine neoplasms, medullary thyroid cancer, systemic therapy, and randomized controlled trial. We only included placebo-controlled RCTs comparing a targeted therapy with placebo reporting adverse-effect incidence with special focus in cardiovascular toxicities. Three of the authors (C.A., M.Y. and K.D.) worked in duplicates independently and screened all potentially eligible titles and abstracts and subsequently the full-text manuscripts to finalize eligibility. Disagreements were resolved by consensus between C.A., M.Y. and K.D.

4.2. Outcomes and Data Extraction

The primary outcomes of this study were biotherapy's and MTTs' safety profiles. In particular, we assessed grade 3 and 4 (severe and life-threatening or disabling) AE, all grade AE, grade 3 and 4 cardiac AE, grade 3 and 4 vascular AE and treatment-related hypertension according to the National Cancer Institute Common Terminology Criteria for Adverse Events (CTCAE) v5.0 [14]. A CTCAE category is a broad classification of AEs based on anatomy and/or pathophysiology (for example, cardiac disorders; vascular disorders etc.) and within each category there are specific CTCAE terms that provide the standards for the description and exchange of safety information in oncology research. A list of serious and not serious treatment-related disorders as well as specific cardiac AEs and vascular AEs including hypertension were mainly obtained from clinicaltrials.gov and are provided in detail in Table S3.

Absolute values of AE were extracted and OR with 95% Confidence Intervals (CI) for PFS rates were calculated. Data on study-, patient- and tumor-characteristics, as well as industry sponsorship were also extracted. C.A., M.Y. and K.D. worked in duplicate and extracted all data independently. Discordances were resolved by consensus.

4.3. Risk of Bias and Quality of Evidence Assessment

We used the Grading of Recommendations Assessment, Development and Evaluation (GRADE) from the Cochrane Risk of Bias Tool to assess the risk of bias for the included RCTs [40]. We applied scores for standard domains: random sequence generation, allocation concealment, blinding of participants and personnel, blinding of outcome assessment, completeness of outcome data, for each domain. M.Y. and K.D. worked in duplicate and assessed the risk of bias and quality of evidence of the included RCTs. Disagreements were resolved by consensus.

4.4. Statistical Analysis

The pooled estimates for the AE in patients with WD-NENS or MTC were assessed for the outcomes of interest and OR were calculated taking into account the correction of Haldane-Anscombe about 0 cells [41]. An OR is a relative measure of effect, which allows the comparison of the intervention group of a study relative to the placebo group. In particular, the OR represents the odds that an outcome will occur given a particular exposure (treatment) in the intervention group, compared to the odds of the outcome occurring in the absence of that exposure (administration of placebo) in the placebo group. The random variance component was estimated using the approach by Der Simonian and Laird [42]. To explore heterogeneity between the studies the I^2 statistics were used. When I^2 was > 0.50% the statistical heterogeneity was considered substantial [43]. Publication bias was assessed by the application of funnel plots and the Egger's test to investigate the asymmetry among the study estimates [44]. All the analyses were performed using the STATA statistical package (version 13.1; StataCorp, College Station, TX, USA)

5. Conclusions

Our systematic review and quantitative meta-analysis have implications for clinical practice and further research in the field of neuroendocrine tumors. It provides a comprehensive overview of the available randomized evidence on the safety profile of biotherapy (somatotatin analogs and tryptophan hydroxylase inhibitors) and that of molecular targeted therapies (mTOR and tyrosine kinase inhibitors) with a special focus on cardiovascular treatment-related toxicities Somatostatin analogs and tryptophan hydroxylase inhibitors appear to be safer as compared to mTOR and tyrosine kinase inhibitors with regards to their overall toxicity profile, and cardiovascular toxicities in particular. In addition, new onset or exacerbation of pre-existing hypertension was often encountered in patients who received tyrosine kinase inhibitors. Apart from evidence on the efficacy of biotherapy and MTTs, data on treatment-related toxicities and the distinct safety profile of each agent could promote a patient-tailored approach guiding clinicians' treatment decisions, but also patient surveillance with early recognition and prompt management of treatment-related toxicities when they appear. Finally, our results highlight the need for further research in assessing long-term real world-data on cardiovascular health as well as effects on quality of life of patients receiving different targeted NEN therapies in order to achieve a balance between antitumor activity and toxicities. This is of course most probably accomplished when NEN patients receiving multimodal treatments are managed in dedicated centers with treatment decisions being taken in the context of a multidisciplinary tumor board.

Supplementary Materials: The following are available online at https://www.mdpi.com/article/10.3390/cancers13092159/s1, Figure S1A: Funnel plot for studies included in the pooled analysis for Grade 3 and 4 Adverse Effects; S1B: Galbraith's plot for studies included in this analysis; S1C: Egger's plot for studies included in this analysis, Figure S2A: Funnel plot for studies included in the pooled analysis for all Grade Adverse Effects; S2B: Galbraith's plot for studies included in this analysis; S2C: Egger's plot for studies included in this analysis, Figure S3A: Funnel plot for studies included in the pooled analysis for Grade 3 and 4 Cardiac Adverse Effects; S3B: Galbraith's plot for studies included in this analysis; S3C: Egger's plot for studies included in this analysis, Figure S4A: Funnel plot for studies included in the pooled analysis for Grade 3 and 4 Vascular Adverse Effects; S4B: Galbraith's plot for studies included in this analysis; S4C: Egger's plot for studies included in this analysis, Figure S5A: Funnel plot for studies included in the pooled analysis for treatment-related Hypertension; S5B: Galbraith's plot for studies included in this analysis; S5C: Egger's plot for studies included in this analysis, Table S1: Patient and tumor characteristics across the included studies. Table S2: Systematic literature search strategy, Table S3: A. List of serious and not-serious disorders B. Specific cardiac adverse effects and C. Specific vascular adverse effects including hypertension assessed in the present study in order to categorize toxicities into different safety profiles (serious toxicities, all grade toxicities, serious cardiac toxicities, vascular toxicities and hypertension) according to the National Cancer Institute Common Terminology Criteria for Adverse Events v5.0.

Author Contributions: Conceptualization, K.D.; methodology, C.A., M.-E.S., M.Y. and K.D.; data curation and quality assessment, C.A., M.Y. and K.D.; software, M.-E.S.; validation, M.Y. and K.D.; statistical analysis. M.-E.S.; writing—original draft preparation, C.A., M.Y., A.K. and K.D.; writing—review and editing, all authors; visualization, M.Y., A.K., E.K., G.W. and G.K.; supervision, K.D. All authors have read and agreed to the published version of the manuscript.

Funding: K.D. was supported by the Royal Swedish Academy of Sciences. The other authors of the study have not received any funding.

Institutional Review Board Statement: Not applicable.

Informed Consent Statement: Not applicable.

Data Availability Statement: Individual patient data from the original studies included in the present meta-analysis is not available and data sharing at this level is not applicable for a systematic review.

Acknowledgments: The authors would like to thank Liz Holmgren and Linda Bejerstrand at the Medical Library of Örebro University for their assistance with systematic literature retrieval.

Conflicts of Interest: The authors declare that there is no conflict of interest.

References

1. Dasari, A.; Shen, C.; Halperin, D.; Zhao, B.; Zhou, S.; Xu, Y.; Shih, T.; Yao, J.C. Trends in the Incidence, Prevalence, and Survival Outcomes in Patients with Neuroendocrine Tumors in the United States. *JAMA Oncol.* **2017**, *3*, 1335–1342. [CrossRef] [PubMed]
2. Roman, S.; Lin, R.; Sosa, J.A. Prognosis of medullary thyroid carcinoma: Demographic, clinical, and pathologic predictors of survival in 1252 cases. *Cancer* **2006**, *107*, 2134–2142. [CrossRef] [PubMed]

3. Alexandraki, K.I.; Kaltsas, G. Gastroenteropancreatic neuroendocrine tumors: New insights in the diagnosis and therapy. *Endocrine* **2012**, *41*, 40–52. [CrossRef] [PubMed]
4. Pavel, M.; Valle, J.W.; Eriksson, B.; Rinke, A.; Caplin, M.; Chen, J.; Costa, F.; Falkerby, J.; Fazio, N.; Gorbounova, V.; et al. ENETS Consensus Guidelines for the Standards of Care in Neuroendocrine Neoplasms: Systemic Therapy—Biotherapy and Novel Targeted Agents. *Neuroendocrinology* **2017**, *105*, 266–280. [CrossRef]
5. Kaderli, R.M.; Spanjol, M.; Kollar, A.; Butikofer, L.; Gloy, V.; Dumont, R.A.; Seiler, C.A.; Christ, E.R.; Radojewski, P.; Briel, M.; et al. Therapeutic Options for Neuroendocrine Tumors: A Systematic Review and Network Meta-analysis. *JAMA Oncol.* **2019**, *5*, 480–489. [CrossRef] [PubMed]
6. Oleinikov, K.; Korach, A.; Planer, D.; Gilon, D.; Grozinsky-Glasberg, S. Update in carcinoid heart disease—The heart of the matter. *Rev. Endocr. Metab. Disord.* **2021**. [CrossRef] [PubMed]
7. Liu, M.; Armeni, E.; Navalkissoor, S.; Davar, J.; Sullivan, L.; Leigh, C.; O'Mahony, L.F.; Hayes, A.; Mandair, D.; Chen, J.; et al. Cardiac Metastases in Patients with Neuroendocrine Tumours: Clinical Features, Therapy Outcomes, and Prognostic Implications. *Neuroendocrinology* **2020**. [CrossRef] [PubMed]
8. Alexandraki, K.I.; Daskalakis, K.; Tsoli, M.; Grossman, A.B.; Kaltsas, G.A. Endocrinological Toxicity Secondary to Treatment of Gastroenteropancreatic Neuroendocrine Neoplasms (GEP-NENs). *Trends Endocrinol. Metab.* **2020**, *31*, 239–255. [CrossRef]
9. Heidarpour, M.; Shafie, D.; Aminorroaya, A.; Sarrafzadegan, N.; Farajzadegan, Z.; Nouri, R.; Najimi, A.; Dimopolou, C.; Stalla, G. Effects of somatostatin analog treatment on cardiovascular parameters in patients with acromegaly: A systematic review. *J. Res. Med. Sci.* **2019**, *24*, 29. [CrossRef]
10. Denney, W.D.; Kemp, W.E., Jr.; Anthony, L.B.; Oates, J.A.; Byrd, B.F., 3rd. Echocardiographic and biochemical evaluation of the development and progression of carcinoid heart disease. *J. Am. Coll. Cardiol.* **1998**, *32*, 1017–1022. [CrossRef]
11. Cheng, H.; Force, T. Molecular mechanisms of cardiovascular toxicity of targeted cancer therapeutics. *Circ. Res.* **2010**, *106*, 21–34. [CrossRef] [PubMed]
12. Liu, K.L.; Chen, J.S.; Chen, S.C.; Chu, P.H. Cardiovascular Toxicity of Molecular Targeted Therapy in Cancer Patients: A Double-Edged Sword. *Acta Cardiol. Sin.* **2013**, *29*, 295–303.
13. Hasinoff, B.B. The cardiotoxicity and myocyte damage caused by small molecule anticancer tyrosine kinase inhibitors is correlated with lack of target specificity. *Toxicol. Appl. Pharmacol.* **2010**, *244*, 190–195. [CrossRef]
14. Common Terminology Criteria for Adverse Events v5.0 (CTCAE). Available online: https://ctep.cancer.gov/protocoldevelopment/electronic_applications/ctc.htm (accessed on 1 January 2021).
15. Wells, S.A., Jr.; Asa, S.L.; Dralle, H.; Elisei, R.; Evans, D.B.; Gagel, R.F.; Lee, N.; Machens, A.; Moley, J.F.; Pacini, F.; et al. Revised American Thyroid Association guidelines for the management of medullary thyroid carcinoma. *Thyroid* **2015**, *25*, 567–610. [CrossRef] [PubMed]
16. Schlumberger, M.; Bastholt, L.; Dralle, H.; Jarzab, B.; Pacini, F.; Smit, J.W.; European Thyroid Association Task, F. 2012 European thyroid association guidelines for metastatic medullary thyroid cancer. *Eur. Thyroid. J.* **2012**, *1*, 5–14. [CrossRef] [PubMed]
17. Caplin, M.E.; Pavel, M.; Cwikla, J.B.; Phan, A.T.; Raderer, M.; Sedlackova, E.; Cadiot, G.; Wolin, E.M.; Capdevila, J.; Wall, L.; et al. Lanreotide in metastatic enteropancreatic neuroendocrine tumors. *N. Eng. J. Med.* **2014**, *371*, 224–233. [CrossRef] [PubMed]
18. Rinke, A.; Muller, H.-H.; Schade-Brittinger, C.; Klose, K.-J.; Barth, P.; Wied, M.; Mayer, C.; Aminossadati, B.; Pape, U.-F.; Blaker, M.; et al. Placebo-controlled, double-blind, prospective, randomized study on the effect of octreotide LAR in the control of tumor growth in patients with metastatic neuroendocrine midgut tumors: A report from the PROMID Study Group. *J. Clin. Oncol. Off. J. Am. Soc. Clin. Oncol.* **2009**, *27*, 4656–4663. [CrossRef]
19. Vinik, A.I.; Wolin, E.M.; Liyanage, N.; Gomez-Panzani, E.; Fisher, G.A. Evaluation of lanreotide depot/autogel efficacy and safety as a carcinoid syndrome treatment (elect): A randomized, double-blind, placebo-controlled trial. *Endocr. Prac. Off. J. Am. Coll. Endocrinol. Am. Assoc. Clin. Endocrinol.* **2016**, *22*, 1068–1080. [CrossRef]
20. Kulke, M.H.; Horsch, D.; Caplin, M.E.; Anthony, L.B.; Bergsland, E.; Oberg, K.; Welin, S.; Warner, R.R.P.; Lombard-Bohas, C.; Kunz, P.L.; et al. Telotristat Ethyl, a Tryptophan Hydroxylase Inhibitor for the Treatment of Carcinoid Syndrome. *J. Clin. Oncol. Off. J. Am. Soc. Clin. Oncol.* **2017**, *35*, 14–23. [CrossRef]
21. Pavel, M.; Gross, D.J.; Benavent, M.; Perros, P.; Srirajaskanthan, R.; Warner, R.R.P.; Kulke, M.H.; Anthony, L.B.; Kunz, P.L.; Horsch, D.; et al. Telotristat ethyl in carcinoid syndrome: Safety and efficacy in the TELECAST phase 3 trial. *Endocr. Relat. Cancer* **2018**, *25*, 309–322. [CrossRef] [PubMed]
22. Kulke, M.H.; O'Dorisio, T.; Phan, A.; Bergsland, E.; Law, L.; Banks, P.; Freiman, J.; Frazier, K.; Jackson, J.; Yao, J.C.; et al. Telotristat etiprate, a novel serotonin synthesis inhibitor, in patients with carcinoid syndrome and diarrhea not adequately controlled by octreotide. *Endocr. Relat. Cancer* **2014**, *21*, 705–714. [CrossRef] [PubMed]
23. Pavel, M.E.; Baudin, E.; Oberg, K.E.; Hainsworth, J.D.; Voi, M.; Rouyrre, N.; Peeters, M.; Gross, D.J.; Yao, J.C. Efficacy of everolimus plus octreotide LAR in patients with advanced neuroendocrine tumor and carcinoid syndrome: Final overall survival from the randomized, placebo-controlled phase 3 RADIANT-2 study. *Ann. Oncol. Off. J. Eur. Soc. Med. Oncol.* **2017**, *28*, 1569–1575. [CrossRef] [PubMed]
24. Yao, J.C.; Shah, M.H.; Ito, T.; Bohas, C.L.; Wolin, E.M.; Van Cutsem, E.; Hobday, T.J.; Okusaka, T.; Capdevila, J.; de Vries, E.G.E.; et al. Everolimus for advanced pancreatic neuroendocrine tumors. *N. Eng. J. Med.* **2011**, *364*, 514–523. [CrossRef] [PubMed]

25. Yao, J.C.; Fazio, N.; Singh, S.; Buzzoni, R.; Carnaghi, C.; Wolin, E.; Tomasek, J.; Raderer, M.; Lahner, H.; Voi, M.; et al. Everolimus for the treatment of advanced, non-functional neuroendocrine tumours of the lung or gastrointestinal tract (RADIANT-4): A randomised, placebo-controlled, phase 3 study. *Lancet* **2016**, *387*, 968–977. [CrossRef]
26. Raymond, E.; Dahan, L.; Raoul, J.-L.; Bang, Y.-J.; Borbath, I.; Lombard-Bohas, C.; Valle, J.; Metrakos, P.; Smith, D.; Vinik, A.; et al. Sunitinib malate for the treatment of pancreatic neuroendocrine tumors. *N. Eng. J. Med.* **2011**, *364*, 501–513. [CrossRef] [PubMed]
27. Wells, S.A., Jr.; Robinson, B.G.; Gagel, R.F.; Dralle, H.; Fagin, J.A.; Santoro, M.; Baudin, E.; Elisei, R.; Jarzab, B.; Vasselli, J.R.; et al. Vandetanib in patients with locally advanced or metastatic medullary thyroid cancer: A randomized, double-blind phase III trial. *J. Clin. Oncol. Off. J. Am. Soc. Clin. Oncol.* **2012**, *30*, 134–141. [CrossRef]
28. Schlumberger, M.; Elisei, R.; Müller, S.; Schöffski, P.; Brose, M.; Shah, M.; Licitra, L.; Krajewska, J.; Kreissl, M.C.; Niederle, B.; et al. Overall survival analysis of EXAM, a phase III trial of cabozantinib in patients with radiographically progressive medullary thyroid carcinoma. *Ann. Oncol. Off. J. Eur. Soc. Med. Oncol.* **2017**, *28*, 2813–2819. [CrossRef]
29. Xu, J.; Shen, L.; Bai, C.; Wang, W.; Li, J.; Yu, X.; Li, Z.; Li, E.; Yuan, X.; Chi, Y.; et al. Surufatinib in advanced pancreatic neuroendocrine tumours (SANET-p): A randomised, double-blind, placebo-controlled, phase 3 study. *Lancet Oncol.* **2020**, *21*, 1489–1499. [CrossRef]
30. Rocio Garcia-Carbonero, M.B.; Fonseca, P.J.; Castellano, D.; Alonso, T.; Teule, A.; Custodio, A.; Tafuto, S.; Munoa, A.L.; Spada, F.; López-López, C.; et al. A phase II/III randomized double-blind study of octreotide acetate LAR with axitinib versus octreotide acetate LAR with placebo in patients with advanced G1-G2 NETs of non-pancreatic origin (AXINET trial-GETNE-1107). *J. Clin. Oncol.* **2021**. [CrossRef]
31. Bergsland, E.K.; Mahoney, M.R.; Asmis, T.R.; Hall, N.; Kumthekar, P.; Maitland, M.L.; Niedzwiecki, D.; Nixon, A.B.; O'Reilly, E.M.; Schwartz, L.H.; et al. Meyerhardt. Prospective randomized phase II trial of pazopanib versus placebo in patients with progressive carcinoid tumors (CARC) (Alliance A021202). *Am. Soc. Clin. Oncol.* **2019**. [CrossRef]
32. Xu, J.; Shen, L.; Zhou, Z.; Li, J.; Bai, C.; Chi, Y.; Li, Z.; Xu, N.; Li, E.; Liu, T.; et al. Surufatinib in advanced extrapancreatic neuroendocrine tumours (SANET-ep): A randomised, double-blind, placebo-controlled, phase 3 study. *Lancet Oncol.* **2020**, *21*, 1500–1512. [CrossRef]
33. Dam, G.; Gronbaek, H.; Sorbye, H.; Thiis Evensen, E.; Paulsson, B.; Sundin, A.; Jensen, C.; Ebbesen, D.; Knigge, U.; Tiensuu Janson, E. Prospective Study of Chromogranin A as a Predictor of Progression in Patients with Pancreatic, Small-Intestinal, and Unknown Primary Neuroendocrine Tumors. *Neuroendocrinology* **2020**, *110*, 217–224. [CrossRef]
34. Wedin, M.; Mehta, S.; Angeras-Kraftling, J.; Wallin, G.; Daskalakis, K. The Role of Serum 5-HIAA as a Predictor of Progression and an Alternative to 24-h Urine 5-HIAA in Well-Differentiated Neuroendocrine Neoplasms. *Biology* **2021**, *10*, 76. [CrossRef] [PubMed]
35. Hall, P.S.; Harshman, L.C.; Srinivas, S.; Witteles, R.M. The frequency and severity of cardiovascular toxicity from targeted therapy in advanced renal cell carcinoma patients. *JACC Heart Fail.* **2013**, *1*, 72–78. [CrossRef] [PubMed]
36. Schmidinger, M.; Zielinski, C.C.; Vogl, U.M.; Bojic, A.; Bojic, M.; Schukro, C.; Ruhsam, M.; Hejna, M.; Schmidinger, H. Cardiac toxicity of sunitinib and sorafenib in patients with metastatic renal cell carcinoma. *J. Clin. Oncol.* **2008**, *26*, 5204–5212. [CrossRef]
37. Richards, C.J.; Je, Y.; Schutz, F.A.; Heng, D.Y.; Dallabrida, S.M.; Moslehi, J.J.; Choueiri, T.K. Incidence and risk of congestive heart failure in patients with renal and nonrenal cell carcinoma treated with sunitinib. *J. Clin. Oncol.* **2011**, *29*, 3450–3456. [CrossRef]
38. Cumpston, M.; Li, T.; Page, M.J.; Chandler, J.; Welch, V.A.; Higgins, J.P.; Thomas, J. Updated guidance for trusted systematic reviews: A new edition of the Cochrane Handbook for Systematic Reviews of Interventions. *Cochrane Database Syst. Rev.* **2019**, *10*, ED000142. [CrossRef]
39. Moher, D.; Liberati, A.; Tetzlaff, J.; Altman, D.G.; Group, P. Preferred reporting items for systematic reviews and meta-analyses: The PRISMA statement. *BMJ* **2009**, *339*, b2535. [CrossRef] [PubMed]
40. Guyatt, G.H.; Oxman, A.D.; Vist, G.E.; Kunz, R.; Falck-Ytter, Y.; Alonso-Coello, P.; Schunemann, H.J.; Group, G.W. GRADE: An emerging consensus on rating quality of evidence and strength of recommendations. *BMJ* **2008**, *336*, 924–926. [CrossRef] [PubMed]
41. Lawson, R. Small sample confidence intervals for the odds ratio. *Commun. Stat. Simul. Comput.* **2004**, *33*, 1095–1113. [CrossRef]
42. DerSimonian, R.; Laird, N. Meta-analysis in clinical trials. *Control. Clin. Trials* **1986**, *7*, 177–188. [CrossRef]
43. Higgins, J.P.; Thompson, S.G. Quantifying heterogeneity in a meta-analysis. *Stat. Med.* **2002**, *21*, 1539–1558. [CrossRef] [PubMed]
44. Sterne, J.A.; Sutton, A.J.; Ioannidis, J.P.; Terrin, N.; Jones, D.R.; Lau, J.; Carpenter, J.; Rucker, G.; Harbord, R.M.; Schmid, C.H.; et al. Recommendations for examining and interpreting funnel plot asymmetry in meta-analyses of randomised controlled trials. *BMJ* **2011**, *343*, d4002. [CrossRef] [PubMed]

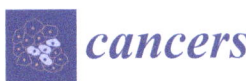

Systematic Review

Neuroendocrine Carcinomas with Atypical Proliferation Index and Clinical Behavior: A Systematic Review

Tiziana Feola [1,2], Roberta Centello [1], Franz Sesti [1], Giulia Puliani [1,3], Monica Verrico [4], Valentina Di Vito [1], Cira Di Gioia [4], Oreste Bagni [5], Andrea Lenzi [1], Andrea M. Isidori [1], Elisa Giannetta [1] and Antongiulio Faggiano [6,*]

[1] Department of Experimental Medicine, "Sapienza" University of Rome, 00161 Rome, Italy; tiziana.feola@uniroma1.it (T.F.); roberta.centello@uniroma1.it (R.C.); franz.sesti@uniroma1.it (F.S.); giulia.puliani@uniroma1.it (G.P.); valentina.divito@uniroma1.it (V.D.V.); andrea.lenzi@uniroma1.it (A.L.); andrea.isidori@uniroma1.it (A.M.I.); elisa.giannetta@uniroma1.it (E.G.)
[2] Neuroendocrinology, Neuromed Institute, IRCCS, 86077 Pozzilli (IS), Italy
[3] Oncological Endocrinology Unit, Regina Elena National Cancer Institute, IRCCS, 00144 Rome, Italy
[4] Department of Radiological, Oncological and Pathological Sciences, "Sapienza" University of Rome, 00161 Rome, Italy; monica.verrico@uniroma1.it (M.V.); cira.digioia@uniroma1.it (C.D.G.)
[5] Radiology Unit, "Santa Maria Goretti" Hospital, 04100 Latina, Italy; oreste.bagni@uniroma1.it
[6] Endocrinology Unit, Department of Clinical and Molecular Medicine, Sant'Andrea Hospital, Sapienza University of Rome, 00189 Rome, Italy
* Correspondence: antongiulio.faggiano@uniroma1.it; Tel.: +39-06-49972656

Simple Summary: Neuroendocrine carcinomas (NECs) are generally highly proliferative and clinically aggressive neuroendocrine neoplasms, but recent literature data suggested that NECs could be further subdivided into two prognostic distinct categories based on the Ki67 labeling index (LI) cut-off of 55%. However, no clear indication on the clinical management and the specific treatment protocol of NECs with a low Ki67 LI are available. We performed a systematic review of the literature to explore the clinicopathological features and the treatment response according to Ki67 LI cut-off in NECs, which is a "hot topic" in neuroendocrinology. Using evidence from 8 studies, for a total of 268 NEC affected patients, the systematic review showed that NECs with a low Ki67 LI had a better prognosis than the subgroup with higher Ki67 LI but worse than G3 neuroendocrine tumors suggesting that NECs are a heterogeneous disease for the pathology findings, the clinical behavior and the treatment response.

Abstract: Background: Highly proliferative (G3) neuroendocrine neoplasms are divided into well differentiated tumors (NETs) and poorly differentiated carcinomas (NECs), based on the morphological appearance. This systematic review aims to evaluate the clinicopathological features and the treatment response of the NEC subgroup with a Ki67 labeling index (LI) < 55%. Methods: A literature search was performed using MEDLINE, Cochrane Library, and Scopus between December 2019 and April 2020, last update in October 2020. We included studies reporting data on the clinicopathological characteristics, survival, and/or therapy efficacy of patients with NECs, in which the Ki67 LI was specified. Results: 8 papers were included, on a total of 268 NEC affected patients. NECs with a Ki67 LI < 55% have been reported in patients of both sexes, mainly of sixth decade, pancreatic origin, and large-cell morphology. The prevalent treatment choice was chemotherapy, followed by surgery and, in only one study, peptide receptor radionuclide therapy. The subgroup of patients with NEC with a Ki67 LI < 55% showed longer overall survival and progression free survival and higher response rates than the subgroup of patients with a tumor with higher Ki67 LI (≥55%). Conclusions: NECs are heterogeneous tumors. The subgroup with a Ki67 LI < 55% has a better prognosis and should be treated and monitored differently from NECs with a Ki67 LI ≥ 55%.

Keywords: neuroendocrine neoplasm; neuroendocrine carcinoma; Ki67 labeling index; Ki67 proliferation index

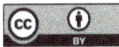

1. Introduction

Neuroendocrine neoplasms (NENs) are a heterogeneous group of neoplasms arising from the neuroendocrine system, expressing markers of neuroendocrine differentiation as well as hormones and tissue-specific transcription factors [1]. The 2010 World Health Organization (WHO) classification of gastroenteropancreatic (GEP)-NENs divided NENs on the basis of the mitotic count and/or the Ki67 labeling index (LI) in low-intermediate grade (G1-G2) and well differentiated (WD) morphology forms, named "neuroendocrine tumors" (NETs), and high grade (G3) and poorly differentiated (PD) morphology ones, named "neuroendocrine carcinomas" (NECs). According to this classification, G1 NETs are characterized by a mitotic count <2/10 high power fields (HPFs) and/or a Ki67 LI <3%; G2 NETs are characterized by a mitotic count 2–20/10 HPFs and/or a Ki67 LI 3-20%; NECs are characterized by a mitotic count >20/10 HPFs and/or a Ki67 LI >20%. Recently, the 2017 and 2019 WHO classifications of NENs introduced the definition of G3 NET, a WD high grade tumor [2,3]. On this basis, G3 NENs are todays divided into NETs and NECs, based on the morphological appearance. NECs include a small cell (SC) type and a large cell (LC) type, which differ for the cytological details (Figure 1 for NENs nomenclature).

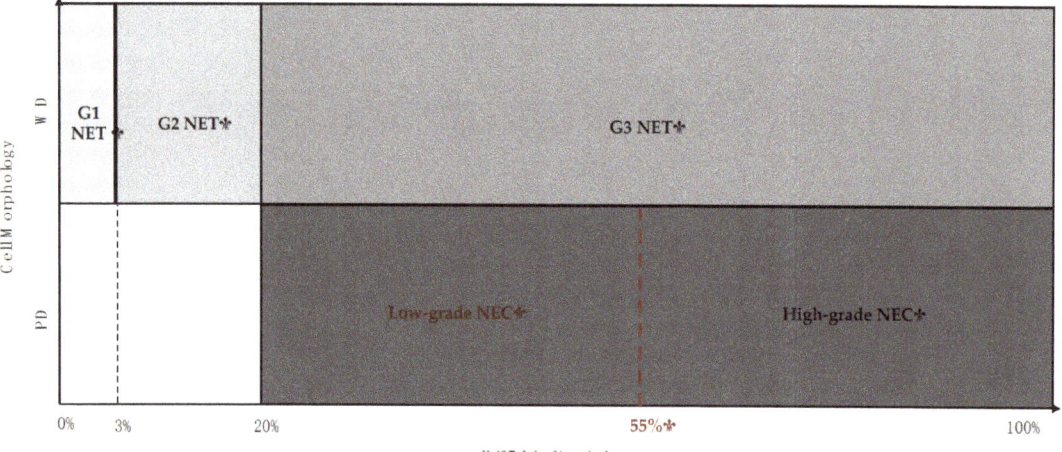

Figure 1. Current World Health Organization (WHO) gastroenteropancreatic neuroendocrine neoplasms (GEP-NENs) classification based on both cell morphology and Ki67 labelling index (LI). G1 neuroendocrine tumor (NET): a well-differentiated (WD) tumor characterized by a mitotic count <2/10 high power fields (HPFs) and/or a Ki67 LI <3%; G2 NET: a WD tumor characterized by a mitotic count 2–20/10 HPFs and/or a Ki67 LI 3–20%; G3 NET: a WD tumor characterized by a mitotic count >20/10 HPFs and/or a Ki67 LI >20%; G3 neuroendocrine carcinoma (NEC): a poorly-differentiated (PD) tumor characterized by a mitotic count >20/10 HPFs and/or a Ki67 LI >20%. As recent literature data suggested, NECs could be further subdivided into two distinct prognostic categories based on the Ki67 LI cut-off of 55%.

NENs of the lung (Lu-NENs) maintained the 2015 WHO classification into four different variants, based on mitotic count, necrosis areas, and local/distant invasion: typical carcinoid (TC) and atypical carcinoid (AC) as low grade tumors; SC lung carcinoma (SCLC) and LC neuroendocrine carcinoma (LCNEC) as high grade tumors [4].

PD-NECs both from GEP and lung origin are highly proliferative and clinically aggressive NENs, generally characterized by a high rate of the Ki67 LI. These tumors well respond to platinum-based chemotherapy, but the tumor response duration is short. Some literature data suggested that PD-NECs could be subdivided into two prognostic distinct categories based on the Ki67 LI cut-off of 55%, with a better prognosis in patients with a tumor with a Ki67 LI <55%, showing an intermediate behavior between the G3 NETs and the typical NECs [5,6]. Limited evidence supports treatment recommendations specific to

NECs, most likely secondary to the lack of sufficient patients numbers to conduct large phase II or III clinical trials [7]. While cisplatin or carboplatin-etoposide treatment regimens are a well-defined first-line therapeutic approach, based on therapy responses reported in SCLC studies [8], the combinations of 5-FU, leucovorin and irinotecan (FOLFIRI) and 5-FU, leucovorin and oxaliplatin (FOLFOX) have shown promising results in GEP-NECs as second line therapy [9,10]. Moreover, temozolomide and capecitabine may be used for patients who failed on first-line chemotherapy [11,12]. The peptide receptor radionuclide therapy (PRRT) also has been proposed as an alternative treatment approach for GEP-NECs [13,14], while immunotherapy is promising, but its effectiveness has not been demonstrated yet in GEP-NECs [15]. At now, effective treatment options alternative to platin-based chemotherapy are very limited.

Recently, it has been reported that NECs with relatively low Ki67 LI better respond to standard therapy than NECs with higher Ki67 LI [6]. However, no clear indication on the treatment of NECs with low Ki67 LI are now available.

We present a systematic review of the literature about the clinicopathological features and the treatment response of the NEC subgroup with Ki67 LI <55%, compared with the subgroup of NECs with higher Ki67 LI (≥55%).

2. Materials and Methods

A systematic review was performed following a robust methodology based on the Cochrane Collaboration and PRISMA statements [16,17].

A computerized literature search of MEDLINE and the Cochrane Database of Systematic Reviews revealed that there was no previous publication on G3 NECs with low proliferation rate. English-language original articles were independently searched by two authors (T.F. and R.C.) in several databases (MEDLINE, Cochrane Library, and Scopus) between December 2019 and April 2020. The following key words were used for the study search: ((("cancer" OR "carcinoma" OR "neoplasm" OR "malignant" OR "tumor") AND "neuroendocrine") OR "NEC" OR "poorly differentiated neuroendocrine carcinoma" AND "Ki67" OR "low proliferative rate" OR "low proliferation" AND ("management" OR "therapy"). Additional articles were identified by hand-searching reference lists of all the articles retrieved to identify potentially relevant studies. An update of the search was conducted in October 2020.

The titles and the abstracts of all the identified articles were independently screened by two reviewers (T.F. and R.C.) to assess their relevance. Reviews, editorials, letters, and animal studies were excluded. Full texts of selected, potentially relevant, papers were further evaluated. Suitability of the studies was defined for the purpose of this review as reporting on the clinical or biological characteristics, treatment, or clinical outcomes of patients with GEP-NEC or Lu-LCNEC. We selected all the studies that met all the following eligibility criteria: (i) randomized-controlled trial, prospective or retrospective studies; (ii) NEC population defined, according to the 2017 WHO criteria, by both poor cell differentiation and high proliferation indices; (ii) assessment of different subgroups of Ki67 LI (<55% and ≥55%); and (iii) data on survival and/or therapy efficacy for each subgroup. Additionally, studies exploring treatment of G3 NET exclusively were excluded, as were those that did not contain individual data for patients with NEC or provided no data on survival and response rate (RR). Any differences of opinion were resolved by discussion and consensus.

Two authors (T.F and R.C.) independently extracted the following data from included publications: first author, year of publication, study design, study populations, type of NEN, age, sex, cell differentiation and Ki67 LI, therapy regimens, RR, median overall survival (OS), and/or progression free survival (PFS).

3. Results

3.1. Study Selection

Of 668 potentially relevant studies initially identified, 468 were excluded based on the title and abstract screening. The main reasons for exclusion were reviews, conference abstracts, animal studies, duplicates, not clear histology, lack of group of interest (Ki67 LI <55% vs. ≥55%), and non-relevant outcomes. Of the 200 remaining publications, 191 were excluded after full text assessment because they did not meet all the eligibility criteria. All papers in which G3 NECs were not separated from G3 NETs, according to morphological appearance, were excluded, as were those without Ki67 LI subgroups or individual data on Ki67 LI. This process led to the selection of 8 studies. Figure 2 shows the study selection process.

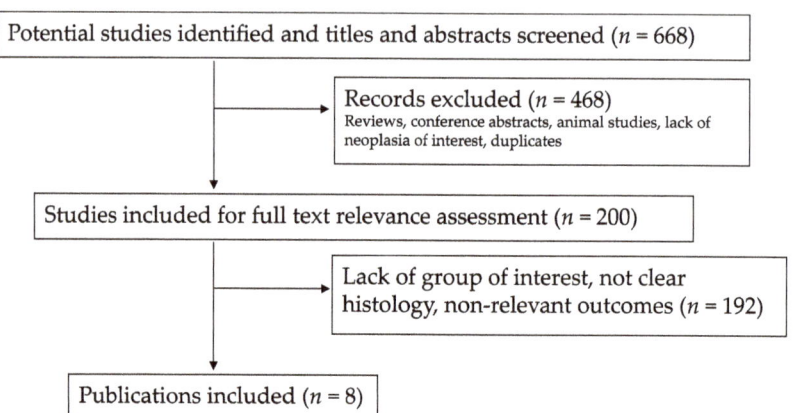

Figure 2. Flow-chart of the literature eligibility assessment process.

3.2. Study Characteristics

The eight studies finally selected were all retrospective studies [6,9,10,18–22] including a total of 268 patients with NECs in which Ki67 LI was specified to distinguish two subcategories: NECs with Ki67 LI <55% and NECs with Ki67 LI ≥55% (Table 1).

Table 1. Characteristics of the included studies.

First Author (Year) (Reference)	Study Design	Population Object of the Study (n)	Primary Site (n) Type of Cells (n)	Therapy Regimen	Summary
O. Hentic, et al. (2012) [9]	R	GEP-NEC (19)	- Pancreas (10) - Liver (6) - Anus (2) - Pelvic (1) • SC (11) • LC (6) • NA (2)	FOLFIRI as second line after platinum-etoposide	FOLFIRI may be an efficient second-line tx in patients with NECs who are in good condition after failure of platinum-based tx/etoposide.
O. Basturk et al. (2014) [18]	R	NEC (44)	- Pancreas (44) • LC (27) • SC (17)	S ± adjuvant CHT (cisplatinum based) ± RTx	PD-NEC of the pancreas is a highly aggressive neoplasm, with frequent metastases and poor survival. There was no survival difference between Ki67 LI <55% NEC patients and Ki67 LI ≥55% ones.

Table 1. Cont.

First Author (Year) (Reference)	Study Design	Population Object of the Study (n)	Primary Site (n) Type of Cells (n)	Therapy Regimen	Summary
J. Hadoux et al. (2015) [10]	R	NEC (20)	- -GEP (12) - Thoracic (4) - -Other (2) - Unknown (2) • SC (7) • LC (12) • NA (1)	FOLFOX as second line after platinum-etoposide	FOLFOX regimen may be an effective second-line tx in NEC patients after platinum-based first-line treatment. There was no difference in terms of RRs according to the 55% Ki67 LI-cutoff. A longer PFS and OS was observed for patients with Ki67 LI <55% NECs.
M. Milione et al. (2017) [6]	R	G3 GEP-NEN (136) -G3 NET (24) -NEC (112)	- Pancreas (22) - Stomach (23) - Esophagus (5) - Duodenum (5) - -Ileum-cecum (13) - -Colon-rectum (42) - Gallbladder (2) • NA	Platinum-etoposide ($n = 59$), Other platinum-based CHT ($n = 31$), Non-platinum-based CHT ($n = 12$), Other non-cytotoxic tx ($n = 8$)	Median OS was best for G3 NET, intermediate for NEC with a Ki67 LI 21–54% and lower for NEC cases with a Ki67 LI ≥55%. The 55% Ki67 LI cut-off is an independent prognostic factor for PD-GEP-NENs.
E. A. Carlsen et al. (2019) [19]	R	G3 GEP-NEN (149) -G3 NET (60) -NEC (62) -NA (27)	-Pancreas (89) - Unknown (26) -Other (34) • NA	PRRT	PRRT can be effective in high-grade GEP-NEN patients. PFS and OS differed significantly in patients according to differentiation and proliferation.
B. C. M. Hermans et al. (2019) [20]	R	LCNEC with a solitary brain metastasis (11)	- Lung (11) • LC (11)	9/11: definitive tx (S ± SRT ± CHT) 2/11: metastasectomy ± SRT brain	Stage IV LCNEC with a solitary brain metastasis and N0/N1 disease show in the majority of cases Ki67 LI ≤40% and prolonged survival, distinguishing them from general LCNEC.
H. Kim et al. (2020) [21]	R	NEN (82) -G1 NET (20) -G2 NET (47) -G3 NET (8) -NEC (7)	- Pancreas (82) • SC (4) • LC (3)	S ± CHT	Histological features supporting the diagnosis of pNECs over G3 pNETs were the absence of a low-grade pNET component, the presence of diffuse marked nuclear atypia, solid growth pattern, frequent apoptosis, and markedly increased proliferative activity. No statistical analysis was performed between the two subgroups (Ki67 LI <55% vs. Ki67 LI ≥55%)
E. Merola et al. (2020) [22]	R	G3 GEP-NEN (15) -G3 NET (7) -NEC (6) -MiNEN (2)	- Pancreas (9) - Colorectal (2) - Gastro-esophageal (1) - Ileum (1) - Appendix (2) • LC (6)	S + CHT (cisplatinum/etoposide)	Radical intended surgery may be considered for very highly selected stage IV GEP-NENs G3, with a LCNEC or a NET G3 histopathology. No statistical analysis was performed between the two subgroups (Ki67 LI <55% vs. Ki67 LI ≥55%).

CHT, chemotherapy; CRS, cytoreductive surgery; FOLFIRI, folinic acid, 5-fluorouracil and irinotecan; FOLFOX, 5-fluorouracil and oxaliplatin; G1, grade 1; G2, grade 2; G3, grade 3; GEP, gastroenteropancreatic; large cell neuroendocrine carcinoma; MiNEN: mixed neuroendocrine-non-neuroendocrine neoplasm; mo, months; NA, not available; NEC, neuroendocrine carcinoma; NEN, neuroendocrine neoplasm; NET, neuroendocrine tumor; OS, overall survival; PD, poorly differentiated; PFS, progression-free survival; pNEC, pancreatic neuroendocrine carcinoma; pNET, pancreatic neuroendocrine tumor; PRRT, peptide receptor radionuclide therapy; px, patients; R, retrospective; RTx, radiotherapy; RR, response rate; S, surgery; SRT, stereotactic radiotherapy; SSA, somatostatin analog; TMZ, temozolomide; tx, therapy.

All studies differed according to types of NEN enrolled and treatments received. Specifically, four studies considered both WD G3 NENs and PD-NENs [6,19,21,22], while four studies [9,10,18,20] included only patients presenting the specific subgroup of NECs. NENs derived from different primary sites, the most frequent one being the GEP tract.

As far as NENs treatment is concerned, three studies considered patients treated with different chemotherapy regimens. The studies of Hentic et al. and Hadoux et al. evaluated FOLFIRI and FOLFOX regimens respectively, as second-line treatment but no details were provided about the first-line therapy with platinum-etoposide according to the Ki67 LI [9,10]. The study of Milione et al. considered patients treated with chemotherapy: platinum-etoposide ($n = 59$), other platinum-based regimen ($n = 31$), non-platinum-based chemotherapy ($n = 12$), and other non-cytotoxic therapy ($n = 8$), but unfortunately when the authors stratified the tumors according to the Ki67 LI, they did not provide specific data on the chemotherapy regimen [6]. In four studies, chemotherapy was used combined with other treatment strategies (radiotherapy and/or surgery), specific data on use and outcome of standard first line therapy cannot be extracted from these studies [18,20–22]. One study evaluated PRRT efficacy [19].

3.3. Clinicopathological Features of Patients with NEC with Ki67 LI <55%

Among all the subjects with NEC, 112 with a Ki67 LI <55% were identified vs. 156 with a Ki67 LI ≥55%, reported in this review as control group. Table 2 summarizes the main demographic and pathological characteristic.

Table 2. Demographic and pathological features of patients with neuroendocrine carcinoma (NEC) and low Ki67 labeling index (LI) vs. high Ki67 LI.

NEC Features	Ki67 LI < 55%	Ki67 LI ≥ 55%
n/tot (%)	112/268 (41.8)	156/268 (58.2)
Median age, yrs (range)	51 (41.3–52.6)	64.6 (53.4–71)
Sex, n	49	96
Male:Female	26:23	59:37
Primary site, n (%)	62	127
Pancreas	32 (51.6)	48 (37.8)
Colon-rectum	8 (12.9)	35 (27.5)
Small bowel	6 (11.1)	13 (10.2)
Stomach	6 (9.7)	17 (13.4)
Lung	6 (9.7)	5 (3.9)
Liver	3 (4.8)	2 (1.6)
Esophagus	1 (1.6)	4 (3.1)
Gallbladder	–	2 (1.6)
Anus	–	1 (0.78)
Type of cells, n (%)		
LC GEP-NECs	8/12 (66.7)	6/14 (42.8%)
SC GEP-NECs	4/12 (33.3)	8/14 (57.1%)
LC Lung-NECs	6/11 (54.5)	5/11 (45.5%)

LC, large cell; LI, labeling index; GEP, gastroenteropancreatic; mo, months; n, number; NEC, neuroendocrine carcinoma; OS, overall survival; PFS, progression-free survival; SC, small cell; yrs, years.

Three studies [9,20,21] reported on patients' age: the median age was 51 years (range 41.3–52.6) vs. 64.6 (53.4–71) in the subgroup with Ki67 LI ≥55%. Four studies [6,9,20,21] reported on gender: males were 26/49 (53%) among patients with a Ki67 LI <55% NEC, while 59/96 (61.4%) among those with a Ki67 LI ≥55%.

Data about primary NEC site for each Ki67 LI-based subgroup could be extracted from five studies [6,9,18,21,22] ($n = 189$). Pancreas was the prevalent site: among the 62 tumors with a Ki67 LI <55%, 32 had a pNEC (50.8%), whereas 48 out of 127 tumors with a Ki67 LI ≥55% had a pNEC (37.8%). The other GEP primary sites were colon-rectum ($n = 8$, 12.9% vs. $n = 35$, 27.5%), small bowel ($n = 7$, 11.1% vs. $n = 13$, 10.2%), stomach ($n = 6$, 9.7% vs. $n = 17$, 13.4%), liver ($n = 3$, 4.8% vs. $n = 2$, 1.6%), and esophagus ($n = 1$, 1.6% vs. $n = 4$, 3.1%). The remaining GEP cases with Ki67 LI ≥55% were in gallbladder ($n = 2$, 1.6%) and anus ($n = 1$, 0.8%) no Ki67 LI <55% NECs were observed in these sites. Carlsen at al. enrolled only G3 GEP-NECs (44 with Ki67 LI <55% and 11 with Ki67 LI ≥55%), but no further details on primary site were provided. In the study of Hadoux et al., a heterogeneous population of G3 NECs (12 GEP, 4 thoracic, 2 others, 2 unknown) were included. Anyway, when the authors stratified the results according to the Ki67 LI, the site of the tumor was not specified.

Regarding Lu-NENs, in the study of Hermans et al., only 11 patients were included: 6 of them were affected by a NEC with a Ki67 LI <55%, while 5 with a Ki67 LI ≥55% [20].

Four studies reported on morphology of the different subgroups of patients [9,20–22] (n = 37): among 12 GEP-NECs with a Ki67 LI <55%, 8 were LC carcinomas (66.7%) while 4 had a SC morphology (33.3%); instead, in the subgroup with a Ki67 LI ≥55%, there were 6/14 GEP-NECs with a LC morphology (42.8%) and 8/14 cases with a SC morphology (57.14%). We only considered lung NECs with a LC morphology (n = 11, 100%).

As far as survival and efficacy data is concerned, median OS ranged from 13 months of Basturk et al., to 24.5 months of Milione et al. In the former, there was no survival difference between NEC with Ki67 LI <55% (13 months) vs. ≥55% (16 months) [18]. In the latter, one of the largest studies on pNEC [6], the median OS was the best for G3 NETs (43.6 months), intermediate for NECs with a Ki67 LI ranging 21–54% (24.5 months), and lower for NECs with a Ki67 LI ≥55% (5 months) [6]. The 55% Ki67 LI cut-off was demonstrated as an independent prognostic factor for PD-GEP-NENs [6].

According to the study of Milione et al., PFS and OS differed significantly between patients with different morphology and LI (OS: 44 months vs. 22 months vs. 9 months, PFS: 19 months vs. 11 months vs. 4 months for NETs G3, NECs with Ki67 LI <55%, NECs with Ki67 LI ≥55%, respectively). This was the largest study assessing the outcomes of patients with advanced high-grade GEP-NEN after PRRT [19].

In the study of Hentic et al., in which FOLFIRI regimen was used as second-line therapy after platinum-etoposide in GEP-NECs, the median OS was longer for the subgroup with a Ki67 LI <55% (19.5 vs. 16 months), while the median PFS did not vary between subgroups (4 months) [9]. A longer median PFS characterized the Ki67 LI <55% pNEC compared with the Ki67 LI ≥55% NECs (13 vs. 8 months) in the study of Merola et al., in which a radical intended surgery was proposed for very highly selected stage IV G3 GEP-NENs, with a LCNEC or a G3 NET histopathology [22].

In the study of Hadoux et al., including both GEP and Lu-NENs, there was no difference in terms of RRs according to the 55% Ki67 LI-cutoff, but a longer OS (19.5 months vs. 8.5 months) and PFS (6.2 months vs. 3.6 months) was observed for patients with Ki67 LI <55% [10].

Regarding only Lu-NECs, a prolonged OS (17 months vs. 5 months) and PFS (12 months vs. 3.5 months) was observed in patients with Lu-LCNECs with solitary brain metastases and a Ki67 LI ≤40%, suggesting a prognostic role of the proliferative index [20]. Table 3 summarizes the results on treatment response and outcomes in patients with NEC and low Ki67 LI vs. high Ki67 LI.

Table 3. Treatment response and outcomes in patients with neuroendocrine carcinoma (NEC) and low Ki67 labeling index (LI) vs. high Ki67 LI.

Authors (Year) (Reference)	NEC Subgroups for Ki67 LI					
	Ki67 LI < 55%			Ki67 LI ≥ 55%		
	RR, %	Median OS, mo (Range)	Median PFS, mo (Range)	RR, %	Median OS, mo (Range)	Median PFS, mo (Range)
O. Hentic et al. (2012) [9]	6 DC 4 PD (2 px still alive, >30 mo)	19.5 (12–28)	4 (1–8)	3 DC 2 PD	16 (11–26)	4 (2–7)
O. Basturk et al. (2014) [18]	NA	13 (6–20)	NA	NA	16 (6–24)	NA

Table 3. Cont.

Authors (Year) (Reference)	NEC Subgroups for Ki67 LI					
	Ki67 LI < 55%			Ki67 LI ≥ 55%		
	RR, %	Median OS, mo (Range)	Median PFS, mo (Range)	RR, %	Median OS, mo (Range)	Median PFS, mo (Range)
J. Hadoux et al. (2015) [10]	NA	19.5	6.2	NA	8.5	3.6
M. Milione et al. (2017) [6]	NA	24.5 (16.9–29.0)	NA	NA	5.3 (3.3–8.9)	NA
E. A. Carlsen et al. (2019) [19]	CR: 3 PR: 41 SD: 31 PD: 26	22 (16.0–28.0)	11 (5.4–16.6)	CR: 0 PR: 45 SD: 9 PD: 45	9 (1.6–16.4)	4 (0.8–7.2)
B. C. M. Hermans et al. (2019) [20]	NA	17 (11–23) (2 px still alive, >5 yrs)	12 (5–51)	NA	5 (0.7–9.3)	3.5 (2–4)
H. Kim et al. (2020) [21]	NA	15 (4–60)	8 (3–15)	NA	8 (2–17)	5.5 (2–17)
E. Merola et al. (2020) [22]	NA	23 (1 px still alive)	13	NA	14.5 (8–35) *	8 (5–16)

CR, complete response; DC, disease control; LI, labeling index; mo, months; n, number; NA, not available; OS, overall survival; PD, progressive disease; PFS, progression-free survival; PR, partial response; px, patient(s); RR, response rate; SD, stable disease; yrs, years; * Data of 4 pts out 5.

4. Discussion

We performed a systematic review of the literature to explore the clinicopathological features and the treatment response according to the Ki67 LI cut-off in NECs. A further subclassification of NECs based on this marker is a still debated topic in neuroendocrinology [5]. The current clinical guidelines do not provide specific treatment algorithms for NECs with a low proliferative rate [23]. The most recent WHO classification is designed to guide NENs treatment and prognosis, but unfortunately, because of heterogeneity of these neoplasms, physicians are challenged to treat patients with tumors that cannot be defined to any of the known NEN subtypes [24]. Literature data suggest that the NECs with a low Ki67 LI respond differently to the standard therapy of NECs, showing intermediate features between the G3 NETs and the typical NECs [6]. We found that PD-NECs with a Ki67 LI <55% affected mainly patients of the sixth decade and both sexes, most of them of pancreatic origin with a predominance of LC morphology. The prevalent treatment choice was chemotherapy, followed by surgery with or without chemo- and radiotherapy and only one study evaluated PRRT [19]. The latter study demonstrated that PRRT could be effective in G3 GEP-NEN patients. Most studies showed longer OS and PFS and higher RRs in this category of patients comparing to PD-NECs with higher Ki67 LI, confirming that the Ki67 LI could be a prognostic factor helpful to guide patient management together with the cell morphology. Moreover, in the two studies that evaluated the G3 NETs together with the NECs with a Ki67 LI <55%, this latter had a worse prognosis, confirming that it represents an intermediate category between the G3 NETs and the G3 NECs with a Ki67 LI ≥55%. A recent meta-analysis on the second-line treatment for patients with advanced extra-pulmonary NECs found that studies with a higher proportion of patients with a Ki67 LI >55% had lower RR and shorter OS [25]. Indeed, the relevance of Ki67 LI in NENs has long been reflected in the GEP-NENs classification system, and is also known to be prognostic in the Nordic NEC study, in which a poorer RR to platinum-based chemotherapy in patients with a Ki67 LI <55% compared to patients with a Ki67 LI ≥55% was observed [26]. Otherwise, a recently published retrospective observational French study evaluating platinum- and fluorouracil-based chemotherapy effect on survival in resected GEP-NECs, assessed the role of the Ki67 LI as a prognostic factor and did not find any impact on OS considering 55%, 70%, and 80% threshold while stated that the Ki67 LI ≥80% had a negative prognostic impact on disease-free survival [27].

For what Lu-NENs classification is concerned, the current WHO guidelines do not include Ki67 LI due to some overlap of cut-off thresholds among different tumors [28]. However, the Ki67 LI has been shown to be ≤20% for low- to intermediate-grade pulmonary NETs and >40% for high-grade tumors [29]. A new proposal for a diagnostic algorithm is emerging for Lu-NEN that is, just as for the GEP-NENs, an integration of morphology (necrosis and mitoses) and proliferation (Ki67 LI), aimed at identifying a three-tiers grading system: Lu-NET G1, Lu-NET G2, and Lu-NET G3 [30]. The Ki67 LI effectively separates carcinoids from SCLC and could help for the clinical management and the therapeutic decision-making process of metastatic disease [7]. In the study of Hermans et al., patients with Lu-LCNECs with a solitary brain metastasis and N1 or N0 disease showed in most of the cases a Ki67 LI ≤40% with a prolonged survival compared to patients with a tumor with higher Ki67 LI. Nine of eleven patients were treated with definitive therapy (resection or stereotactic radiotherapy) for both primary and metastatic lesions, instead of standard treatment for stage IV LCNEC with palliative chemotherapy. This study suggests that stage IV Lu-LCNEC is a biological heterogeneous disease and that in some selected cases, a curative treatment could be attempt instead of standard palliative treatment to improve OS. Further prospective studies with larger study populations are needed to confirm these data.

Of note, one Phase II study investigating the efficacy and safety of the second-line FOLFIRI or CAPTEM regimens after failure of the first-line platinum-based chemotherapy in patients with Lu- and GEP-NECs is currently registered at ClinicalTrials.gov (National Clinical Trial identifier NCT03387592). It has been planned to perform a subgroup analysis according to Ki67 LI (21–55% vs. >55%) other than primary tumors site (lung vs. GEP), so it will be hopefully able to carry out useful results for the management of this heterogeneous and rare disease [31].

Our systematic review has some limitations due to the low number of studies on this topic, the heterogeneity of tumor origin and treatment regimens, the small number of patients enrolled in the studies. However, for the best of our knowledge, it is the first systematic review on the "hot topic" of NECs with a low Ki67 LI, according to the latest WHO classification that separated G3 NETs from NECs and indicates the need of further prospective studies with the aim of a better categorization of NECs to improve patients survival outcomes.

5. Conclusions

The current systematic review of the literature on NECs with a low Ki67 LI demonstrated that NECs are a rare and heterogeneous disease for the pathology findings, the clinical behavior, and the treatment response. In this context, the 55% cut-off of Ki67 LI could be an important prognostic factor, which is not included in the current NEC WHO classification and consequently, guidelines recommend the same treatment for both low and high Ki67 LI NECs. The systematic review confirmed that NECs with a low Ki67 LI had a better prognosis than the subgroup with higher Ki67 LI but worse than the G3 NETs. Moreover, this subgroup of NECs could benefit more from different treatment strategies that should be validated in prospective, clinical studies.

Author Contributions: T.F. is the first author for this systematic review of literature. A.F. is the corresponding author that concepted and designed the study. R.C. contributed to study search, study selection and data extraction. F.S., G.P., M.V. and V.D.V. contributed to the manuscript, tables and figures preparation. E.G., C.D.G., O.B., A.L. and A.M.I. revised critically this work. All authors contributed to manuscript revision, read, and approved the submitted version. All authors have read and agreed to the published version of the manuscript.

Funding: This study was partially supported by the ministerial research project PRIN2017Z3N3YC.

Institutional Review Board Statement: Not applicable.

Informed Consent Statement: Not applicable.

Data Availability Statement: No new data were created or analyzed in this study. Data sharing is not applicable to this article.

Acknowledgments: We wish to thank the NETTARE Unit—NeuroEndocrine Tumor TAsk foRcE of "Sapienza" University of Rome, Italy, led by Andrea Lenzi, Andrea M. Isidori and Elisa Giannetta, for integrating the patient's multidisciplinary clinical, diagnostic and therapeutic management and follow-up.

Conflicts of Interest: The authors declare that the research was conducted in the absence of any commercial or financial relationships that could be construed as a potential conflict of interest.

References

1. Rindi, G.; Wiedenmann, B. Neuroendocrine neoplasms of the gut and pancreas: New insights. *Nat. Rev. Endocrinol.* **2011**, *8*, 54–64. [CrossRef] [PubMed]
2. Lloyd, R.V.; Osamura, R.Y.; Klöppel, G.N.; Rosai, J.; World Health Organization; International Agency for Research on Cancer. *WHO Classification of Tumours of Endocrine Organs*; IARC: Lyon, France, 2017.
3. Lokuhetty, D.; White, V.A.; Watanabe, R.; Cree, I.A.; World Health Organization; International Agency for Research on Cancer. *Digestive System Tumours*; WHO: Geneva, Switzerland, 2019.
4. Travis, W.D.; Brambilla, E.; Burke, A.P.; Marx, A.; Nicholson, A.G. *WHO Classification of Tumours of the Lung, Pleura, Thymus and Heart*; IARC: Lyon, France, 2015; Volume 4.
5. Zatelli, M.C.; Guadagno, E.; Messina, E.; Lo Calzo, F.; Faggiano, A.; Colao, A.; NIKE Group. Open issues on G3 neuroendocrine neoplasms: Back to the future. *Endocr. Relat. Cancer* **2018**, *25*, R375–R384. [CrossRef]
6. Milione, M.; Maisonneuve, P.; Spada, F.; Pellegrinelli, A.; Spaggiari, P.; Albarello, L.; Pisa, E.; Barberis, M.; Vanoli, A.; Buzzoni, R.; et al. The Clinicopathologic Heterogeneity of Grade 3 Gastroenteropancreatic Neuroendocrine Neoplasms: Morphological Differentiation and Proliferation Identify Different Prognostic Categories. *Neuroendocrinology* **2017**, *104*, 85–93. [CrossRef]
7. Thomas, K.E.H.; Voros, B.A.; Boudreaux, J.P.; Thiagarajan, R.; Woltering, E.A.; Ramirez, R.A. Current Treatment Options in Gastroenteropancreatic Neuroendocrine Carcinoma. *Oncologist* **2019**, *24*, 1076–1088. [CrossRef]
8. Garcia-Carbonero, R.; Sorbye, H.; Baudin, E.; Raymond, E.; Wiedenmann, B.; Niederle, B.; Sedlackova, E.; Toumpanakis, C.; Anlauf, M.; Cwikla, J.B.; et al. ENETS Consensus Guidelines for High-Grade Gastroenteropancreatic Neuroendocrine Tumors and Neuroendocrine Carcinomas. *Neuroendocrinology* **2016**, *103*, 186–194. [CrossRef]
9. Hentic, O.; Hammel, P.; Couvelard, A.; Rebours, V.; Zappa, M.; Palazzo, M.; Maire, F.; Goujon, G.; Gillet, A.; Levy, P.; et al. FOLFIRI regimen: An effective second-line chemotherapy after failure of etoposide-platinum combination in patients with neuroendocrine carcinomas grade 3. *Endocr. Relat. Cancer* **2012**, *19*, 751–757. [CrossRef] [PubMed]
10. Hadoux, J.; Malka, D.; Planchard, D.; Scoazec, J.Y.; Caramella, C.; Guigay, J.; Boige, V.; Leboulleux, S.; Burtin, P.; Berdelou, A.; et al. Post-first-line FOLFOX chemotherapy for grade 3 neuroendocrine carcinoma. *Endocr. Relat. Cancer* **2015**, *22*, 289–298. [CrossRef]
11. Welin, S.; Sorbye, H.; Sebjornsen, S.; Knappskog, S.; Busch, C.; Oberg, K. Clinical effect of temozolomide-based chemotherapy in poorly differentiated endocrine carcinoma after progression on first-line chemotherapy. *Cancer* **2011**, *117*, 4617–4622. [CrossRef]
12. Thomas, K.; Voros, B.A.; Meadows-Taylor, M.; Smeltzer, M.P.; Griffin, R.; Boudreaux, J.P.; Thiagarajan, R.; Woltering, E.A.; Ramirez, R.A. Outcomes of Capecitabine and Temozolomide (CAPTEM) in Advanced Neuroendocrine Neoplasms (NENs). *Cancers* **2020**, *12*, 206. [CrossRef] [PubMed]
13. Garske, U.; Sandstrom, M.; Johansson, S.; Granberg, D.; Lundqvist, H.; Lubberink, M.; Sundin, A.; Eriksson, B. Lessons on Tumour Response: Imaging during Therapy with (177)Lu-DOTA-octreotate. A Case Report on a Patient with a Large Volume of Poorly Differentiated Neuroendocrine Carcinoma. *Theranostics* **2012**, *2*, 459–471. [CrossRef]
14. Montanier, N.; Joubert-Zakeyh, J.; Petorin, C.; Montoriol, P.F.; Maqdasy, S.; Kelly, A. The prognostic influence of the proliferative discordance in metastatic pancreatic neuroendocrine carcinoma revealed by peptide receptor radionuclide therapy: Case report and review of literature. *Medicine* **2017**, *96*, e6062. [CrossRef] [PubMed]
15. Weber, M.M.; Fottner, C. Immune Checkpoint Inhibitors in the Treatment of Patients with Neuroendocrine Neoplasia. *Oncol. Res. Treat.* **2018**, *41*, 306–312. [CrossRef]
16. Moher, D.; Liberati, A.; Tetzlaff, J.; Altman, D.G.; PRISMA Group. Preferred reporting items for systematic reviews and meta-analyses: The PRISMA statement. *J. Clin. Epidemiol.* **2009**, *62*, 1006–1012. [CrossRef] [PubMed]
17. Liberati, A.; Altman, D.G.; Tetzlaff, J.; Mulrow, C.; Gotzsche, P.C.; Ioannidis, J.P.; Clarke, M.; Devereaux, P.J.; Kleijnen, J.; Moher, D. The PRISMA statement for reporting systematic reviews and meta-analyses of studies that evaluate health care interventions: Explanation and elaboration. *J. Clin. Epidemiol.* **2009**, *62*, e1–e34. [CrossRef]
18. Basturk, O.; Tang, L.; Hruban, R.H.; Adsay, V.; Yang, Z.; Krasinskas, A.M.; Vakiani, E.; La Rosa, S.; Jang, K.T.; Frankel, W.L.; et al. Poorly differentiated neuroendocrine carcinomas of the pancreas: A clinicopathologic analysis of 44 cases. *Am. J. Surg. Pathol.* **2014**, *38*, 437–447. [CrossRef] [PubMed]

19. Carlsen, E.A.; Fazio, N.; Granberg, D.; Grozinsky-Glasberg, S.; Ahmadzadehfar, H.; Grana, C.M.; Zandee, W.T.; Cwikla, J.; Walter, M.A.; Oturai, P.S.; et al. Peptide receptor radionuclide therapy in gastroenteropancreatic NEN G3: A multicenter cohort study. *Endocr. Relat. Cancer* **2019**, *26*, 227–239. [CrossRef]
20. Hermans, B.C.M.; Derks, J.L.; Groen, H.J.M.; Stigt, J.A.; van Suylen, R.J.; Hillen, L.M.; van den Broek, E.C.; Speel, E.J.M.; Dingemans, A.C. Large cell neuroendocrine carcinoma with a solitary brain metastasis and low Ki-67: A unique subtype. *Endocr. Connect.* **2019**, *8*, 1600–1606. [CrossRef]
21. Kim, H.; An, S.; Lee, K.; Ahn, S.; Park, D.Y.; Kim, J.H.; Kang, D.W.; Kim, M.J.; Chang, M.S.; Jung, E.S.; et al. Pancreatic High-Grade Neuroendocrine Neoplasms in the Korean Population: A Multicenter Study. *Cancer Res. Treat.* **2020**, *52*, 263–276. [CrossRef]
22. Merola, E.; Falconi, M.; Rinke, A.; Staettner, S.; Krendl, F.; Partelli, S.; Andreasi, V.; Gress, T.M.; Pascher, A.; Arsenic, R.; et al. Radical intended surgery for highly selected stage IV neuroendocrine neoplasms G3. *Am. J. Surg.* **2020**. [CrossRef]
23. Partelli, S.; Bartsch, D.K.; Capdevila, J.; Chen, J.; Knigge, U.; Niederle, B.; Nieveen van Dijkum, E.J.M.; Pape, U.F.; Pascher, A.; Ramage, J.; et al. ENETS Consensus Guidelines for Standard of Care in Neuroendocrine Tumours: Surgery for Small Intestinal and Pancreatic Neuroendocrine Tumours. *Neuroendocrinology* **2017**, *105*, 255–265. [CrossRef]
24. Nikiforchin, A.; Peng, R.; Sittig, M.; Kotiah, S. A Rare Case of Metastatic Heterogeneous Poorly Differentiated Neuroendocrine Carcinoma of Ileum: A Case Report and Literature Review. *J. Med. Cases* **2020**, *11*, 6–11. [CrossRef]
25. McNamara, M.G.; Frizziero, M.; Jacobs, T.; Lamarca, A.; Hubner, R.A.; Valle, J.W.; Amir, E. Second-line treatment in patients with advanced extra-pulmonary poorly differentiated neuroendocrine carcinoma: A systematic review and meta-analysis. *Ther. Adv. Med. Oncol.* **2020**, *12*, 1758835920915299. [CrossRef] [PubMed]
26. Sorbye, H.; Welin, S.; Langer, S.W.; Vestermark, L.W.; Holt, N.; Osterlund, P.; Dueland, S.; Hofsli, E.; Guren, M.G.; Ohrling, K.; et al. Predictive and prognostic factors for treatment and survival in 305 patients with advanced gastrointestinal neuroendocrine carcinoma (WHO G3): The NORDIC NEC study. *Ann. Oncol.* **2013**, *24*, 152–160. [CrossRef] [PubMed]
27. Pellat, A.; Walter, T.; Augustin, J.; Hautefeuille, V.; Hentic, O.; Do Cao, C.; Lievre, A.; Coriat, R.; Hammel, P.; Dubreuil, O.; et al. Chemotherapy in Resected Neuroendocrine Carcinomas of the Digestive Tract: A National Study from the French Group of Endocrine Tumours. *Neuroendocrinology* **2020**, *110*, 404–412. [CrossRef]
28. Travis, W.D.; Brambilla, E.; Burke, A.P.; Marx, A.; Nicholson, A.G. Introduction to The 2015 World Health Organization Classification of Tumors of the Lung, Pleura, Thymus, and Heart. *J. Thorac. Oncol.* **2015**, *10*, 1240–1242. [CrossRef]
29. Pelosi, G.; Sonzogni, A.; Harari, S.; Albini, A.; Bresaola, E.; Marchio, C.; Massa, F.; Righi, L.; Gatti, G.; Papanikolaou, N.; et al. Classification of pulmonary neuroendocrine tumors: New insights. *Transl. Lung Cancer Res.* **2017**, *6*, 513–529. [CrossRef] [PubMed]
30. Rindi, G.; Klersy, C.; Inzani, F.; Fellegara, G.; Ampollini, L.; Ardizzoni, A.; Campanini, N.; Carbognani, P.; De Pas, T.M.; Galetta, D.; et al. Grading the neuroendocrine tumors of the lung: An evidence-based proposal. *Endocr. Relat. Cancer* **2014**, *21*, 1–16. [CrossRef]
31. Bongiovanni, A.; Liverani, C.; Pusceddu, S.; Leo, S.; Di Meglio, G.; Tamberi, S.; Santini, D.; Gelsomino, F.; Pucci, F.; Berardi, R.; et al. Randomised phase II trial of CAPTEM or FOLFIRI as SEcond-line therapy in NEuroendocrine CArcinomas and exploratory analysis of predictive role of PET/CT imaging and biological markers (SENECA trial): A study protocol. *BMJ Open* **2020**, *10*, e034393. [CrossRef]

MDPI
St. Alban-Anlage 66
4052 Basel
Switzerland
Tel. +41 61 683 77 34
Fax +41 61 302 89 18
www.mdpi.com

Cancers Editorial Office
E-mail: cancers@mdpi.com
www.mdpi.com/journal/cancers

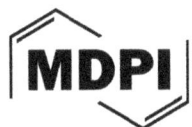

www.ingramcontent.com/pod-product-compliance
Lightning Source LLC
LaVergne TN
LVHW070720100526
838202LV00013B/1133